DIAGNOSTIC AND INTERVENTIONAL CATHETERIZATION IN CONGENITAL HEART DISEASE

SECOND EDITION

DIAGNOSTIC AND INTERVENTIONAL CATHETERIZATION IN CONGENITAL HEART DISEASE

edited by

James E. Lock, M.D.
John F. Keane, M.D.
Stanton B. Perry, M.D.

Department of Cardiology
Children's Hospital, Boston

KLUWER ACADEMIC PUBLISHERS
Boston / Dordrecht / London

Distributors for North, Central and South America:
Kluwer Academic Publishers
101 Philip Drive
Assinippi Park
Norwell, Massachusetts 02061 USA

Distributors for all other countries:
Kluwer Academic Publishers Group
Distribution Centre
Post Office Box 322
3300 AH Dordrecht, THE NETHERLANDS

Library of Congress Cataloging-in-Publication Data

Lock, James E.
    Diagnostic and interventional catheterization in congenital heart
disease / by James E. Lock, John F. Keane, Stanton B. Perry. -- 2nd
ed.
      p. cm. -- (Developments in cardiovascular medicine ; v. 221)
    Includes bibliographical references and index.
    ISBN 0-7923-8597-7 (alk. paper)
    1. Cardiac catheterization in childen. 2. Congenital heart
diseases.   I. Keane, John F., 1934- . II. Perry, Stanton B.
III. Title.   IV. Series.
    [DNLM: 1. Heart Defects, Congenital--diagnosis--Child. 2. Heart
Catheterization--Child.   3. Heart Catheterization--methods.
4. Heart Defects, Congenital --therapy--Child.   WS 290 L813d 2000}
RJ423.5.C36L63 2000
617.4'12--dc21
DNLM/DLC
for Library of Congress   99-27712
                                                CIP

Printed on acid-free paper.

Printed in the United States of America

198. Antoine Lafont, Eric Topol (eds.): *Arterial Remodeling: A Critical Factor in Restenosis.* 1997 ISBN 0-7923-8008-8
199. Michele Mercuri, David D. McPherson, Hisham Bassiouny, Seymour Glagov (eds.):*Non-Invasive Imaging of Atherosclerosis* ISBN 0-7923-8036-3
200. Walmor C. DeMello, Michiel J. Janse(eds.): *Heart Cell Communication in Health and Disease* ISBN 0-7923-8052-5
201. P.E. Vardas (ed.): *Cardiac Arrhythmias Pacing and Electrophysiology.* The Expert View. 1998 ISBN 0-7923-4908-3
202. E.E. van der Wall, P.K. Blanksma, M.G. Niemeyer, W. Vaalburg and H.J.G.M. Crijns (eds.) *Advanced Imaging in Coronary Artery Disease, PET, SPECT, MRI, IVUS, EBCT. 1998* ISBN 0-7923-5083-9
203. R.L. Wilensky (ed.) *Unstable Coronary Artery Syndromes, Pathophysiology, Diagnosis and Treatment. 1998.* ISBN 0-7923-8201-3
204. J.H.C. Reiber, E.E. van der Wall (eds.): *What's New in Cardiovascular Imaging?* 1998 ISBN 0-7923-5121-5
205. Juan Carlos Kaski, David W. Holt (eds.): *Myocardial Damage Early Detection by Novel Biochemical Markers. 1998.* ISBN 0-7923-5140-1
207. Gary F. Baxter, Derek M. Yellon, *Delayed Preconditioning and Adaptive Cardioprotection. 1998.* ISBN 0-7923-5259-9
208. Bernard Swynghedauw, *Molecular Cardiology for the Cardiologist, Second Edition* 1998. ISBN 0-7923-8323-0
209. Geoffrey Burnstock, James G.Dobson, Jr., Bruce T. Liang, Joel Linden (eds): *Cardiovascular Biology of Purines.* 1998. ISBN: 0-7923-8334-6
210. Brian D. Hoit, Richard A. Walsh (eds): *Cardiovascular Physiology in the Genetically Engineered Mouse.* 1998. ISBN: 0-7923-8356-7
211. Peter Whittaker, George S. Abela (eds.): *Direct Myocardial Revascularization: History, Methodology, Technology* 1998. ISBN: 0-7923-8398-2
212. C.A. Nienaber, R. Fattori (eds.): Diagnosis and Treatment of Aortic Diseases. 1999. ISBN: 0-7923-5517-2
213. Juan Carlos Kaski (ed.): *Chest Pain with Normal Coronary Angiograms: Pathogenesis, Diagnosis and Management.* 1999. ISBN: 0-7923-8421-0
214. P.A. Doevendans, R.S. Reneman and M. Van Bilsen (eds): *Cardiovascular Specific Gene Expression.* 1999 ISBN:0-7923-5633-0
215. G. Pons-Lladó, F. Carreras, X. Borrás, Subirana and L.J. Jiménez-Borreguero (eds.): *Atlas of Practical Cardiac Applications of MRI.* 1999 ISBN: 0-7923-5636-5
216. L.W. Klein, J.E. Calvin, *Resource Utilization in Cardiac Disease.* 1999. ISBN:0-7923-8509-8
217. R. Gorlin, G. Dangas, P. K. Toutouzas, M.M Konstadoulakis, *Contemporary Concepts in Cardiology, Pathophysiology and Clinical Management.*1999 ISBN:0-7923-8514-4
218. S. Gupta, J. Camm (eds.): *Chronic Infection, Chlamydia and Coronary Heart Disease.* 1999. ISBN:0-7923-5797-3
219. M. Rajskina: *Ventricular Fibrillation in Sudden Coronary Death.* 1999. ISBN:0-7923-8570-5
220. Z. Abedin, R. Conner: *Interpretation of Cardiac Arrhythmias: Self Assessment Approach.* 1999. ISBN:0-7923-8576-4
221. J. E. Lock, J.F. Keane, S. B. Perry: *Diagnostic and Interventional Catheterization In Congenital Heart Disease.* 2000. ISBN: 0-7923-8597-7

Previous volumes are still available

KLUWER ACADEMIC PUBLISHERS - DORDRECHT/BOSTON/LONDON

DIAGNOSTIC AND INTERVENTIONAL CATHETERIZATION IN CONGENITAL HEART DISEASE

CONTENTS

CONTRIBUTING AUTHORS

Patricia E. Burrows, M.D.
Professor of Radiology
Harvard Medical School
Children's Hospital
300 Longwood Avenue
Boston, Massachusetts

Taylor Chung, M.D
Instructor of Radiology
Harvard Medical School
Children's Hospital
300 Longwood Avenue
Boston, Massachusetts

Michael F. Flanagan, M.D.
Assistant Professor in Pediatrics
Dartmouth Medical School
Dartmouth Hitchcock Med. Ctr.
One Medical Center Drive
Lebanon, New Hampshire

Dolly D. Hansen, M.D.
Associate Professor of Anaesthesia
(Pediatrics)
Harvard Medical School
Children's Hospital
300 Longwood Avenue
Boston, Massachusetts

John F. Keane, M.D.
Professor of Pediatrics
Harvard Medical School
Children's Hospital
300 Longwood Avenue
Boston, Massachusetts

Jacqueline Kreutzer, M.D.
Instructor in Pediatrics
Harvard Medical School
Children's Hospital
300 Longwood Avenue
Boston, Massachusetts

Michael J. Landzberg, M.D.
Instructor in Pediatrics
Instructor in Medicine
Harvard Medical School
Children's Hospital
300 Longwood Avenue
Boston, Massachusetts

Peter Lang, M.D.
Associate Professor of Pediatrics
Harvard Medical School
Children's Hospital
300 Longwood Avenue
Boston, Massachusetts

Peter C. Laussen, MB, BS
Assistant Professor in Anaesthesia
Harvard Medical School
Children's Hospital
300 Longwood Avenue
Boston, Massachusetts

James E. Lock, M.D.
Chair, Alexander S. Nadas
Professor of Pediatrics
Harvard Medical School
Department of Cardiology
Children's Hospital
300 Longwood Avenue
Boston, Massachusetts

John E. Mayer, M.D.
Professor of Surgery
Harvard Medical School
Children's Hospital
300 Longwood Avenue
Boston, Massachusetts

Phillip Moore, M.D.
Assistant Clinical Professor of
Pediatrics.
U.C.S.F.
Box 0544, House 1403
505 Parnassuss Avenue
San Francisco, California

Stanton B. Perry, M.D.
Assistant Professor of Pediatrics
Harvard Medical School
Children's Hospital
300 Longwood Avenue
Boston, Massachusetts

Albert Rocchini, M.D.
Professor of Pediatrics
Univ. of Michigan Health System
Director of Pediatric Cardiology
C.S. Mott Children's Hospital
Box 0204
Ann Arbor, Michigan

Johnathan Rome, M.D.
Assistant Professor of Pediatrics
Univ. of Penn. School of Medicine
Children's Hospital of Philadelphia
324 South 34th Street
Philadelphia, Pennsylvania

Mary E. Van der Velde, M.D.
Assistant Professor of Pediatrics
Harvard Medical School
Children's Hospital
300 Longwood Avenue
Boston, Massachusetts

Edward P. Walsh, M.D.
Associate Professor of Pediatrics
Harvard Medical School
Children's Hospital
300 Longwood Avenue
Boston, Massachusetts

Scott B. Yeager, M.D.
Associate Professor in Ped. Card.
University of Vermont
Fletcher Allen Health Care
McClure 1, MCHV
Burlington, Vermont

PREFACE

By all appearances, the field of cardiac catheterization for congenital heart disease is nearing the end of a period of rapid expansion, change, and diversification. Now is a good time to identify and assess many of these changes. This kind of retrospective view serves more purposes than self-congratulation: it allows a clearer prediction of where the field is likely to go, and how it gets there.

The first and most obvious change is the continued rapid growth of catheter-directed interventional procedures. Balloon valvotomies are well established, as are coil closure of PDA's and stent enlargement of central pulmonary arteries. Even the more exotic procedures such as closure of VSD and paravalvar leaks, and coil embolization of coronary fistula have become commonplace in some centers. The next decade will see a consolidation of these gains, with incremental improvements in devices and sharpening of indications, patient selection, and follow up studies.

A less dramatic but equally pervasive change has been the improvement in non-invasive diagnosis, primarily by ultrasound but increasingly via magnetic resonance imaging. Diagnostic studies account for fewer than 40% of our catheterizations. That percentage will continue to shrink, but the pace of change will slow until we provide much better non-invasive assessments in two areas which have resisted change: the non-invasive measurement of intracavitary pressure, and the non-invasive diagnosis of rejection following cardiac transplantation. One non-invasive diagnostic arena that does seem poised for a rapid change is the use of magnetic resonance angiography to measure instantaneous flows and velocities. This will not only obviate the need to measure cardiac output, it may provide accurate measurements of regurgitant volumes, and hence accurate evaluations of procedures that produce or relieve valve regurgitation.

A much less obvious but highly revolutionary change has been the consolidation and shrinkage of cardiologists who perform interventional procedures. Higher standards, more demanding technical skills, and an increased awareness of institutional and individual learning curves for complex procedures has made the part-time invasive cardiologist an endangered species. An interesting converse of this trend has been the emergence of the outpatient specialist for congenital heart disease, a development that has major implications for training programs and departmental organization.

Where will the next decade take the catheterizer and his or her colleagues? Perhaps into catheter delivery of gene therapy to treat inherited myopathies or vasculopathies. Even likelier is the use of catheters to implant pulmonary valves made from a patient's own tissue. Likelier still will be the demise of film and the continued emergence of the multimedia laboratory.

Underlying the success of any and all of these changes will be a commitment to rigorous self-criticism and unbiased analysis. A renewed commitment to these values is especially important at this time for the field of diagnostic and interventional catheterization in congenital heart disease.

ACKNOWLEDGEMENTS

This book is dedicated to the cardiology fellows-in-training, technicians and nurses at the catheterization laboratories where these diagnostic and interventional studies were undertaken and to Drs. Alexander S. Nadas, Donald C. Fyler, John A. Kelly, Arthur M. Levy and Burton. S. Tabakin. We are grateful for manuscript preparation to Joni D'Annolfo, Julie Fedorwich, Minet Mitchell, Tara O'Regan, Carol Richardson, Carol Vey and Eileen Walsh, for proof reading (among many other things) to Clare Keane and for all figures and art work to Emily and Bill Flynn McIntosh. Finally we are deeply indebted to Deirdre O'Donnell whose skill, humor, tolerance and enthusiasm have made this book possible.

INTERVENTIONAL CATHETERIZATION: A SURGEON'S PERSPECTIVE

John E. Mayer, Jr., M.D.

Innovations in interventional catheterization techniques and the availability of multiple devices which can be delivered through catheters have significantly altered the management of certain forms of congenital heart disease in many centers. This expanding role for interventional catheterization has the potential for creating a competitive atmosphere between surgeons and interventional cardiologists over the treatment of some of these forms of congenital heart disease. From one perspective, the use of interventional catheterization techniques could be interpreted as a presenting a threat to the practices of congenital heart surgeons since, when viewed in isolation, they appear to result in a reduction in the number of cases referred for surgical intervention. In addition, for defects such as atrial septal defects, pulmonary valvar stenosis, patent ductus arteriosus, and coarctation of the aorta, the "lost" surgical procedures are relatively straightforward, "bread and butter" procedures which have a low surgical risk and which are important cases for the education and training of surgical fellows. From a different perspective, however, it is short-sighted to view surgical interventions and interventional catheterization techniques as "competing" therapeutic approaches to the treatment of congenital heart defects. In many forms of congenital heart disease, the data are quite convincing that an interventional catheterization approach is less invasive, equally effective, and frequently less costly than a classical surgical procedure. The treatment of pulmonary valvar stenosis by balloon dilation of the pulmonary valve is an example of a situation in which the interventional catheterization approach is associated with such desirable outcomes. As a consequence, surgical pulmonary valvotomy for pulmonary valvar stenosis has become a rare entry on the surgical case log here at Children's Hospital. As experience has been gained with both surgical and interventional catheterization approaches to more complex congenital cardiac defects, it has become clear that the techniques are more often complementary than competing. It is the purpose of this discussion to outline at least some of the ways in which surgical and interventional catheterization approaches complement one another so that the ability to treat patients with more complex forms of congenital heart disease is enhanced.

VENTRICULAR SEPTAL DEFECT

The large majority of ventricular septal defects which require closure seem to be best managed by a surgical approach. For defects in the paramembranous area, the inlet septum, the posterior muscular septum, and the outlet septum, surgical results are quite good, and non-surgical device approaches place adjacent valve structures at significant risk for entanglement or injury by a device delivered via a catheter. Since surgical therapy is highly successful in achieving both defect closure and avoiding injury to adjacent structures, surgical approaches seem preferable for defects in these areas. The more problematic patients are those with multiple VSDs, particularly when one or more of the VSDs are at the apex of the heart below the moderator band, where the extensive trabeculations can make surgical exposure of the defects via the right atrium or infundibulum more difficult. Ideal surgical exposure can be obtained via a left ventriculotomy, but there is some evidence to suggest that a significant number of patients having a left ventriculotomy will have significant depression of left ventricular function as a result.[1] Therefore, for some defects in the apical area of the septum, a catheterization laboratory approach has proven to be of significant value.[2] We have utilized an apical right ventricular approach with some success for isolated apical ventricular septal defects, and the appropriate selection criteria for surgical vs. interventional catheterization approaches remain to be determined.

A second situation where a surgical approach seems to be less successful is that of residual ventricular septal defects following attempted surgical closure, particularly in patients with double outlet right ventricle and tetralogy of Fallot. These defects seem to be frequently located behind muscle bands in the infundibular area which can be difficult to identify surgically. Some success has been reported with interventional catheterization approaches to these "intramural" ventricular septal defects.[3] The indications for surgical vs. interventional device closure of ventricular septal defects will likely continue to evolve as improvements in both surgical and interventional catheterization techniques are refined.

TETRALOGY OF FALLOT

In most cases of tetralogy of Fallot, standard surgical therapy yields extremely good results with a low mortality and complication rate.[4] The more difficult cases to manage with an exclusively surgical approach are those with tetralogy of Fallot, severely hypoplastic central pulmonary arteries, and multiple aorto-pulmonary collaterals. In these patients we have found that a combined interventional catheterization and surgical approach has resulted in a significant number of these patients being able to undergo closure of the ventricular septal defect with right ventricular pressures which are less than 2/3 of systemic.[5] The interventional catheterization techniques which are used in these patients include balloon dilation and stenting of the hypoplastic pulmonary arteries and coil occlusion of aorto-pulmonary collaterals which are supplying segments that are also supplied by the central pulmonary arteries.

The timing and staging of surgical and catheterization laboratory interventions in these patients must be individualized due to the significant variations within the spectrum of this disorder, and close communication and planning by both the surgeon and interventional catheterization team is essential. A typical pattern of interventions for a patient with tetralogy of Fallot, diminutive central pulmonary arteries, and multiple aorto-pulmonary collateral vessels would entail an initial diagnostic catheterization to establish the diagnosis and then placement of a small (8-11mm) right ventricle to pulmonary artery homograft conduit in the first year of life, leaving the VSD open. Subsequently, a repeat catheterization is carried out several months later to more completely establish the anatomy of the pulmonary circulation. It has been our experience that angiography carried out antegrade by direct injection into the true pulmonary arteries has frequently demonstrated that the central pulmonary arteries are distributed to more segments of lung parenchyma than could be demonstrated on the initial diagnostic catheterization where dye entered the pulmonary circulation only through systemic to pulmonary artery collaterals. At this same follow-up catheterization, those aortopulmonary collaterals which supply segments of the lung which are also supplied from the true pulmonary arteries can be occluded with coils. Hypoplastic pulmonary arteries can be dilated and/or stented at the same catheterization. After 2-3 months, a repeat catheterization is carried out to assess the results of the surgical and catheterization interventions, and when a net left to right shunt is found at the ventricular level, the ventricular septal defect can generally be successfully closed and the right ventricular to pulmonary artery conduit is replaced. In some patients we have placed a ventricular septal defect patch with a restrictive "fenestration" of 3-4 mm diameter and have been able to close this fenestration at a subsequent catheterization. The treatment of patients with tetralogy and diminutive pulmonary arteries has been an important area where the collaborations between interventional catheterization techniques and surgical interventions have significantly increased the possibility of achieving a more favorable result than either discipline could offer alone.

SINGLE VENTRICLE:

The management of patients with single ventricle is a third area in which the combination of surgical and interventional catheterization techniques has significantly improved the outcome for patients and has expanded the population of patients who can achieve a circulation in which the systemic and pulmonary venous return can be separated to achieve full oxygenation. Nearly ten years ago the concept of creating a fenestration in the partition between the systemic and venous return as part of the Fontan procedure and then closing this fenestration with a device delivered in the catheterization laboratory was described by Bridges et al.[6] There is reasonably good evidence that the use of the fenestration has allowed higher risk patients to undergo this procedure with comparable mortality and morbidity (primarily pleural effusions) to a lower risk group of patients.[7]

However, there are a number of other problems that are encountered in patients with single ventricle where interventional catheterization techniques augment and simplify the surgical approach to constructing a Fontan circulation. Pulmonary artery distortions have been demonstrated to have a negative impact on the outcome after Fontan operations,[8] and balloon dilations and stenting have been successfully employed in patients with hypoplastic or distorted pulmonary arteries. In addition, patients may develop connections between the systemic venous system and either the pulmonary veins or the atrium which will serve as the pulmonary venous atrium after the Fontan procedure. These collaterals between the systemic veins and the pulmonary venous atrium will result in arterial desaturation after the Fontan procedure, and may be difficult to identify at surgery, particularly in patients with prior surgical procedures. Therefore it is our current practice to attempt occlusion of these collaterals either prior to or following the Fontan procedure. Single ventricle patients also have a tendency to develop collateral vessels between the systemic arterial and the pulmonary arterial circulations. These collaterals often arise from the internal thoracic (mammary) arteries and from the intercostal arteries, and are not uncommon in patients who have had prior palliative surgical procedures. These collaterals will provide pulmonary blood flow which can potentially "compete" with systemic venous return for access to the pulmonary circulation and thereby raise pulmonary artery pressure following the Fontan circulation. It has been our practice to attempt to identify these collateral vessels at preoperative catheterization and to occlude them with coils since these collaterals can also be difficult to identify at the time of surgery.

CONCLUDING COMMENTS:

The intent of this brief discussion of the interactions between congenital heart surgeons and interventional cardiologists has been to demonstrate some of the ways in which these interactions can improve and expand the therapeutic options open to patients with more complex forms of congenital heart disease. In these situations, surgical and interventional catheterization techniques are clearly complementary rather than competitive therapies, and better patient outcomes are the result, and the number of patients who can be effectively treated is increased. In other situations outlined in the introduction, the therapies might be viewed as competitive with only one of the two options being employed in the therapy of a given defect. However, when viewed from the perspective of the patient, the availability of more than one option is potentially a benefit, since the patient receives the additional value of having a choice of therapeutic options. Patients will not always choose "less invasive" catheterization techniques when presented with all of the known information. It should be the goal of a program for congenital heart disease management that patients be provided with the highest quality care and the highest value interventions. It is only the patients and their families who can determine what is of value to them, and the overall value of a program is enhanced when the patients have "choice."

There are other benefits of a strong interventional catheterization program to the congenital heart surgeon. To the extent that there is "competition" between various therapies surgeons are prompted to refine and improve surgical techniques such as the use of thoracoscopy for ligation of patent ductus arteriosus, and use of limited or "mini-" sternotomy approaches for the repair of certain intracardiac defects. It is critically important that an open intellectual atmosphere be maintained within a congenital cardiac program, and there must be a willingness on the side of both surgeons and cardiologists to allow for the development and trial of new techniques. It is in this type of atmosphere that many advances have occurred in our own institution, and future advances in the management of congenital heart disease seem more likely to occur when an open, intellectually challenging, and collaborative atmosphere is maintained.

BIBLIOGRAPHY

1. Hanna B, Colan SD, Bridges ND, Mayer JE, Castaneda A. Clinical and myocardial status after left ventriculotomy for ventricular septal defect closure. J Am Coll Cardiol 1991; 17: Suppl: 110A. Abstract.

2. Bridges ND, Perry SB, Keane JF, Goldstein SAN, Mandell V, Mayer JE Jr, JonasRA, Castaneda AR, and Lock JE. Preoperative transcatheter closure of congenital muscular ventricular septal defects. New Eng J Med 1991;324:1312-1317.

3. Preminger TJ, Sanders SP, van der Velde ME, Castaneda AR, Lock JE: "Intramural" Residual intraventricular defects after repair of conotruncal malformations. Circulation 1994; 89: 236-242.

4. Kirklin JW, Blackstone EH, Jonas RA, Shimazaki Y, Kirklin JK, Mayer JE Jr, Pacifico AD, Castaneda AR. Morphologic and surgical determinants of outcome events after repair of tetralogy of Fallot and pulmonary stenosis. A two-institution study. J Thorac and Cardiovasc Surgery, 1992;103:706-723.

5. Rome JJ, Mayer JE Jr, Castaneda AR, Lock JE. Tetralogy of Fallot with pulmonary atresia. Rehabilitation of diminutive pulmonary arteries. Circulation 1993;88 (part 1):1691-1698.

6. Bridges ND, Lock JE, Castaneda AR. Baffle Fenestration with Subsequent Transcatheter Closure. Modification of the Fontan Operation for Patients at Increased Risk. 1990;82:1681-1689.

7. Bridges ND, Mayer JE Jr, Lock JE, Castaneda AR: Effect of fenestration on outcome of Fontan repair. Circ 1991;84:Suppl II:II-120-II-120.

8. Mayer JE Jr, Bridges ND, Lock JE, Hanley FL, Jonas RA, Castaneda AR: Factors associated with marked reduction in mortality for Fontan operations in patients with single ventricle. J Thorac Cardiovasc Surg 1992;103:444-452.

1. EVALUATION AND MANAGEMENT PRIOR TO CATHETERIZATION

James E. Lock, M.D.

For the last three decades, improvements in the diagnosis and management of congenital heart disease have resulted in some of the most astounding survival increases in all of medical science. Despite this progress, deciding whether to catheterize a particular child remains a difficult, uneven, and poorly predictable event. Testimony to the difficulty of this decision is provided by a recent study by Kreutzer et al [1]. Using administrative data bases from several states, and assuming that the indications for surgery are roughly equivalent across multiple centers, the frequency of catheterizations per open heart surgeries varies enormously (Fig. 1-1).

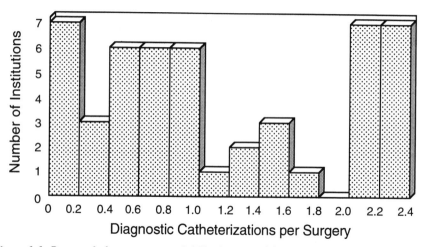

Figure 1-1: Bar graph demonstrates variability in rates of diagnostic cardiac catheterizations per surgical repair for ventricular septal defect among institutions from 9 states in 1992 (data obtained from analysis of hospital discharge administrative data).

The precise sources of this variability are not known, and understanding it would undoubtedly improve clinical decision making and resource allocation decisions. Nonetheless, several factors are likely responsible, at least in part, for this marked variability in the utilization of cardiac catheterization.

THE MEDICAL AND PYSCHOLOGICAL RISKS OF CARDIAC CATHETERIZATION.

Efforts to reduce the risks and pain of cardiac catheterization, including improved catheter tools, contrast agents, imaging systems, and limitations on credentialing of cardiologists to perform catheterizations, have succeeded. The mortality rate for diagnostic cardiac catheterizations has fallen as has the complication rate, even for patients thought to be at the highest risk (i.e. neonates and patients with primary pulmonary hypertension)[2]. Thus, a low risk procedure that may improve management will be utilized more frequently.

THE ACCURACY OF NON-INVASIVE TESTING.

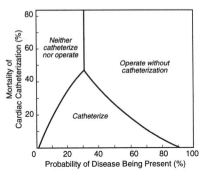

Improved echocardiographic and magnetic resonance imaging techniques significantly reduce the need for cardiac catheterization and run counter to improvements in catheterization results. This simple relation was first described by McCartney et al (Fig. 1-2), and helps explain some of the variability.

Figure 1-2: The decision of whether or not to catheterize an infant with coarctation of the aorta depends on the risks of the catheterization and the accuracy of the non-invasive testing. (Printed from MaCartney et al., Br. Heart J. 51:330, 1984).

THE SUCCESS OF MANAGEMENT OF THE DISEASE IN QUESTION.

If medical or surgical management is almost always successful (e.g., the silent PDA, or arterial switch for simple TGA), improving diagnostic accuracy seems a bit superfluous. On the other hand, catheterization may very well be justified in very dangerous conditions (e.g., primary pulmonary hypertension or HLHS s/p Stage 1) even when the results of catheterization are often of limited value.

THE ECONOMIC COSTS OF CATHETERIZATION.

Among the most frequently lamented influences on medical decision-making is the impact of financial considerations on the consumption of medical care. Such considerations will have more of an impact on procedures such as cardiac catheterization in congenital heart disease, where the medical indications are changing rapidly and are ill-defined. Some economic forces serve to artificially increase cath lab utilization (hospital profitability, professional reimbursements), while others (capitated care, insurance disallowances) artificially reduce it. A healthy, reasonable and balanced alignment of financial incentives has yet to come to the management of congenital heart disease. Until it does, giving the proper weight to financial considerations depends primarily on the integrity and wisdom of the physicians involved.

Ten years ago, we described the decision-making process of whom to catheterize as a series of "collaborative, floating, ad hoc decisions by clinical cardiologists, surgeons, ultrasonographers, radiologists and catheterizing cardiologists". That process hasn't changed, but the results have: there are, in general, fewer diagnostic catheterizations and more frequent interventional studies (Fig. 1-3).

It must seem disappointing that this process is so unscientific. One might well expect that two or three studies, similar to the well-designed prospective trials so common in coronary artery disease, would compare echo results, cath results,

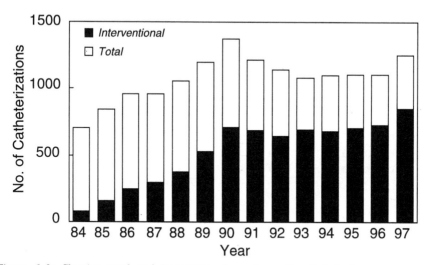

Figure 1-3: Showing total and interventional numbers of catheterization per year at Children's Hospital Boston 1984 – 1997.

and surgical outcomes to arrive at a much more precise understanding of the indications for cardiac catheterization in children or adults with congenital heart disease. Such studies are unlikely to become widely utilized in the decision analysis of congenital heart disease for several reasons: the diseases are rare, making statistically meaningful data sets for any given disease difficult to acquire. In addition, the indications for cardiac catheterization are very strongly dependent on the skill of the operating catheterizer, as well as the skills of the operating surgeon and the operating ultrasonographer.

This operator dependence is a confounding variable in many medical disciplines, but is most important in procedurally dominated disciplines taking care of rare anatomic disease, and is perhaps best exemplified in the case of patients with congenital heart disease. Until effective statistical tools to assess and control for operator skill become available, such prospective multicenter trials will be rare and difficult to interpret.

We have, nonetheless, prepared a modified table of the indications for cardiac catheterization that embodies the current practice at the Children's Hospital in Boston (Table 1-1). When compared to a decade ago, the changes are obvious: diagnostic studies are becoming increasingly rare, with fewer indications. Interventions are now becoming commonplace, and widely accepted. Although many of the indications are straightforward, some deserve further comment.

4

TABLE 1-1

Diagnosis	Cath Usually Indicated?	Potential or Real Indication for Catheterization
1. ASD secundum	Yes and No	Catheter closure in appropriate cases
2. ASD primum	No	Rule out suspected associated defects
3. CAVC	No	Rule out suspected associated defects
4. Aortic stenosis	Yes	Valvuloplasty
5. Aortic stenosis and regurgitation, pre Ross	Yes and No	Confirm hemodynamics, assess LV compliance
6. Coarctation, native	Yes and No	Angioplasty/Stent
7. Coarctation, post-op	Yes	Angioplasty/Stent
8. Mitral stenosis, pre-op	Yes	Valvuloplasty
9. Mitral valve replacement	Yes	Hemodynamic assessment
10. PDA	Yes and No	Device closure
11. Tetralogy of Fallot, pre-op	No	Close muscular VSD, aortopulmonary collaterals
12. Tetralogy of Fallot, pulmonary atresia	Yes	Define PA anatomy
13. Tetralogy of Fallot and PA, post-op	Yes	Angioplasty & Stents of PAs, conduit
14. Truncus, TGA/VSD/PS, S/P conduit repair	Yes	Close intramural VSD, stent conduit
15. TGA	Yes	Balloon septostomy
16. Single Ventricle, pre-op	No	Rule out suspected associated defects
17. Single Ventricle, pre-Glenn	Yes	Hemodynamics, close venous and arterial collaterals
18. Single Ventricle, pre-Fontan	Yes	Hemodynamics, close collaterals, dilate PA's
19. Single Ventricle, post-Fontan	Yes	Correct residual abnormalities
20. TAPVR	No	Assess intraparenchymal pulmonary veins
21. Pulmonary Atresia, Intact Septum	Yes	Define coronary anatomy

4

Table 1-1 (continued)		
22. PFO, S/P Neurologic event	Yes	Device closure
23. Peripheral Pulmonary Stenosis	Yes	Angioplasty, stents
24. VSD, Simple	No	Assess elevated PVR
25. VSD, Multiple Muscular		Catheter closure

INDICATIONS FOR CARDIAC CATHETERIZATION

ASD secundum: The significant advances in transcatheter closure technology, and the favorable late results of at least one device (see Chapter 7) makes it increasingly likely that catheter closure will become the treatment of choice for many patients. More precise indications will be possible as further data accumulate on device follow up [3], results of minimal sternotomy surgery and the neurologic effects of cardiopulmonary bypass [4].

Coarctation, Pre-op and Post-op: The increasingly successful results of stents in both native and recurrent coarctations, coupled with accumulating evidence that even mild residual gradients have adverse effects [5], will increase the indications for intervention in this group of patients.

Tetralogy of Fallot, Prior to Repair: Advances in echocardiography have made this a rare indication for diagnostic study at our hospital. Nonetheless, one must have heightened awareness of the potential for abnormalities (e.g. muscular VSDs, aortopulmonary collaterals) that will cause left-to-right shunts post-operatively: such shunts will be poorly tolerated.

Pulmonary Atresia, Intact Septum: Precise pre-operative definition of coronary anatomy is mandatory.

Total Anomalous Pulmonary Venous Return: The subgroup of patients with mixed drainage and/or obstruction continue to have a distressingly high incidence of post-operative progressive obstruction. We no longer attribute this problem to surgical effects: it appears to be, somehow, an intrinsic problem of parenchymal pulmonary veins in many patients. Although it is hard to see how pre-operative catheterizations would improve our understanding of these patients, gathering more data makes some sense.

Single Ventricle, Status Post Fontan: The Fontan circulation is inherently unstable, and even minor hemodynamic abnormalities in asymptomatic patients can insidiously destabilize the circulation to the point that devastating and largely irreversible complications ensue. A policy of catheterizing all post-op Fontan patients and correcting even minor abnormalities in asymptomatic patients makes considerable sense.

Large Patent Ductus Arteriosus: Although small (< 3 mm) PDAs are easily, safely and cheaply closed with coils, device closure for larger PDAs is in stiff competition with video assisted thoracic surgery. Both procedures are improving relatively rapidly; either could emerge as superior.

Tetralogy with Pulmonary Atresia, Truncus Arteriosus or TGA, S/P Conduit Repair: These patients have a combination of a right ventriculotomy and a conduit that will deteriorate into progressive stenosis and regurgitation over time. This combination seems to be bad for long-term right ventricular function; even subsystemic right ventricular pressures can produce considerable late right ventricular dysfunction. Aggressive use of stents to minimize right ventricular pressure throughout childhood would seem only prudent.

Patent Foramen Ovale After a Single Neurologic Event: PFOs are so common in the normal population that special efforts to close all of them would be foolhardy. However, since the initial report of PFO closure following an initial event [6], considerable attention has focussed on this problem. Although many of the current uncertainties will only be resolved by a trial comparing Coumadin with device closure, young patients are exposed to a larger cumulative lifelong risk from medical therapy. Device closure in these patients would make considerable sense.

HISTORY AND PHYSICAL EXAMINATION

Each patient must have a thorough general history and physical examination prior to cardiac catheterization, as well as a complete cardiac examination. In addition to this routine evaluation, one must seek some information that relates directly to the technical aspects of performing a routine cardiac catheterization.

Prior History
Family or patient history of bleeding disorder, allergy to drugs, or contrast reactions.

Intercurrent illness or recent fever. A recent illness does not completely preclude a safe cardiac catheterization, depending to some extent on how "elective" the catheterization is. For infants with severe congestive heart failure and frequent infections, it may prove difficult to find a two-week fever-free period during the winter. In general, however, it is wise to avoid catheterization in someone who is febrile (38.0 degrees or higher) or who is likely to be bacteremic during the procedure.

Last menstrual period or possible pregnancy in adolescent or adult females. One needs a powerful reason to expose such a patient to radiation.

Prior catheterizations or cardiac operations. Pay particular attention to unsuccessful prior catheterization attempts or operations (Glenn procedure, Blalock-Taussig shunts) that might limit vascular access.

Physical Examination

Right or left thoracotomy scars. Such scars may be due to prior Blalock-Taussig or Glenn shunts; either may preclude access to the heart from the arms.

Groin or antecubital fossa scars. Previous vascular cutdowns may make subsequent percutaneous study difficult, but by no means impossible. A saphenous cutdown scar will migrate distally with growth, allowing percutaneous vascular entry proximal to the scar but distal to the inguinal ligament. A long (4-6 inch) vertical groin scar will result from a prior cardiac operation during which cardiopulmonary bypass using large bore cannulae was instituted from the common femoral arteries and veins. These vessels are repaired at the end of the procedure, generally remain patent, and can usually be entered percutaneously. However, extensive scar tissue will make passage of dilators and sheaths difficult.

Abdominal, thoracic, or neck vein distension. Patients who have had a Mustard or Senning operation, or infants with prolonged ICU courses and indwelling central lines, will occasionally develop obstruction of the vena cava or either limb of the systemic venous baffle. If severe, these obstructions will cause cutaneous veins to engorge over the anterior thorax. One can generally deduce from physical examination the location of the obstruction.

Peripheral arterial pulses and pressures. Aortic coarctation is the most common but not the only congenital lesion (e.g., subclavian artery isolation) that may limit arterial access to the heart.

LABORATORY TESTS

Every patient with congenital heart disease about to be catheterized needs several routine tests. These tests should include a standard EKG, both frontal and lateral chest films, a two-dimensional echocardiogram, urinalysis and a complete blood count. These tests may be obtained the day of the catheterization or, if the patient is stable, they may be obtained days or weeks in advance of the study. In addition, a number of special tests may need to be obtained prior to catheterization.

Deeply cyanosed older children (hemoglobin over 20 grams%, older than 5 years) may need to have baseline coagulation studies and a platelet count obtained to assess the degree of coagulopathy of the cyanotic heart disease [7,8].

All infants (less than 5 kg) undergoing cardiac catheterization should have a unit of blood typed and cross-matched because of the relatively higher blood loss associated with catheterization. Blood should also be available for patients in whom a transseptal puncture, pericardial tap, septostomy, angioplasty, balloon valvotomy, cardiac biopsy, or transcatheter PDA, atrial (ASD) or eventual septal defect (VSD) closure is planned. All patients undergoing catheterization should have a reliable intravenous line for sedation, resuscitation, or volume replacement.

The hemoglobin level in cyanotic children should be known more than one day prior to catheterization. If the hemoglobin level exceeds 19-20 grams%, intravenous fluids should be given overnight to reduce the risks of dehydration-induced thrombosis [9], hypotension, and further systemic desaturation.

If aortic, mitral, or pulmonary valvotomy is planned at catheterization, the valve annulus diameter should be estimated from a pre-catheterization echocardiogram, and clots in the left atrium or ventricle must be excluded by echo.

Digitalis should be held beginning the night prior to catheterization in order to reduce the risks of catheterization-induced arrhythmias. Quantitative lung scans are needed prior to catheterization in those patients (mostly with tetralogy of Fallot) in whom a significant branch pulmonary artery stenosis is suspected. All other things being equal, one should dilate the artery to the lung receiving the smallest blood flow.

Finally, transesophageal echocardiography has proven to be invaluable in patient selection for catheter closure of ASDs and many VSDs.

PRECATHETERIZATION SEDATION AND FEEDING

Sedation

The optimum sedation for catheterization studies in children (or adults) with congenital heart disease has not been established. The most commonly used sedative/analgesia/anesthetic regimens include Demerol, Phenergan, and Thorazine given as a intramuscular injection (DPT cocktail) [10], morphine and secobarbital [11], droperidol and fentanyl [12], ketamine [13], chloral hydrate, or Valium (see Chapter 12).

Most sedative drugs are known to be vasoactive themselves at various doses, each can have unwanted side effects, and several (especially the DPT cocktail) can alter electrophysiologic properties of heart tissue. The most reasonable approach is to develop an extensive clinical experience, hemodynamic data base, and electrophysiologic data base with only one form of sedation. Our current practices are outlined in Chapter 12.

Feeding

Adolescent or adult patients who undergo elective catheterization procedures are held n.p.o. after midnight, although a small clear liquid breakfast can be given to patients whose case will start late in the day. More attention is needed for infants and young children if dehydration and hypoglycemia are to be avoided (Table 1-2).

TABLE 1-2 Precatheterization Feeding Order

Age	First Case	Second Case
Infants (1 year)	Full diet until 4 A.M. Clear liquids at 6 A.M.	Full diet until 7 A.M. Clear liquids at 9 A.M.
Children (1-5 yr)	Full diet until midnight Clear liquids at 4 A.M.	Full diet until 7 A.M. Clear liquids at 8 A.M.

EXPLAINING CARDIAC CATHETERIZATION BEFORE THE PROCEDURE

Risks

Before informed consent for a catheterization can be obtained from parents and patients, a clear understanding of the risks and benefits of the procedure is required. Mortality from a cardiac catheterization in an older child is exceedingly rare and, when seen, is usually related to very poor precatheterization clinical status or angiography in patients with severe pulmonary hypertension. Mortality is higher in catheterization of the newborn, but even then it is less than 1% (2,14).

Common complications include low-grade fever for 4-8 hours, hematoma at the catheterization site, transient (1-48 hours) occlusion of the catheterized vessel, or transient arrhythmias. Much rarer complications (less than 1% frequency) include strokes, cardiac perforation, permanent pulse loss, seizures, contrast induced transient loss of visual acuity, and allergic reactions to contrast. Specific interventional procedures have their own risks that must be described on an individual basis. The consenting parent or child needs to be informed of the risk of death, the relatively common problems of hematoma and pulse loss, and much rarer but serious complications of stroke and seizures.

Experienced medical and nursing personnel have known for some time that efforts to reduce precatheterization fear will make the procedure less stressful for all concerned. Several books and tapes are available [15] that are designed to explain the catheterization procedure in preschool terms. We have found them helpful.

When discussing a cardiac catheterization with parents and the child who has congenital heart disease (and indeed while planning for catheterization laboratory facilities), it is important to estimate the duration of the procedure. For several reasons, catheterization laboratory procedures in adults, children, and especially infants with congenital heart disease require more time than do procedures in adults with acquired disease. Procedures are longer because many patients have had previous studies and have limited access sites; in infants the vessels are smaller and more difficult to cannulate; the presence of intracardiac shunts obviates the use of quick thermodilution methods for measuring cardiac output; catheter courses are frequently more complicated, and multiple angiograms in several cardiac chambers, using different catheters and views, are often needed. While a 1998 catheterization of the left heart and coronaries in an adult may last 20 to 60 minutes, a time study done at the Children's Hospital, Boston, demonstrated that the average congenital catheterization lasted 4 hours and 3 minutes (Fig. 1-4). A concerted attempt to make the laboratory more efficient reduced that time to 3 hours and 40 minutes. While Children's has a diagnostic/therapeutic patient mix skewed toward complicated cases, many requiring interventional procedures, and while the hospital is a training center, these data indicate that the proper catheterization of patients with congenital heart disease is a time-consuming affair.

OUTPATIENT CARDIAC CATHETERIZATION

Catheterization without admission is now widespread in many pediatric cardiology centers [16]. We estimate that as many as 10-15% of patients scheduled to undergo an outpatient study may need subsequent overnight admission for poor fluid intake, fever, or pulse loss, but if patients known to be at risk are still routinely admitted, there appear to be few disadvantages and many advantages to a program of outpatient catheterization in congenital heart disease (Table 1-3).

TABLE 1-3 Candidates for outpatient cardiac catheterization in congenital heart disease.

1. Over 1 year of age.
2. Acyanotic or mild cyanosis (Hemoglobin < 20 grams %).
3. Less than severe heart failure.
4. Not scheduled for major therapeutic catheterization.

PLANNING THE CATHETERIZATION

Catheterization preparations are not complete until the procedure has been carefully mapped in advance. The diagnostic and therapeutic options in congenital heart disease are quite broad, and the range of patient sizes, angiographic catheters, injection sites and rates, angiographic views, types of hemodynamic variables to be measured, and the potential for unexpected findings is extensive. To make this procedure more efficient, to reduce the possibility that important steps and information will be neglected, and to identify all potential therapeutic procedures in advance, each case should be discussed in a precatheterization conference with cardiologists, radiologists, and trainees. All data should be reviewed, especially previous echocardiograms and angiograms. The review of previous cines orients the catheterizer to the case at hand, and helps prevent the accumulation of redundant information. Such a conference serves the additional role of exposing each decision to catheterize a patient to open peer review.

After the case presentation, the catheterizing cardiologist(s) must identify in considerable detail a plan of approach. The most likely findings, the contingency plans for the unexpected and the therapeutic pitfalls, should all be identified in advance (Table 1-4). After these preparations have been completed, one enters the laboratory.

TABLE 1-4   Planning the catheterization

1.	Preferred, and backup site or sites of vascular access.
2.	Method for obtaining vascular entry, size of sheath(s).
3.	Initial venous catheter, and intended catheter course.
4.	Initial arterial catheter (if needed) and intended catheter course.
5.	Method of choice (and backup) for measuring cardiac output and resistances.
6.	Particular important hemodynamic measurements, and alternate plans for obtaining them.
7.	Other physiologic studies (electrophysiology, oxygen, exercise, etc.) to be obtained prior to any angiography.
8.	First (and hence most important) angiogram. Catheter position, catheter type, flow rate, patient position.
9.	Subsequent angiography.
10.	Potential types of transcatheter therapy, criteria for performing therapy.
11.	Vascular entry site for therapeutic catheter, type of catheter and how to choose it, method for performing procedure.
12.	Follow-up hemodynamics and angiography.
13.	Postcatheterization management.

REFERENCES

1. Kreutzer J, Jenkins KJ, Gavreau K, et al. Variability in use of diagnostic cardiac catheterization for common congenital heart defects in children. Book of Abstracts "The 2nd World congress of Pediatric Cardiology and Cardiac Surgery", 1997, P514.
2. Vitello R., McCrindle BW, Nykanen D, et al. Complications associated with Pediatric Cardiac Catheterization. J Am Coll Cardiol 1998:32 1433-1440.
3. Jenkins KJ, Newburger, JW, Faherty C, et al: Midterm follow-up using the original Bard clamshell septal occluder; complete experience at one center. Circulation 1995: 92(8): 1-308 (abstr).

12

4. Bellinger DC, Jonas RA, Rappaport LA, et al: Developmental and Neurologic Status of Children After Heart Surgery with Hypothermic Circulatory Arrest or Low Flow Cardiopulmonary Bypass. N Engl J Med 1995: 332:549-555.

5. Chung AM, Perry SB, Keane JF, et al: Late Hemodynamic and Anatomic Results of Balloon-Expanded Stent Implantation for Coarctation of the Aorta. Circ 1997, Vol. 96; Suppl 1- 568(A).

6. Bridges ND, Hellenbrand W, Latson et al: Transcatheter Closure of Patient Foramen Ovale After Presumed Paradoxical Embolism. Circ 1992: 86: 1902-1908.

7. Komp DM, Sparrow AW. Polycythemia in cyanotic congenital heart disease – a study of altered coagulation. J Pediatr 1970: 7:231-236.

8. Wedemeyer AL, Lewis JH. Improvement in hemostasis following phlebotomy in cyanotic patients with heart disease. J Pediatr 1973: 83:46-50.

9. Cottrill CM, Kaplan S. Cerebral vascular accidents in cyanotic congenital heart disease. Am J Dis Child 1973: 125:484-487.

10. Ruckman RN, Keane JF, Freed MD, et al. Sedation for cardiac catheterization: A controlled study. Pediatr Cardiol 1980: 1:263-268.

11. Moller JH, Rao S, Lucas RV. Exercise hemodynamics of pulmonary valvar stenosis. Circulation 1972: 46:864-874.

12. Graham TP Jr, Atwood GF and Werner BW. Use of Droperidol-fentanyl sedation for cardiac catheterization in children. Am Heart J 1974: 87:287-293.

13. Faithfull NS, Harder R. Ketamine for cardiac catheterization. An evaluation of its use in children. Anesthesia 1971: 26:318.

14. Cohn HE, Freed MD, Hellenbrand WE, et al. Complications and mortality associated with cardiac catheterization in infants under one year. Pediatr Cardiol 1986.

15. Stevie has his heart examined. Biomedical Graphic Communications, University of Minnesota Hospitals, Minneapolis 1983.

16. Waldman JD, Young TS, Pappelbaum SJ, et al. Pediatric cardiac catheterization with same day discharge. Am J Cardiol 1982: 50:800-80.

2. MANUAL TECHNIQUES OF CARDIAC CATHETERIZATION: VESSEL ENTRY AND CATHETER MANIPULATION.

Stanton B. Perry, MD

VASCULAR ACCESS

For years, most pediatric catheterizations were performed using the umbilical or femoral vessels. Over the last several years use of the subclavian, internal jugular and hepatic veins has become more common, not only as backups for the femoral vein, but as the preferred site for some procedures. Though uncommonly used, the axillary and carotid arteries provide alternatives to the femoral artery.

The importance of proper positioning of the patient and use of local anesthesia in gaining vascular access cannot be overemphasized. Positioning exposes the vessel and helps immobilize even uncooperative patients. Proper use of local anesthesia effectively reduces pain without distorting the anatomy. When injected into the most sensitive tissues, the skin and periosteum, small volumes of local anesthetic will effectively alleviate the pain whereas larger volumes in the subcutaneous tissue will not alleviate pain and may distort the anatomy. Giving the local anesthesia well in advance of attempting access allows it to take effect and gives the patient a chance to calm down after the pain of the injection. This is most efficiently accomplished by giving the local after draping the patient and prior to setting up the rest of the table.

The success of the Seldinger technique for percutaneous access[1] in children [2-4] combined with the increased number of vessels available has eliminated the need for surgical cutdowns. Several needles can be used for percutaneous access including the short-bevelled Cook needle (Cook, Inc., Bloomington, IN.) without an obturator and the Cournand needle with a blunt bevel and a pointed obturator with a lumen. Non-obturator needles are advanced bevel up in short, quick jabs in an attempt to puncture only the anterior or superficial wall. The needle should be removed every 2 to 3 passes and flushed. When the Cook needle is used for internal jugular and subclavian veins, a syringe should be used to aspirate. Due to the blunter tip of the Cournand needle, the skin is first nicked with a scalpel blade. Arterial blood return is often noted through the small lumen in the oburator during advancement. For venous access, the obturator is removed prior to withdrawing the needle very slowly to check for blood return. The Cook needle is generally favored because one is more likely to gain access without puncturing the posterior vessel wall and it can be used with or without a syringe.

Once blood return is noted, attempts are made to pass a guidewire through the needle into the vessel. Keeping the tip of the needle in the vessel lumen during these attempts, especially in an uncooperative patient, requires a combination of firmness and flexibility. When attempting femoral access, for example, the proximal tip of the needle is held between the thumb and index finger of the left hand while resting the edge of the hand gently on the patient. If the patient moves the hand and needle will move with the patient. If the wire meets resistance the angle and depth of the needle should be varied slightly. Forcing the wire almost never results in access and, by creating a false channel, may make access impossible. If the distal end of the wire gets bent during these attempts, one is pushing too hard. Although J-wires are commonly provided, the increased manipulation required to get the wire into the needle may hinder success. Putting a slight curve on the soft end of a standard guidewire allows easy entry into the needle and increases flexibility of the wire as it exits the needle and enters the vessel. The very soft ends of torque-controlled wires are ideal although expensive. On the other hand, failure to get access can be expensive.

Prior to introducing sheaths or catheters, it is wise to check the wire position fluoroscopically. An unusual wire course could be due to a side branch or to an extravascular location. Repositioning the wire or introducing an angiocath over the wire to check for blood return or to perform a contrast injection will clarify this. Contrast injections can also be performed through the introducing needle, but these are much more likely to result in extravasation of contrast than use of an angiocath. A small nick is made in the skin prior to introducing the sheath or catheter; more extensive dissection is rarely required in pediatric patients. The dilator or, more commonly, the tip of the sheath can hang up at the skin, the fascia, or in scar tissue. Rotating the dilator and sheath as they are advanced will help overcome this but if the tip of the dilator or sheath becomes gnarled a new set should be used. Passing the dilator alone or using a larger dilator will be helpful in some cases.

Femoral Access

Beyond the newborn period, the femoral vessels remain the most commonly used for several reasons. First, the same site provides arterial and venous access. Second, most hemodynamic and interventional procedures can be performed using these vessels. Finally, it is relatively easy to position and immobilize even uncooperative patients for femoral access.

Positioning the patient includes extending the legs using soft ties at the ankles and securing the arms above the head using ties at the wrists. During prolonged procedures, especially in anesthetized patients, the arms should be moved and repositioned regularly to avoid brachial plexus injury. The groin is elevated and immobilized by placing pads or an inflatable cushion under the hips and a strap securely around the table and over the thighs just proximal to the knees. Removing the pads once access is obtained loosens the strap.

Both groins should be prepared with betadine. The inguinal skin crease, the femoral artery pulse, and the inguinal ligament, which runs between the anterior superior iliac spine and pubic tubercle are used as landmarks (Fig. 2-1).

Gently placing the index and middle fingers of the left hand just lateral to the femoral pulse localizes and demonstrates the course of the artery without distorting the anatomy and allows the fingers to remain in place while probing with the needle. Although most texts suggest puncturing the skin at or below the skin crease, the more important issue is where the vessel is entered. If the vessels are entered above the ligament, compression after catheter removal will not result in hemostasis and may result in pseudoaneurysms or concealed hematomas. The vessels are larger and covered by fewer layers of fascia between the skin crease and the inguinal ligament in the fossa ovalis. Therefore, it is neither necessary, nor desirable to puncture the skin below the crease. If the skin is punctured above the skin crease, one needs to use a steeper angle with the needle to avoid entering the vessels above the ligament.

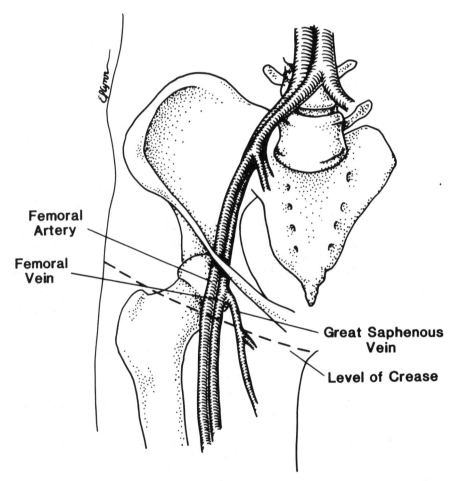

Figure 2-1: Inguinal vascular anatomy in infants and children. The dotted line is the approximate level of the inguinal crease.

The artery runs between the vein medially and the femoral nerve laterally. To access the vein the skin is punctured 2 to 10 mm medial to the arterial pulse depending on the size of the patient and the needle is advanced parallel to the artery in the direction of the umbilicus. Aspirating with a syringe to obtain blood return from the femoral vein is rarely necessary and the manipulation of removing the syringe may result in loss of access. If the needle reaches the inguinal ligament or hits bone without blood return the needle should be slowly withdrawn looking for blood return. After every 2 or 3 passes with the needle it should be removed and flushed. Once blood return is obtained a guidewire is advanced through the needle into the femoral vein, wire position is confirmed fluoroscopically and the needle is exchanged for a sheath and dilator after the skin has been nicked with a scalpel.

If the wire cannot be advanced despite having blood return, the common iliac vein may be occluded. This should be confirmed with a contrast injection. Injecting contrast through the needle risks injecting dye into the femoral sheath or surrounding tissue. We prefer to exchange the needle over a wire for an angiocath. A small hand injection of contrast will demonstrate the anatomy. We prefer to use biplane and the AP field should be large enough to include the contralateral iliac vein. The table should be moved during the injection to follow the contrast to the IVC. A plexus of collaterals will be seen if the vessel is occluded or stenotic. If collaterals fill the contralateral iliac vein it is likely the contralateral femoral vein is also patent. The angiograms should be carefully inspected because access to the inferior vena cava can occasionally be obtained through collaterals or stenotic veins even if normal femoral and iliac vessels are absent. The lateral view is vital for identification of normal venous location. The presence of these collaterals explains why one often gets blood return when the femoral vein is occluded, and much less frequently when the vein is patent. Thus, if there has been no blood return despite multiple passes with the needle, it is still likely that the vein is patent. In seeking the vein, one should start medially and gradually move towards the arterial pulse.

The femoral artery is accessed using similar techniques except that with an artery, it is never necessary to aspirate with a syringe. When the artery is entered, beginners commonly attempt to cover the end of the needle with their finger to minimize blood loss and end up jostling the needle and losing access. Immediately inserting the guidewire wire will prevent significant blood loss. It is rarely possible to advance the wire if flow from the needle is not pulsatile. Prolonged attempts to insert the wire into the artery should be avoided due to propensity for developing hematomas and arterial spasm.

The most common complications of femoral access are hematomas, arteriovenous fistulae, pseudoaneurysms, retroperitoneal hemorrhages, venous thrombosis[5] and loss of the arterial pulse[6,7]. Retroperitoneal hemorrhages are due to tearing vessels with manipulation of large catheters during the catheterization or to puncturing the vessel above the ligament. The rest are most commonly due to improper removal of catheters or incorrect application of pressure to the vessel once catheters are removed. Protamine is rarely, if ever, needed or used. Removing the arterial and venous catheters separately avoids arteriovenous fistulae. Although large patients require more pressure than infants, the need for excessive pressure usually means it is being applied in the wrong place. Compression should be applied where the vessel, not the skin, was punctured and compression should only be forceful enough to prevent bleeding. This can usually be achieved while still maintaining an arterial pulse in the foot. Most vessels stop bleeding within 20 minutes. Absence of the arterial pulse is not uncommon immediately following compression[8]. If it has not returned within 2 to 4 hours the patient is heparinized with 100 units/kg followed by an infusion of 20 units/kg/hour for up to 24 hours or until the pulse returns. If still absent at 24 hours, streptokinase is started at 1,000 units/kg followed by 1,000 units/kg/hour[9]. Bleeding commonly accompanies return of the pulse and infants need to be monitored closely to avoid significant blood loss. Surgery is reserved for patients with signs of ischemia, which is very rare, and not used routinely for pulse loss without signs of ischemia. For patients who have had relatively large catheters in the femoral artery it is not a bad idea to start a prophylactic heparin infusion as soon as hemostasis is achieved. The infusion is stopped if the pulse is present 4 hours later.

Umbilical Access

The major advantage of using the umbilical vessels is that it spares other vessels. Most routine hemodynamic studies and many interventions can be performed from the umbilical vein and artery. The umbilical vein directs the catheter posteriorly in the right atrium towards the foramen ovale and left atrium. It is, therefore, ideal for balloon atrial septostomy in patients with d-transposition of the great arteries. However, the catheter course makes entry into the right ventricle more difficult and crossing a critically stenotic pulmonary valve, which is relatively easy from the femoral vein, is difficult from the umbilical vein. The umbilical arteries descend to the iliac arteries and add an additional curve to the catheter compared with the femoral arteries. This increases the difficulty of maneuvers such as crossing stenotic aortic valves.

The baby is positioned on the table as for femoral access and the umbilicus and both groins are prepared with betadine. If umbilical catheters are in place, they are cut near the skin and exchanged over a guidewire for the appropriate catheters or sheaths. If no catheters are in place, umbilical tape is tied at the base of the umbilicus, the umbilical cord is cut horizontally near the skin and the arteries and vein are identified.

Initially, we attempt to advance a 5 F umbilical catheter through the vein and into the right atrium. The umbilical vein connects to the portal vein and then via the ductus venosus to the inferior vena cava. The ductus venosus is almost always patent the first 24 hours of life but rarely beyond 3 to 4 days of life. Because the ductus venosus dips posteriorly to the inferior vena cava, catheters advanced blindly tend to follow the portal vein into the liver. Using fluoroscopy and tiny hand injections of dye, the patency of the ductus venosus can be demonstrated (Fig. 2-2) and the catheter guided posteriorly by a tip defecting wire or, more likely, a torque-controlled wire can be advanced through the ductus.

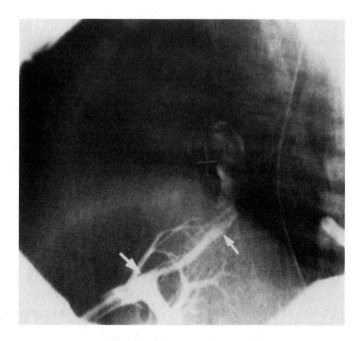

Figure 2-2: Lateral angiogram of umbilical vein (large arrow) as it courses posteriorly, through the ductus venous (small arrow) into the inferior vena cava. Umbilicus is at left, spine at right.

Once the catheter is in the atrium, it is exchanged over a wire for a sheath. Care should be taken to insure the sheath reaches the inferior vena cava before removing the wire or access can be lost. The sheath should have a backstop to prevent air embolism during spontaneous inspiration.

The umbilical arteries can occasionally be accessed up to 7-10 days of age. The umbilical arteries are usually accessed with 3.5 or 5 F umbilical catheter, but as with the vein, if initial attempts fail, tiny contrast injections and torque-controlled wires will assist in gaining access. The umbilical catheter is exchanged over a wire for a pigtail. Sheaths are not commonly used in the umbilical artery.

At the end of the procedure, the umbilical catheters are replaced and hemostasis is achieved using the umbilical tape. Vascular complications of using the umbilical vessels are rare, but we have seen endocarditis after prolonged catheterizations using the umbilical vessels.

Internal Jugular Vein

The internal jugular vein, a large vein even in babies, can be used for right-sided hemodynamics and interventions. Attempting to advance long sheaths and balloon dilation catheters over wires to the pulmonary arteries from the femoral vein often results in a loop in the right atrium rather than forward motion of the catheter tip due to the S-shaped curve through the right atrium and ventricle. The single,

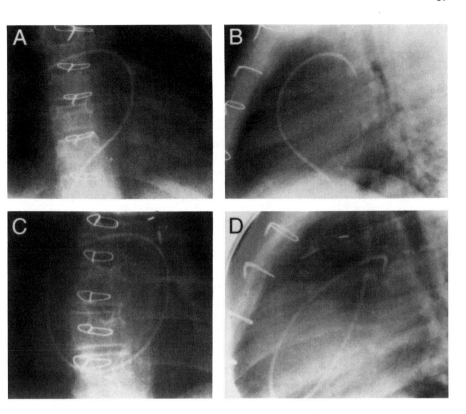

Figure 2-3: Catheter course from inferior vena cava to right pulmonary artery. (A= FRONTAL), (B =LATERAL): from superior vena cava to right pulmonary artery (C= FRONTAL) (D=LATERAL).

continuous curve from the internal jugular or subclavian vein to the pulmonary arteries avoids this problem (Fig. 2-3).

Because the upright position reduces pressure in the internal jugular, patients do not need to remain supine following catheterization. Disadvantages of the internal jugular vein include the difficulty of crossing a patent foramen ovale and the inability to do a transseptal puncture. It is difficult to immobilize uncooperative patients and more sedation or general anesthesia may be required.

There are two approaches to the internal jugular vein, the anterior and the posterior. The internal jugular, running in the triangle formed by the clavicle and the sternal and clavicular bellies of the sternocleidomastoid, enters the chest under the head of the clavicle. The carotid is medial and deeper than the internal jugular. For the anterior approach the ipsilateral arm is placed at the patient's side and the head is rotated to the contralateral side. Having the patient lift his head identifies the sternocleidomastoid. The carotid is palpated and the skin punctured lateral to the carotid near the apex of the triangle. The needle is advanced toward the head of the clavicle and ipsilateral nipple. A syringe with constant aspiration should be used to avoid air embolism when the vessel is entered. Short jabs with the needle are used to increase the chances of puncturing only the anterior wall of the vessel. If there is femoral access, one can advance the femoral venous catheter up the superior vena cava to the internal jugular and, using fluoroscopy, aim the needle at the catheter. This allows the vessel to be entered much lower where it is larger while reducing the risk of pneumothorax. This is especially useful for procedures requiring large sheaths.

For the posterior approach, the needle is inserted in the groove lateral to the clavicular belly of the sternocleidomastiod and advanced parallel to the floor towards the suprasternal notch while aspirating. The needle is usually inserted just caudal or cephalad to the intersection of the external jugular and the groove.

With either approach, the syringe rapidly fills with blood when the vessel is entered and the occasional trickle from small vessels should not be confused with the internal jugular. The right internal jugular vein is more commonly used, but these techniques work as well for the left.

Complications include pneumothorax, and puncture of the trachea or the carotid artery. Pneumothorax is more common with the anterior or a low lateral approach due to the proximity of the apex of the lung. If the carotid artery is punctured the needle should be removed and compression applied. This is more common with the lateral approach but has not resulted in complications if it is recognized prior to inserting the sheath.

At the end of the case, the catheters are removed and pressure applied to the entry site. It is wise to check for a pneumo- or hemothorax before removing the patient from the table. If the patient is awake, it is best to have them sit up while compressing to lower the pressure in the vessel.

Subclavian Vein

The subclavian vein can be used for right-sided hemodynamics and interventions and, like the internal jugular vein, is ideal for some pulmonary artery dilations and stents [10,11]. The subclavian vein is used routinely for patients with Glenn anastomoses. They are also an excellent choice for patients in whom one wants to leave an indwelling catheter at the end of the case. Most catheter manipulations seem easier from the left as compared with the right subclavian vein but either can be used. The subclavian requires less immobilization than the internal jugular. As with the internal jugular it is difficult to cross a patent foramen ovale from the subclavian vein.

With the patient flat or in Trendelenburg position, the patient is positioned with the ipsilateral arm at the side and the head turned to the opposite side. A roll is often placed under the spine but this is not critical. Landmarks are the clavicle and the suprasternal notch. The vein is superficial to the artery and enters the chest at the junction of the clavicle and first rib. The needle with syringe attached is inserted at the junction of the medial and middle third of the clavicle in adults and more laterally in infants and children. In adults, some advance the needle postero-medially until the vessel is accessed or it hits the first rib, but we do not use this approach. Rather, the needle is advanced under the clavicle and then advanced parallel to the floor and towards the suprasternal notch. We commonly put a 10 to 30° upward bend on the distal end of the needle to keep the tip relatively superficial. Care should be taken to avoid passing the needle through the periosteum, as this will make introduction of the sheath nearly impossible. As with the internal jugular vein, it is not subtle when the needle enters the vein; the syringe rapidly fills with blood. If access is not obtained after several attempts, one should consider a contrast injection through an I.V. in the hand or arm to document vessel patency and location.

Complications include pneumo- and hemothorax, and subclavian artery or aortic arch puncture. All of these complications are more common when the anatomy is distorted by previous surgery including Blalock-Taussig shunts and arch repairs. Hemostasis is achieved by compression and by having the patient sit.

Hepatic Vein

Percutaneous hepatic venous access has been used by radiologists for years but only recently by pediatric cardiologists. It is an excellent alternative to the femoral vein, especially in cases where it is necessary to cross an atrial septal defect or perform a Brockenbrough transseptal puncture. Large sheaths can be used without complications.

The Chiba needle is introduced into the skin at the costal margin around the anterior axillary line. It is advanced posteriorly and cephalad towards the intra-hepatic inferior vena cava or just caudal to the inferior vena cava and right atrial junction. The needle is advanced to within a few centimeters of the right border of the spine, the obturator is withdrawn and a syringe with contrast is attached. The syringe is aspirated as the needle is slowly withdrawn. When blood return is obtained a small amount of contrast is injected to determine if the needle is in a hepatic vein. The syringe is removed and a guidewire inserted. An alternative and attractive approach to accessing the hepatic vein is to use ultrasound guidance. At the end of the case, hemostasis is achieved with gelfoam or coils in the tract made through the liver. This is accomplished by placing a catheter at least 1 F size smaller than the sheath through the sheath. While injecting tiny amounts of contrast, the sheath is withdrawn leaving the catheter in the hepatic vein until the sheath is just outside the liver. The catheter is then withdrawn, injecting tiny amounts of contrast until it is out of the vein and lies in the tract through the liver. The tract between the catheter tip and sheath can then be filled with gel-foam or coils. Patients who leave the cath lab following hepatic vein catheterization often complain of abdominal pain during the subsequent 24 hours, presumably due to irritation from peritoneal blood.

22

CATHETER MANIPULATION:

Catheters

In order to decide which vessels to access and which sheaths and catheters to use, one needs to know the anatomy, which vessels are likely to be patent, the patient's size and what needs to be done. For routine diagnostic studies involving measurements of pressures and oxygen saturations and angiography we use a sheath in the vein and a pigtail catheter in the artery. Although an arterial catheter is not essential for many cases as the left side can be accessed with the venous catheter either through septal defects or using transseptal puncture, we prefer an arterial catheter for most cases. It allows simultaneous right and left hemodynamics, allows pressure monitoring during right sided interventions and is essential for some left sided interventions. An arterial sheath is used only when catheter exchanges are anticipated. Sheaths with back-stop valves are used to prevent air embolism through venous sheaths with the tip in the thorax and to prevent blood loss, especially through arterial sheaths. The smallest French size that will accomplish the goals of the catheterization is chosen.

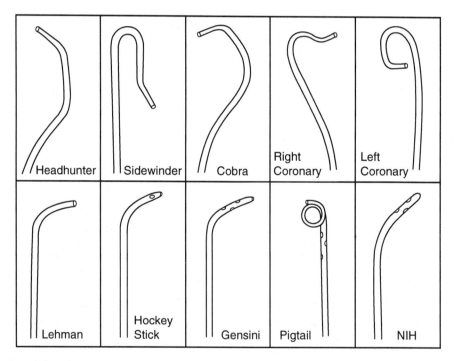

Figure 2-4: Catheter configurations we have found useful in congenital heart disease.

The French size is usually determined by the volume and rate of contrast injections required rather than by the ability to obtain adequate pressure tracings. We commonly use a 4 or 5 F venous sheath and a 3 F pigtail in newborns and 7 F catheters in adult-sized patients. However, for example, if a large patient does not require left-sided angiography, a 3 or 4 F pigtail will be adequate to monitor arterial pressure. If larger sheaths are found to be necessary for interventions, they can be inserted once the diagnostic part of the study is completed.

Catheter manipulation requires hand-eye coordination, knowledge of the anatomy and an understanding of how catheters and guidewires move. A great variety of catheters and guidewires are available. Catheters may be flow-directed, torque-controlled or designed to be advanced over guidewires. Flow-directed catheters are soft shafted, balloon-tipped catheters with relatively poor torque-control and include pulmonary artery wedge (single end-hole) catheters, Berman angiographic (multiple side-holes) catheters and thermodilution catheters. These catheters are manipulated primarily by inflating the balloon and pushing combined with some torquing. Torque-controlled catheters, many with woven nylon or wire mesh skeletons, have stiffer shafts and are manipulated by rotating (torquing) the shaft until the tip is pointed in the right direction and then advancing the catheter. Catheters in this group come with a variety of preformed shapes including those shown in Fig. 2-4.

Many were developed for peripheral vascular or coronary work but can be useful, with or without modification, for difficult maneuvers such as entering arterial or venous collaterals, shunts, or abnormal pulmonary arteries. Almost all catheters or sheaths can have their shapes modified by hand if the shaft is first heated for a minute or so in steam. The different types of catheters are not mutually exclusive; flow directed catheters can be torqued and advanced without the balloon. Each has advantages and disadvantages. Flow-directed catheters, with their relatively soft shafts and balloon tips, minimize the risk of cardiac or vessel perforation especially with the balloon inflated. Torque-controlled catheters are commonly needed for more difficult maneuvers, but increase the risk of complications.

Guidewires

The increased variety of guidewires available over the last 10 years has dramatically changed cardiac catheterization. Standard guidewires with relatively stiff shafts and soft tips are available with or without J-tips and are usually 140 cm long. Exchange wires, 180 to 300 cm in length, are now available with extra-stiff shafts and very short soft tips. Torque-controlled wires have made it much easier and, due to the floppy tips, safer, to enter stenotic branch pulmonary arteries, shunts, collaterals and other difficult sites. "Slime-coated" (Turumo) wires combined with "slime-coated" catheters have made it relatively easy to access sites which, due to multiple curves, could not be entered previously. Tip-deflector wires (Cook, Inc) remain invaluable for certain maneuvers such as entering the pulmonary arteries in d-transposition of the great arteries, unrepaired or following atrial switch procedure.
The following examples include commonly performed maneuvers as well as more

advanced techniques. Rather than memorizing maneuvers, such as when to rotate the catheter clock-wise, one should try to understand why clock-wise rotation works. In general, one should start with the safest maneuvers and progress to riskier alternatives only as needed. The risk of any maneuver is, of course, related to the experience of the catheterizer. Experience is also important in knowing when to try another technique, but if a particular maneuver has not worked the first 10 times, it probably will not work the next. Never forget that it is easier to enter a structure if one knows where it is. For example, small hand injections of contrast will show an unusual origin of the right pulmonary artery or the levo-phase of a pulmonary artery injection will show the pulmonary veins. Also remember to use the optimal view. For example, entering the right middle lobe pulmonary artery is essentially a random event using AP fluoro whereas it is much easier and more directed when using lateral fluoro. When planning a catheterization it is important to consider all the options for entering a certain structure. For example, depending on the patient, the pulmonary arteries can be entered from the outflow tract, a Glenn anastomosis (or a persistent right atrial to pulmonary artery connection following a Glenn), an aortic to pulmonary artery shunt or collateral, or a patent ductus arteriosus. The catheterizer who combines a little imagination and a lot of perseverance with an attitude that any structure or vessel can be entered will seldom be disappointed.

Superior Vena Cava

The easiest way to get to the superior vena cava (SVC) from the femoral vein is to advance a straight wire or catheter from the inferior vena cava (IVC). A curved catheter, which tends to move anteriorly as it enters the right atrium, makes entry into the posterior SVC more difficult. With the catheter in the right atrium, it is easiest to work the catheter posteriorly by rotating the shaft in small increments counterclockwise along the lateral border of the right atrium. At the same time the catheter is repeatedly advanced until it hits the atrial wall and then withdrawn to free the tip. Eventually the catheter will advance smoothly to the SVC. This maneuver works most consistently when accomplished without repositioning the fingers on the catheter. Thus, the shaft is gradually rolled between the thumb and index finger which are positioned 2 to 3 inches from the hub; far enough to advance to the SVC without hitting the sheath but close enough to maintain control of the catheter. This maneuver illustrates one of the fundamentals of catheter manipulation and one of the most common errors made by beginners; torque-control of a catheter is optimal when the tip is free. With the tip entrapped, torque-control is lost and rotation of the shaft builds up potential energy in the shaft until the catheter tip suddenly comes loose and the shaft unwinds several turns, the catheter kinks, or the tip perforates the heart.

Right Atrium

Assuming one has venous access, the right atrium is hard to miss. The classic exception to this is an interrupted IVC with azygos continuation. As a femoral venous catheter is advanced on AP fluoroscopy it appears to enter the right atrium but lateral fluoroscopy shows that it is actually posterior in the azygos. Many fellows, not recognizing this, have been surprised how easy it was to get to the SVC and how hard it was to get to the right ventricle.

Right Ventricle

The tricuspid valve is anterior and leftward in the right atrium. From an anterior position, the catheter is rotated clockwise and, thus, leftward across the anterior wall of the right atrium. A balloon-tipped, flow directed catheter will usually bounce as it nears the valve and should be advanced sharply as it dips towards the right ventricle in diastole. Slowing advancing the catheter tends to direct it over the top of the valve. If several attempts fail, bending the catheter against the superior atrial wall for a few seconds will increase the curve. Removing a flow-directed catheter from the body, bending it and the reinserting it rarely works because the catheter does not hold the shape through the IVC. The presence of severe tricuspid regurgitation makes it harder to cross the valve with a flow-directed catheter. In general, it is preferable to cross an atrio-ventricular valve with the balloon inflated, because the catheter is less likely to cross between chordae. This is particularly critical if one plans to dilate the valve.

In pulmonary atresia with intact ventricular septum, crossing the small tricuspid valve using a flow-directed catheter rarely works. Preformed catheters with a curve that can be aimed at the valve, with or without a torque-controlled wire are more likely to work. Bending the stiff-end of a guidewire or using a tip-deflector wire and advancing it to the end, but not out of the catheter, can be used to "shape" a soft catheter that can be aimed at the valve. Rather than advancing the wire and catheter as a unit, it is easier to fix the wire and advance the catheter off the wire and through the valve. The wire-catheter arrangement has some advantages over preformed catheters. The curve on the preformed catheter is obviously fixed, whereas the length and radius of curvature of the wire-catheter unit can be changed by varying the distance between the end of the wire and the end of the catheter.

Although balloon-tipped catheters are generally quite safe, a word of warning is in order. Inflation of the balloon when the tip is entrapped will injure the heart. This could be in the atrial appendage, right ventricular trabeculations or a small vein such as a normal coronary sinus. We have seen rupture of a coronary sinus and creation of a left ventricular aneurysm from this maneuver. Therefore, one should always be sure the tip is free before inflating the balloon.

Pulmonary Artery

A balloon-tipped catheter in the right ventricle can occasionally be advanced directly to the pulmonary artery, but more commonly it advances to the right ventricular apex (Fig. 2-5A). If this happens, the catheter tip, with the balloon

26

inflated, should be positioned freely in the inflow portion of the right ventricle. The catheter is gradually rotated clockwise until the tip flips up towards the outflow tract. At that point, the catheter should be quickly advanced to the pulmonary artery. A counter-clockwise rotation will also work. Occasionally, as the catheter is advanced it will hang up laterally in the outflow tract. Quickly advancing the catheter will cause it to loop in the right atrium. Continued pushing, combined with the altered catheter course through the right atrium and ventricle, usually advances the catheter to the pulmonary artery. Forming and removing a loop in the right atrium is a maneuver that seems to give beginners problems. The problem is that while a full loop will help advance a catheter, a half loop will actually cause the catheter tip in the right ventricle to retract. Thus, the loop needs to be formed quickly, ideally with a single move. Once the catheter is in the pulmonary artery the loop can be removed. This also needs to be done with a rapid single movement. Alternatively, the balloon can be wedged in the distal pulmonary artery to fix the tip while the loop is removed.

If these maneuvers fail, the catheter can be looped in the right atrium prior to entering the right ventricle (Fig. 2-5B). The loop is formed by advancing the catheter to the roof of the atrium, down along the right (lateral) border of the atrium and through the tricuspid valve. This loop tends to direct the catheter tip up towards the right ventricular outflow tract rather than towards the apex. If, however, the catheter does become directed towards the RV apex, insertion of a stiff wire with a tight curve will pull the catheter toward the main pulmonary artery.

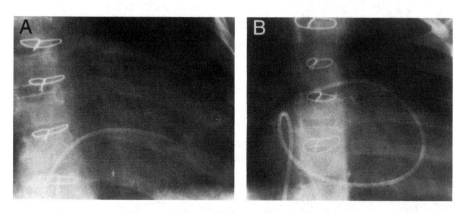

Figure 2-5: (A) Catheter course from right atrium to apex of right ventricle and (B) with right atrial loop to right pulmonary artery.

When advanced, a catheter in the main pulmonary artery will go to the right or left pulmonary artery or through a patent ductus arteriosus. Clockwise rotation will increase the odds of entering the right pulmonary artery and counter-clockwise rotation the odds of entering the left. Entering both pulmonary arteries, when normal, is usually easy. Entering abnormal pulmonary arteries and their branches are among the most challenging catheter manipulations. To avoid prolonged semi-random probing, hand injections of small volumes of contrast will demonstrate the anatomy, allowing appropriate catheters and wires to be chosen and aimed in the correct direction. Shaping the stiff-end of a guidewire with compound clockwise or counter-clockwise loop and advancing it to the end of the catheter will direct the catheter to the right or left. The catheter can then be advanced off the end of the wire into the branch pulmonary artery. Although this technique is very effective, we tend to prefer preformed catheters and torque-controlled guidewires. The catheter with an appropriate curve, based on the angiogram, is advanced to the pulmonary artery over an exchange-length guidewire. The catheter is aimed at the orifice of the branch pulmonary artery and the torque-controlled wire is manipulated into the vessel. Thus, one is advancing, withdrawing and rotating the catheter while simultaneously torquing and probing with the wire. The object is to get the guidewire into the branch pulmonary artery. Often the stiff, preformed catheter used to direct the wire cannot be advanced over the wire into the branch. If not, it can be exchanged for a softer catheter, or the firmer more proximal part of the torque wire can be bent before it enter the pulmonary artery, facilitating subsequent tracking of a stiffer catheter.

Left ventricle

As a pigtail catheter is advanced from the ascending aorta it either crosses the aortic valve or hangs up in one of the cusps. In the latter case, further pushing is unlikely to succeed and may kink the catheter or even injure the valve. Rather, the catheter should be withdrawn until free and readvanced until successful. High-flow, thin-walled pigtail catheters should always be advanced with a guidewire at the tip to avoid kinking the catheter. Advancing the wire out the end of the pigtail will increase the radius of curvature of the pigtail and will usually aid in crossing the valve. The wire should be removed quickly once the catheter is in the left ventricle to decrease the risk of ventricular ectopy.
A straight wire, rather than a loop of wire or catheter, is needed to cross a stenotic aortic valve. In congenital aortic stenosis, the commissure between the left and non-coronary cusp is almost always open; the wire should be directed towards this commissure. A catheter, sometimes a partially cut-off pigtail, with a 90 to 180° curve is used to direct the wire. With the catheter advanced close to the valve the wire will be aimed to the patient's left toward the left coronary artery. While probing in and out with the wire, the catheter is rotated back and forth and gradually withdrawn causing the wire to sweep across the valve toward the patient's right. Once the wire is in the right coronary cusp, the catheter should be readvanced and the process repeated. Further pushing once the wire contacts the valve will not succeed in crossing the valve and may perforate a leaflet, especially in neonates. For this reason we routinely use soft, torque-controlled wires in these patients. When the wire eventually advances beyond the valve it could either be in the left ventricle behind the mitral apparatus, in a coronary artery, or

free in the LV cavity. The experienced catheterizer can usually differentiate these possibilities by the subtle differences in wire course and by the movement of a wire advanced in the confined space of a coronary artery. The beginner rarely recognizes the difference. The easiest method to differentiate these possibilities is to gently advance the wire. If the wire is in a coronary, no loop will form. If it is trapped behind the mitral valve, the tip will remain fixed but a loop will form below the aortic valve and travel through the LV cavity into the LV apex. This maneuver is especially important when positioning a wire prior to aortic valve dilation, to avoid mitral valve injury.

From the left atrium, simply advancing a balloon-tipped catheter may result in crossing the mitral valve. Commonly, however, the balloon gets stuck in the left atrial appendage. The catheter tip can be directed down towards the mitral valve using a compound LPA curve on the stiff-end of a guidewire or a tip-deflector wire and rotating the catheter counter-clockwise (anterior). Once aimed at the valve, the catheter is advanced off the end of the wire and into the ventricle. A balloon-tipped catheter with the balloon inflated is less likely to cross between chordae. This is especially important if one is planning to dilate the mitral valve.

Left Atrium

From the femoral vein, the left atrium is entered via a patent foramen ovale or atrial septal defect. Starting low and anterior in the right atrium, the catheter is rotated clockwise to aim it leftward and posterior and advanced. If the catheter continues leftward on the AP fluoroscopy it could be in the right ventricle, coronary sinus, right atrial appendage or left atrium. If it is posterior on the lateral it is in the coronary sinus or left atrium. With experience, these locations can be differentiated using flouro, but if there is any question the combination of pressure and oxygen saturation will help. The coronary sinus is lower than a patent foramen ovale and is rarely entered from the femoral vein unless larger than normal, as in the presence of a left superior vena cava. Biplane fluoroscopy, though usually not necessary for the experienced catheterizer, can be helpful. While biplane fluoroscopy increases radiation, a brief period of biplane fluoroscopy may provide less radiation than prolonged single plane fluoroscopy. If this maneuver fails after several attempts, the catheter should be advanced to the SVC. It is then withdrawn slowly, maintaining a posterior and leftward orientation. The catheter commonly jumps slightly to the left as it comes over the superior limbic band, the superior margin of the PFO. The catheter should then be advanced. Another useful maneuver is to bend the stiff end of an appropriate guide (e.g. 0.025" for 5F balloon wedge catheter) in a transseptal needle configuration, advance it to the end of the catheter and then probe the septum. The most common error among beginners is to look too high in the atrial septum for the PFO. If there is no PFO or ASD, a Brockenbrough transseptal puncture can be performed (Chapter 10).

Similar to blood flow in a fetus, a catheter is easily advanced from the umbilical vein to the left atrium. On the other hand, crossing a PFO from the subclavian or internal jugular vein is much more difficult. Given the morphology of the PFO, it is much easier to cross from below than above. Thus, the catheter should be advanced from the SVC down to the mouth of the IVC and then turned up and aimed leftward and posterior using the curved end of a stiff guidewire or tip-deflector wire. Once the catheter tip is hooked in the PFO it is advanced off the wire into the left atrium.

Crossing the mitral valve retrograde from the left ventricle is not only difficult but commonly associated with significant ventricular ectopy. It should be attempted only if the information to be gained is important. A catheter with a 180° tight curve, e.g. a cut-off pigtail catheter, is placed in the left ventricular apex and used to direct a torque-controlled wire back toward the mitral orifice. Advancing, withdrawing and rotating the catheter while probing with the wire eventually succeeds in getting the wire into the left atrium or pulmonary vein. It is usually necessary to exchange for a softer catheter to get it to follow the wire into the left atrium. Alternatively, one can enter the left ventricle with a soft, balloon-tipped catheter, and then advance a stiff wire with a compound curve resembling a Judkin's left coronary catheter. The wire will direct the catheter tip toward the left atrium.

Pulmonary Veins

Normal pulmonary veins enter the back of the left atrium near the spine. The veins are most easily entered using access from the femoral, umbilical or hepatic veins. Once in the left atrium the catheter should be rotated posteriorly (clockwise). With the catheter tip in the center of the spine on the AP flouro the catheter is advanced. It is almost always easier to enter the left pulmonary veins. If the catheter enters the veins it will usually advance easily outside the shadow of the heart on the AP view. Position can be confirmed using the lateral fluoroscopy or a small hand injection of contrast. To enter the right veins, the catheter must be rotated clockwise until the tip is to the right of the spine and then advanced. It tends to go to the right upper lobe vein or pops back into the right atrium with the extreme clockwise rotation. To enter the right lower pulmonary vein, it is commonly easier to put a tight 180° curve on the catheter with the stiff end of a guidewire, aim the catheter at the vein with clockwise rotation and then advance the catheter off the wire.

Patent Ductus Arteriosus (PDA)

A large PDA can be easily crossed with either the venous or arterial catheter. A small PDA is usually easier to cross from the arterial side because the aortic ampulla funnels down to the narrowest part of the PDA, which is almost always at the pulmonary end. A pre-shaped catheter such as a Cobra or right coronary artery catheter will either advance directly into the ampulla and through the PDA or can be used to direct a guidewire through the PDA. When crossing from the venous side, it is easiest to use a straight catheter in the main pulmonary artery to direct a straight wire towards and through the PDA.

Blalock-Taussig Shunts

Blalock-Taussig shunts can be crossed using either venous or arterial access. The difficulty of crossing the shunt from the venous side depends primarily on the intracardiac anatomy and the catheter course through the heart. Crossing the shunt from the femoral artery is almost always easier than from the vein. The occasional BT shunt with proximal atresia of the innominate or subclavian artery is one of the few absolute indications for axillary or brachial artery access. The most common patient in whom we cross the shunt is the 4 to 6 month old with single ventricle who is undergoing a pre-Glenn catheterization. In these small patients, a 3 F pigtail with the tail cut to 180° is ideal. With the catheter in the descending aorta, an 0.018 inch torque-controlled wire is advanced out the catheter and both are advanced into the ascending aorta. The catheter is pulled back over the wire until both are straight with the wire extending out the end of the catheter. Both are now withdrawn together. As the catheter is pulled around the arch the wire is gradually aimed more superiorly and can be advanced into the innominate artery and up the carotid or preferably the subclavian artery. The catheter is then advanced over the wire into the innominate artery. The wire is withdrawn which allows the curve in the catheter to reform. As the catheter is slowly withdrawn, the tip will fall into the shunt, the wire can be advanced to the distal pulmonary arteries and the catheter then advanced over the wire to the pulmonary arteries. Again, if not successful after 1 or 2 attempts, a hand injection through the pigtail in the innominate artery will show the location of the shunt and simplify entry.

Occasionally it is useful to enter a Blalock-Taussig shunt from the pulmonary end. For example, a balloon-tipped wedge catheter in the distal end of the shunt can be used to occlude the shunt while coils are delivered from the arterial side. It is easiest to enter the shunt using a pre-formed catheter with a short sharply angled tip such as a cut-off Amplatz right coronary catheter and a torque-controlled wire.

Central Shunts

Central shunts tend to be harder to enter than BT shunts. Their location is variable, but they usually come off the right or left side of the ascending aorta. The most common error is probably to probe too posteriorly in the aorta. An ascending aortogram is rarely as helpful as anticipated in localizing the origin of the shunt and a lot of dye is wasted. Small hand injections, similar to the techniques used for coronary arteries, are more likely to be useful. An Amplatz right coronary artery catheter with the distal tip removed may be used, probing the side of the aorta with a torque-controlled wire and intermittent contrast injections. An alternative approach is to use a balloon tipped catheter, retrograde, with the tip kinked, and pushed to loop against the aortic valve. Another technique is to maneuver the inflated balloon along the side of the aorta using a tip-deflector

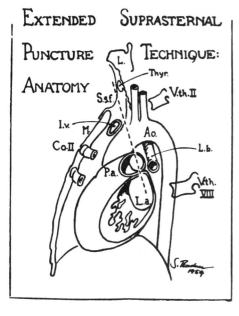

EXTENDED SUPRASTERNAL PUNCTURE TECHNIQUE: ANATOMY

wire. With the balloon inflated the catheter will rarely enter the pulmonary artery. Rather, one watches for the balloon to get stuck, due to blood flow, in the origin of the shunt. If a wire will not enter the pulmonary artery, it is probably because the side rather than the end of the balloon is stuck in the shunt. An attempt is made to gently reorient the catheter tip. One can also deflate the balloon in the hope that the catheter will pop through the shunt. Central shunts are often as easy to enter with the venous as with the arterial catheter.

Figure 2-6: Suprasternal puncture technique, as described by Radner. Although used in a number of conditions including transposition in the 1950s and 1960s, it has been supplanted by less daunting catheter techniques. (Reprinted from Acta Med. Scand. 151:223).

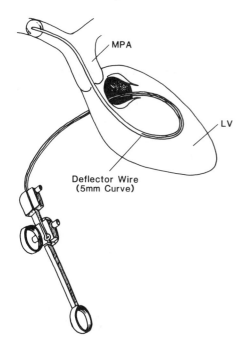

Other

Entering the pulmonary arteries from the left ventricle in d-transposition of the great arteries was commonly performed in the past, but the advent of the arterial switch and the tendency to operate in the newborn period without catheterization has all but eliminated the need for this maneuver. The Radner technique (Fig. 2-6) involved advancing a long needle through the thoracic wall and aorta into the pulmonary artery[12].

Figure 2-7: Use of a tip-deflecting wire and balloon catheter to enter the pulmonary arteries in transposition of the great arteries.

To the disappointment of many, this technique is no longer recommended. Currently, the easiest technique employs a balloon-tipped catheter positioned near the left-ventricular apex. A tip-deflector wire is used to curve the catheter tip towards the base of the heart. The catheter is then advanced off the end of the wire into the pulmonary artery (Fig.2-7). There are two keys to this maneuver. First, the catheter tip must be free in the apex of the ventricle to allow it to curve back up toward the base of the heart.

Second, when advancing the catheter off the wire, the wire must be held to prevent the wire and catheter from being pushed into the apex of the ventricle. The wire, when held away from the apex, acts as a fulcrum off which the catheter is pushed. This technique has become increasingly important as we increasingly use an antegrade approach to dilate aortic valves in young patients.

Catheter Exchanges Over Guidewires

One of the most common maneuvers is exchanging catheters over guidewires. When removing a catheter over a wire it is helpful to see as much of the wire as possible, but, at a minimum, the distal tip should be watched. With practice, it is possible to remove a catheter without moving the guidewire. Advancing the guidewire can perforate the vessel distally and allowing it to come back can result in loss of position. It is best to fix the wire with the right hand on the table and then pull the catheter with the left hand until it meets the right hand. This is repeated in multiple steps. Advancing catheters over wires seems to give inexperienced catheterizers much more difficulty because they do not handle the wire properly. The wire needs to be taut and released as soon as the tip begins to retract. If the wire is not taut, the slack in wire outside the body will advance with the catheter. This could result in perforation of the distal vessel or formation of a loop in the wire course. A loop can also form, e.g. in the right atrium in a wire positioned in the distal pulmonary artery, if the catheter tip gets stuck as it is being advanced. The loop increases the length of the wire course inside the body and, unless the wire is released, the tip will retract. There are many reasons a catheter may not follow a wire smoothly. If there is a mismatch between the catheter and wire, tissue may become embedded between the wire and catheter tip. If the catheter tip is not tapered it may hang up on valves, stenoses, branch points or stents. If the catheter course has multiple curves, friction is produced by contact with vessel walls at multiple sites. This can be overcome by slightly withdrawing the catheter and wire to minimize contact with vessel walls. A long sheath can also be used to decrease friction and provide support. "Terumo" coated wires and catheters are ideal in these cases. Occasionally it is necessary to loop a femoral venous catheter in the right atrium to get it to follow the wire to the pulmonary arteries. This allows application of more force to the catheter, but the large loop in the right atrium commonly results in bradycardia. Thus, one needs to form the loop, quickly advance the catheter and then remove the loop. As opposed to a full loop, a half loop will actually cause the catheter and wire to retract. Thus, these loops need to be formed and removed with a single rapid action. The wire should not be held while the catheter is advanced to form the loop. Exchanging catheters from the subclavian or internal jugular vein is more difficult than from the femoral vessels because of the extra curve in the wire course outside the body (when working from the standard position at the side of the table).

Catheter and Guidewire Modification

Despite the variety of catheters, sheaths and guidewires available, situations commonly arise in which they prove inadequate or less than ideal. The solution can often be found through modification of existing equipment. Modifications include shaping or cutting catheters and sheaths and bending guidewires. Successful modification of catheters and wires requires an understanding of the anatomy and what modifications need to be made. This is often based on trial and error. In other words, if one understands why the previous catheter and wire failed, one is more likely to choose a better catheter and wire. Does the catheter and or wire need a tighter curve, a shorter curve, a single sharp angle or what?

The shapes of catheter tips can be modified by cutting the catheter, by using guidewires or by shaping the catheters. Partially removing the tip of a preformed catheter changes the curve and angle of the tip. For example, a Judkin's left coronary catheter has 2 curves totaling 270°. Depending on how much of the catheter tip is removed, the remaining catheter will have a long 180° curve or shorter curves of 0° to 180°. The stiff-end of a guidewire can be bent into almost any shape with curves and bends in single or multiple planes and will be stiff enough to reshape most catheter tips although extreme curves and angles may be impossible to traverse via the catheter lumen. The wire is advanced to the end of the catheter but not beyond and used to direct the catheter tip. By varying the distance between the end of the guidewire and catheter, the length of the curve or angle can be changed.

Catheters and sheaths can be reshaped using hot water, steam, hot air or by gently stripping the catheter or sheath between the fingers or between a finger and rigid object such as a clamp. Most catheters and sheaths, however, tend to revert to their original shape once inside the body. The degree to which this occurs depends to a large extent on the catheter material.

The shape of most guidewires can be modified by hand to help enter difficult vessels. Rotating a straight wire has little impact; one should almost always put a gentle (30-60°) curve on the soft end of a torque-controlled wire to allow the tip to be directed in the desirable direction. We have increasingly used curves fashioned in the stiff end of standard wires to modify catheter shapes and behavior. Thus, a 60° curve at a radius of 8-10 cm in a stiff wire can be advanced to 10 cm back from the tip of a Judkin's right coronary catheter, and make it look like a Cobra. Compound curves are especially helpful: an S-shaped compound curve will direct catheters into the right upper lobe pulmonary artery from the main right pulmonary artery, or into the MPA from the RV in patients with severe RPA obstruction. A curve fashioned to fit the RV-MPA sweep can have an additional 90° short curve added to the wire tip: with the wire curve pointed away from your eyes, a secondary 90° curve towards the right at the wire tip will drive a catheter into the LPA.

Modifying pigtail catheters by removing part of the pigtail has become routine in our lab[13]. The tail on a pigtail catheter serves to increase the resistance to flow through the end-hole and, thus, to increase flow through the side-holes during contrast injections. If a power injection is performed with the tail removed, the jet of contrast through the end can infiltrate the vessel or myocardial wall. However, an injection can be safely performed using a Y-adaptor and guidewire to plug the end-hole. In thin-walled, high-flow pigtails (e.g. pigtails from UMI and Cook, Inc.) the lumen in the body of the catheter is larger than the lumen in the tail, which is commonly tapered to accept a 0.035" wire. Thus, although the wire decreases the amount and rate at which contrast that can be injected, adequate angiograms can be obtained. This use of cut-off pigtails greatly increases the efficiency of many interventions. The guidewire, once across a lesion, can remain until the procedure is completed and the pigtail catheter can be used for pressure measurements and angiograms between, for example, balloon dilations. The tail should be cut perpendicular to the curve to prevent a sharp point, which could injure vessel walls. Enough of the tail should be left so that the catheter tip tapers to fit the guidewire. Pre-cut pigtails are now commercially available. As noted above, partially cut-off pigtails are useful for many maneuvers including crossing stenotic aortic valves and BT shunts. Removing different amounts of the tail can produce a catheter with a tight curve of any angle.

Conclusion

Successful catheter manipulation is an activity at the core of interventional cardiology. Imagination, attention to detail and perseverance help, but a deep understanding of normal anatomy in three dimensions and its many variations is perhaps most important of all.

REFERENCES

1. Seldinger S.I., Catheter replacement of the needle in percutaneous arteriography: A new technique. Acta Radiol. 1953: 39:368-376.
2. Lurie P.R., Armer R.M. and Klatte E.C. Percutaneous guide wire catheterization: Diagnosis and therapy. Am. J. Dis. Child. 1963: 106:189-196.
3. Takahashi M., Petry E.L., Lurie P.R., et al. Percutaneous heart catheterization in infants and children: Catheter placement and manipulation with guide wires. Circulation 1970: 42:1037-1048.
4. Carter G.A., Girod D.A. and Hurwitz R.A. Percutaneous cardiac catheterization of the neonate. Pediatrics 19?? 55:662-665.

5. Keane J.F., Lang P., Newburger J. et al. Iliac vein-inferior caval thrombosis after cardiac catheterization in infancy. Pediatr. Cardiol. 1980: 1:257-261.

6. Freed M.D., Keane J.F., and Rosenthal A. The effect of heparinization to prevent arterial thrombosis after percutaneous cardiac catheterization in children. Circulation 1974: 50:565-569.

7. Stanger P., Heymann M.A., Tarnoff H., et al. Complications of cardiac catheterization of neonates, infants, and children. Circulation 1974: 50:595-608.

8. Sequeira F., Girod D.A., Stacki M., et al. Arterial spasm during and following pediatric cardiac catheterization. Pediatr. Cardiol. 1980 : (Abstr) 1:176.

9. Wessel D.L., Keane J.F., Fellows K.E., et al. Fibrinolytic therapy for femoral arterial thrombosis following cardiac catheterization in infants and children. Am. J. Cardiol. 1986: 58:347-351.

10. Linos D.A. Subclavian vein: A golden route. Mayo Clin. Proc. 1980: 55:315-321.

11. Filston H.C. and Grant J.P. A safer system for percutaneous subclavian venous catheterization in newborn infants. J. Pediatr. Surg. 1979: 14:564-570.

12. Radner S. Extended suprasternal puncture technique. Acta Medica Scand. 1955: 151:223-227.

13. Verma R. and Keane J.F. Use of Cutoff Pigtail Catheters With Intraluminal Guidewires in Interventional Procedures in Congenital Heart Disease.

3. HEMODYNAMIC EVALUATION OF CONGENITAL HEART DISEASE

John F. Keane, M.D.
James E. Lock, M.D.

A fundamental understanding of basic instrumentation and cardiovascular physiology is essential to competently assess the hemodynamic status of patients with congenital heart disease. The following is a very superficial view of these topics and readers should consult any of a number of more detailed texts [1-3]. The contents of this chapter are presented in the following sequence.

1. **PRESSURE MEASUREMENTS.**
2. **BLOOD OXYGEN MEASUREMENTS AND SHUNT DETECTION.**
3. **BLOOD GAS MEASUREMENTS.**
4. **CARDIAC OUTPUT MEASUREMENTS.**
5. **SHUNT, RESISTANCE AND VALVE AREA MEASUREMENTS.**

1. PRESSURE MEASUREMENTS

Beautiful pressure tracings, like the Ode to Joy in Beethoven's ninth symphony, stir the heart and soul of the true catheterizer. The pressure at the catheter tip is transmitted via the catheter and tubing to a transducer, converted to an electrical signal which is passed to a multichannel recorder and then by an optical beam to photographic paper. The principles of intravascular pressure measurement were described by Stephen Hale who in 1733 inserted a brass pipe into the femoral artery of a supine mare and connected it to a second pipe nine feet in height [4]. Currently, an inelastic tube, the catheter, is inserted into the vasculature, filled with an incompressible air-free fluid and the pressure generated displaces a fluid column (generally mercury) against gravity. Soft catheters expand and contract slightly with changing pressures thus altering the actual pressure contour. Very small catheters clot at the tip, impairing pressure transmission, as does any blood that adheres to the wall along the length. Heparinization and frequent flushing reduce these problems, as does use of thin walled inelastic catheters with relatively large lumens and short lengths and as few stopcocks as possible. End-hole catheters are used to measure wedged pressures in the pulmonary vascular tree and double lumen catheters to precisely localize gradients. Side-hole and pigtail catheters, used also for angiography are less likely to develop tip obstruction from either blood or tissue and more accurately represent true systemic pressure than end hole catheters.

Transducers are not essential to pressure measurement. One could simply leave the vertical column open to air and, provided that the clear tubing was at least 6 feet high, one could watch the blood move up and down the tubing with each heart beat. For convenience, a transducer is used in which the column of fluid stops at a membrane. This membrane moves only a very small amount (less than 1 - 2 mm) with large changes in pressure. This movement is linear: the movement induced by

38

20mmHg of pressure will be 20% of that produced by 100mmHg. Membrane movement is converted into an electrical signal by a wheatstone bridge and the current is then amplified and recorded. All modern recording systems allow calibration and changes in signal range and paper speeds.

The entire system of catheter/transducer/recorder must meet certain requirements to represent intravascular pressures accurately. It must respond fast enough to inscribe pressures that change 60 to 180 times a minute (1-3 cycles per second or 1 - 3 cps). In fact, it must respond faster; atrial, arterial and ventricular pressure tracings have several contour changes for every heart beat; a simple sine wave curve whose peak occurs at the top of the pressure tracing will reflect pressure tracings very poorly. Fourier demonstrated that if one keeps adding up sine waves whose frequency is higher than that of the previous sine wave, one will eventually represent accurately any complex curve. By convention, the first sine wave curve has the same frequency as the heart rate; for a heart rate of 60 beats/min, that sine wave frequency will be 1 cps. Subsequent frequencies (or harmonics) for this "Fourier analysis" will be multiples of the first frequency, i.e. for a heart rate of one beat per second, the 6th harmonic will have 6 cps (Fig. 3-1).

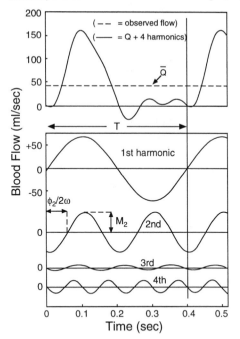

Figure 3-1: An example of a Fourier analysis, or transformation, of a biologic pressure curve. (Reprinted with permission from W.R. Milnor. In Cardiovascular Fluid Dynamics, Vol, 2, Academic Press, New York, 1972.

The first harmonic contributes the most and each subsequent harmonic less and less. For most cardiovascular pressures the 10th harmonic (with a frequency 10 times faster than the heart rate or 35 cps) contributes less than 1% of the pressure curve (Figure 3-1). Thus, a catheter /transducer /recorder system that has a frequency response of 35 cps can accurately reproduce intravascular pressure curves. The natural frequency is directly proportional to the radius of the catheter system lumen and inversely proportional to the catheter length and compliance and density of the fluid filling the system. The highest natural frequency would occur with a short catheter of large lumen filled with low density fluid and connected directly to the transducer. Such a system would be very "underdamped": damping is necessary to keep the frequency response flat.[1] The Fourier transform method of analyzing pressure curves may provide information about the biologic properties of the system that generates the pressure curve as well as define criteria for good measurement systems. For example impedance is an estimate of the opposition to pulsatile flow of a fluid, regardless of net flow. An extreme example is blood moving back and forth across a tricuspid valve in pulmonary atresia; there is "resistance" to this blood flow but, without net forward flow, standard resistance calculations cannot express it. To estimate impedance, a first step is to transform the pressure curve into its component harmonics.

Physiologic recorders have multiple channels for recording not only pressures but

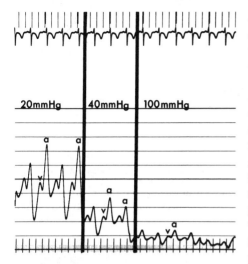

Figure 3-2: A left atrial pressure in a patient with mitral stenosis recorded at high attenuation (right panel), medium, and low attenuation.

also electrocardiographic and occasionally other signals. They have an oscilloscope that allows one to inspect the tracing as it is being generated and decide if it is worth recording. The recording device uses a light beam that is developed onto the paper directly. Paper speeds can be very slow (e.g. 1 mm/sec) to record mean pressure tracings, or to have a permanent record of blood pressure and heart rate during an interventional procedure. They may also be as fast as 100 mm/sec, to record evanescent events such as intracardiac electrocardiograms or instantaneous transvascular pressure gradients. Although most pressures are measured as a continuous "instantaneous " systolic and diastolic pressure, atrial and arterial pressures are also "meaned" in order to calculate resistances (see below).

The mean pressure is derived electrically: the amplifier can damp almost all phasic variability in the tracing. Finally, the scale (or attenuation) at which a pressure can be measured is variable. One can expand the scale (making the top line 20 mm Hg) to record atrial tracings on "low attenuation," (Fig. 3-2) or contract the scale (making the top line 200 mmHg or more) for patients with aortic stenosis.

Calibration

Pressures may be absolute (compared to a vacuum) or relative. Cardiologists compare pressures to the atmospheric pressure in the middle of the heart, defined as

0mmHg. By convention, we assume that the midway point between the back of the thorax and the top of the sternum in a supine neonate, child, or adult is the middle of the heart. The distance from the middle of the chest to the top of the fluoroscopy table is measured. The transducer is positioned such that, when the transducer is filled with saline and the stopcock is opened to air, the tip of the stopcock is at mid-chest. The baseline knob on the multichannel recorder is then adjusted so that the signal from the amplifier is at zero on the oscilloscope. A standard mercury pressure manometer, attached to the transducer is pumped up so that the column of mercury is 100 mm high; the calibration factor knob on the recorder moves the amplifier signal to the 100mmHg line on the oscilloscope. (Water could also be used but, since mercury is 13.6 times denser than water, the column of glass needed is much shorter). One should also calibrate the system at 20 mmHg and 200 mmHg to be certain it is linear. Most recorder amplifiers have 25 Hz filters which will eliminate high frequency oscillatory distortions caused by artifacts such as catheter whipping and wall impact.

Normal Pressures and Tracings

Several studies have documented normal intracardiac pressures in adult men and women. Few such data exist in children; even fewer are available at any given age. Since these few normal pressures came from catheterization of children with uncharacteristic innocent murmurs, and since such children no longer undergo cardiac catheterization, we will need to make do with what little data are currently available.

A review of the literature revealed several papers with normal pressure data from a total of 140 pediatric patients except for left ventricular values [7-13]. A simple arithmetic mean from these 140 pediatric patients, ranging in age from 12 days to 16 years, is listed in table 3-1; the left ventricular values are derived from an additional group of 36 patients of our own, without significant congenital heart disease, the lowest value being 58/5 at age 4 days and 110/5 mmHg in the oldest patient at 24 years.

TABLE 3-1. Normal hemodynamic data in children.

Right atrium	3 mmHg (mean)
Right ventricle	24/5 mmHg (systole/end diastole)
Pulmonary artery	13 mmHg (mean)
PA wedge	8 mmHg (mean)
Left ventricle	96/5 mmHg (systole/end diastole)
Systemic artery	115/67 mmHg (systole/diastole)

These data may be flawed in a number of ways. Specific clinical criteria of "normal" are generally missing; they were collected in different centers over different eras; no effort was made to standardize methodology and the ages of the patients are for the most part unknown. We gathered what data were available on the patients with known ages in these studies and searched the records at Children's Hospital, Boston, for any "normal" hemodynamic data. The results shown as mean values from the combined series at each age level are depicted in Fig. 3-3.

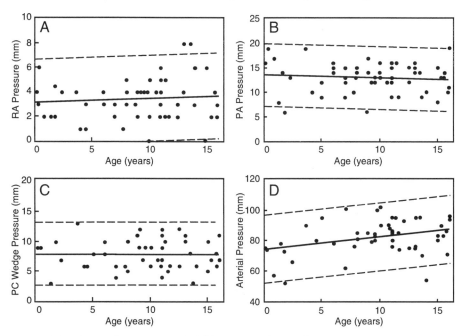

Figure 3-3: Mean values in normal children A= right atrial; B= pulmonary artery; C = pulmonary arterial wedge: D= systemic arterial; hatched lines represent two standard deviations from the mean.

Right Atrium

The normal right atrial pressure tracing is composed of three waves: "a," "c," "v". The "a" wave, thought to represent atrial systole, is the first wave after the "p" wave on the surface EKG and usually peaks at the beginning of the QRS. The "c" wave is a small upward deflection in early systole; we have not found it useful clinically. The "v" wave occurs at the end of systole, and may represent continued atrial filling against a closed tricuspid valve. The fall in pressure that follows the "a" wave is the x descent; that following the "v" wave is the y descent. Normally, the right atrial pressure has a dominant "a" wave that is usually 2-3 mmHg higher than the "v" wave. Neither wave is very tall and they both tend to be within 3-4 mmHg of the mean right atrial pressure (Fig 3-4). Considerable respiratory variability can be seen in the right atrial tracing: in normal children, end inspiratory lung pressures may be minus 7-9 mmHg, and end expiratory pressures are plus 2-4 mmHg. Markedly increased respiratory variability in right atrial pressures is usually due to some form of obstructive airway disease or restrictive lung pathology (Fig 3-5).

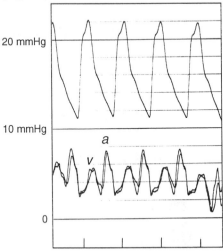

Figure 3-4: Right atrial pressure showing a and v waves at attenuation 20 mmHg: the arterial pressure is at attenuation 100 mmHg

Left Atrium

The same waves seen in the right atrium are present in the normal left atrial pressure trace. In contrast, the mean left atrial pressure is normally higher, and the "v" wave is higher than the "a" wave (Fig. 3-6). In the left atrium, the height of the "v" wave is in part caused by pulmonary vein contraction: "v" waves are usually higher when measured in the pulmonary veins themselves and patients with total anomalous pulmonary venous return have dominant "a" waves in the left atrium.

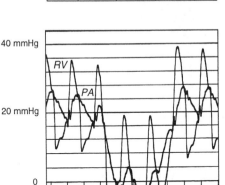

Fig. 3-5: Effects of snoring on right ventricle and pulmonary artery pressures in patient with trivial pulmonary stenosis.

Right Ventricle

The normal right ventricular tracing has a rapid upstroke representing isovolumetric contraction; there follows a ragged downward falling plateau representing isovolumetric relaxation and a slow but steady diastolic rise in pressure (Fig. 3-7). We assume that early diastolic pressure is zero, and only describe end diastolic pressures in the ventricle.

Left Ventricle

The left ventricle tracing is slightly different from that of the right ventricle (Fig. 3-7). Again, early diastolic pressure should be at or near zero.

Normal Mitral Valve
LA - LV

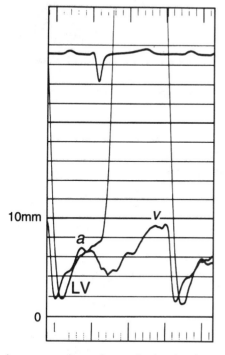

10mm

0

Figure 3-6: Simultaneous left atrial and ventricular pressures showing atrial a and v waves.

In addition, the upstroke is more rapid, the plateau phase is usually flatter and the diastolic rise has an end diastolic hump that is a bit more pronounced.

An often discussed issue is the precise spot where the end-diastolic pressure is. Early workers, using pen and ink recorders, cited the spot where a rapid rise in ventricular pressure caused the ink on the paper to thin. Others cite a small "bump" on the upstroke of the left ventricular tracing, calling that the end diastolic pressure. In adults with slower heart rates, some investigators measure this at 0.052 sec. from the onset of the EKG Q wave. However, end-diastolic pressure is best identified from that spot in patients without mitral stenosis, where the left ventricular and left atrial tracings cross (Fig. 3-6). We therefore try to record, in every patient where mitral valve function or left ventricular performance may be issues, a simultaneous left ventricular and atrial (or pulmonary arterial wedge) pressure at low attenuation.

Pulmonary Artery

This pressure tracing is normally a low amplitude tracing with a slow systolic upstroke, a variable dicrotic notch and a slow fall to end diastole. As with all right heart pressures respiratory variability may be considerable. Normally the pulmonary artery diastolic pressure is similar to the left ventricular end diastolic value: such an observation thus excludes mitral stenosis (Fig. 3-8).

44

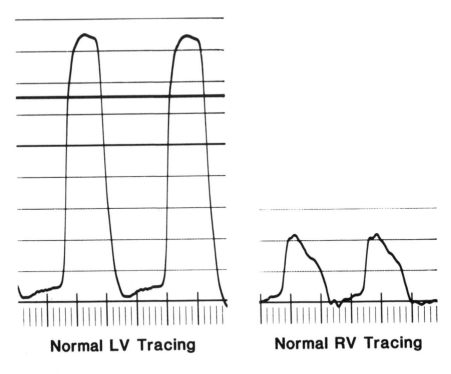

Normal LV Tracing   **Normal RV Tracing**

Figure 3-7: Examples of normal left and right ventricular pressure tracings.

Aorta

The normal aortic tracing varies considerably with the site of measurement near the aortic arch; it has a relatively slow uptake, a broad peak, a relatively subtle dicrotic notch and a nearly linear fall to end diastole.

Although the mean arterial pressure normally falls imperceptibly between the ascending aorta and peripheral arteries, the pressure contour is altered quite a bit: the systolic peak becomes sharper and higher, the dicrotic notch more prominent and diastolic pressure falls a fair bit (Fig. 3-9).

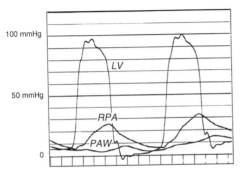

Figure 3-8: Simultaneous right pulmonary artery (RPA) pulmonary arterial wedge (PAW) and left ventricular pressures showing RPA diastolic and PAW pressures similar to the left ventricular end diastolic value, a normal finding.

45

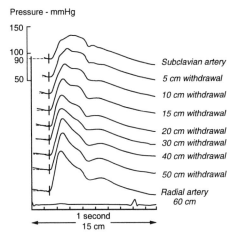

Pressure - mmHg

Subclavian artery
5 cm withdrawal
10 cm withdrawal
15 cm withdrawal
20 cm withdrawal
30 cm withdrawal
40 cm withdrawal
50 cm withdrawal
Radial artery
60 cm

1 second
15 cm

Figure 3-9: "Amplification" of the arterial pulse as it progresses from the central aorta to a more peripheral artery. Pulse amplifications of 15 mmHg are not uncommon in children. (Reprinted from Marshall, H.W. et al.: Physiologic consequences of congenital heart disease. In Hamilton, W.F., and Dow, P. (eds.): Handbook of Physiology, Sect. 2. Circulation, Vol. 1. Washington, DC, American Physiological Society, 1962, p. 417.

Thus, the pulse pressure widens. We therefore do not assume that a femoral or radial artery tracing is identical to that in the ascending aorta.

Wedge Pressures

Systemic arterial or venous wedge pressures are, with few exceptions [14], never used: a wedged arterial catheter will measure a pressure determined partly by downstream atrial pressure, but will be variably lower than that because of one-way venous valves, and variably higher because of arterio-arterial anastomoses. The pulmonary circulation is, however, different: there are no venous valves, no arterio-arterial anastomoses between lung segments and no pulmonary vein-vein anastomoses [15]. Thus, pulmonary artery wedge tracings are good estimates of left atrial pressures, and pulmonary vein wedge pressures can help assess pulmonary artery pressure.

The mean pulmonary artery wedge tracing is usually quite close to mean left atrial tracing, but the phasic contour may be delayed by 50-100 msec., and the amplitude of the waves tends to be a bit lower [16-18].

The pulmonary vein wedge tracing is almost always a damped tracing that has a lower mean than the pulmonary artery pressure itself. When the pulmonary vein wedge is 15 mmHg or less, the pulmonary artery mean is almost always 20 mmHg or below; but when higher one cannot predict the pulmonary artery pressure, except to say that it is usually elevated [19].

Abnormalities of Intracardiac Pressures

Right atrial pressures are depressed by volume depletion; they may be elevated by pericardial tamponade, abnormal connection of the right atrium to a systemic ventricle, large left to right atrial shunts, decreased right ventricular compliance (due either to right ventricular hypertrophy, abnormal systolic or diastolic function), tricuspid stenosis or tricuspid regurgitation. Analysis of the wave pattern is only occasionally helpful: the compliances of the right atrium and attached venae cavae are so high that instantaneous pressure changes tend to be quite small.

Occasionally, one may see a very high "a" wave in functional tricuspid atresia and stenosis of the interatrial septum or mitral valve (Fig. 3-10).

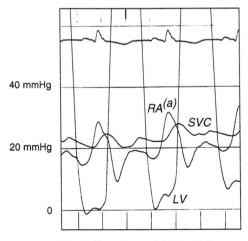

Figure 3-10: Very elevated right atrial A wave in patient with functional tricuspid atresia, open atrial septum, bidirectional Glenn and severe mitral stenosis.

Left atrial pressures may be low because of dehydration or a large interatrial communication. In the latter condition, the atrial pressures equalize (within 2 mmHg mean pressures) with some fall in left atrial pressures. More than a 2 mmHg mean difference (or more than 4mmHg between the "a" or "v" waves) effectively rules out a large atrial hole [21]. Elevated left atrial pressures are due to volume loads, pressure loads (depicted in Fig. 3-11), or left ventricular noncompliance.

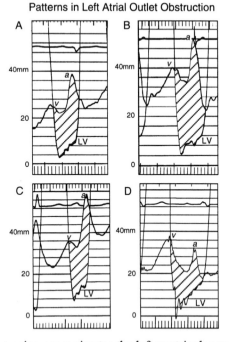

Patterns in Left Atrial Outlet Obstruction

Figure 3-11: Patterns in left atrial outlet obstruction: (A) Congenital mitral stenosis: (B) Prosthetic mitral valve stenosis: (C) Obstructive supravalvar mitral ring: (D) Obstructive supra-annular mitral valve prosthesis.

Since the left atrium is less compliant, pressure changes tend to be large: mitral stenosis produces large "a" waves, and mitral regurgitation large "v" waves. In supra-annular prosthetic stenosis the "v" wave is larger than the "a" wave and the LVED is generally elevated [20].

Right ventricular pressure may be elevated from either pressure or volume loads. The pressure tracings differ: with large ventricular septal defects (VSD) and right ventricular hypertension, the right ventricular tracing approximates the left ventricular pressure, with a broad flat systolic plateau. With a large VSD the two ventricular pressures are equivalent. The pressure tracing in severe pulmonary hypertension is similar. In contrast, in pulmonary valve stenosis, the right ventricular trace is much more peaked; there is an early systolic rise that falls off abruptly (Fig. 3-12).

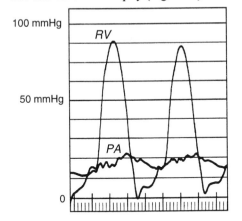

Figure 3-12: Simultaneous right ventricular (RV) and pulmonary artery (PA) pressures in 12 year old patient with valvar pulmonary stenosis.

Left ventricular hypertension will also be associated with a peaked tracing if due to outflow obstruction, and broad if due to systemic hypertension or coarctation. If the stenosis is at the valve, the pullback tracing will have an abrupt pressure fall at the great vessel level (Fig. 3-13).

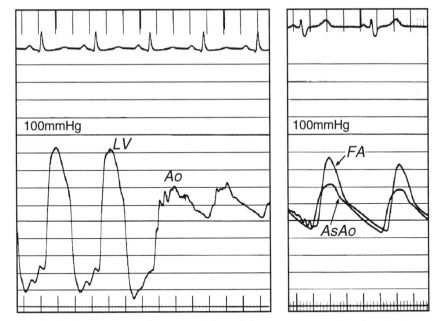

Figure 3-13: A pressure pullback in an infant with aortic stenosis. Note how, in the same patient, pulse amplification between the ascending aorta and femoral artery would cause the gradient to be underestimated if only a femoral arterial tracing were available.

48

In subaortic stenosis, there is a subvalvar ventricular "chamber" with lower pressure than the main ventricular chamber (Fig. 3-14). In supravalvar aortic stenosis, there will be a high pressure great vessel tracing above the aortic valve (Fig. 3-15). Pulmonary hypertension may be due to vascular disease, pulmonary venous or left atrial hypertension, branch pulmonary artery stenosis, or high pulmonary blood flow. In the first two instances, the high pulmonary arterial pressure will have a relatively narrow pulse pressure, with a high diastolic pressure; if due to a large left to right shunt (and hence a large stroke volume) or distal arterial obstructions, the pulse pressure will be wide.

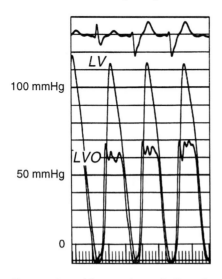

Figure 3-14: Simultaneous left ventricular (LV) and outflow (LVO) pressures in a child with subaortic stenosis, documenting a lower pressure in the left ventricular outflow tract (LVO).

Tamponade/Restrictive Physiology

Elevated filling pressures due to pericardial tamponade or "restrictive" physiology have a characteristic pattern [22, 23]. In tamponade, pericardial fluid serves to equalize pressures throughout the heart during diastole. Both atrial pressures are equal throughout the cardiac cycle, with prominent "a" and "v" waves, and rapid x and y descents. Simultaneous intrapericardial pressures would show a similar, albeit slightly lower, pressure. The ventricular pressures drop in early diastole, but then rise promptly to high levels (the "square-root" sign; Fig. 3-16). Respiratory variability can be exaggerated.

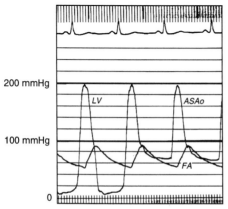

Figure 3-15: A pressure pullback in a child with supravalvar aortic stenosis

The arterial pressure is also altered, causing "pulsus paradoxus". The "paradoxical" finding appears to relate, not to the blood pressure, but to the peripheral pulse rate: normally, blood pressure falls with inspiration and there is a concomitant small but measurable rise in the heart rate. These two effects are more pronounced in tamponade. The systolic pressure fall may be so great that one cannot feel the radial pulse, producing a paradoxical fall in the palpable pulse rate. A fall of up to 10mmHg in the systolic arterial pressure is normal; greater falls should be considered as harbingers of tamponade.

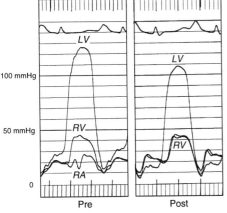

Figure 3-16: Showing simultaneous pre and post pericardiocentesis LV, RV pressures in 12 year old with huge pericardial effusion.

Finally, some patients may have chronic restriction by the pericardium, the myocardium, or both. The distinction is very important: pericardial restriction can be relieved by pericardiectomy (Fig. 3-17). Cardiologists have used both cardiac biopsy and fluid loading [24] to separate the two. The latter study is performed at cardiac catheterization: if atrial pressures are identical, a large (10-20 cc/kg) infusion of warmed saline is administered over a few minutes. If the atrial pressures separate, it supports the notion that the restriction is due to intracardiac (i.e., myocardial) rather than extracardiac (i.e., pericardial) effects.

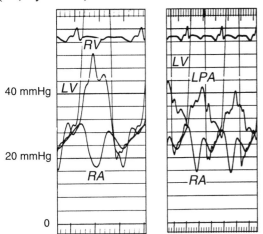

Figure 3-17: Showing simultaneous RA, RV,LPA and LV pressures at attenuation 40 in 14 yr. old patient with late severe postoperative constrictive "pericardial"disease;

Hypertrophic Subaortic Stenosis

After a ventricular extrasystole, the pause results in increased ventricular pressures, both from a longer filling time and from a separate increase in intrinsic inotropy. The two combine to increase stroke volume. In "fixed" left ventricular obstructions (valvar, sub-valvar and supravalvar aortic stenosis) the postextrasystolic beat increases ventricular pressure, aortic pressure, and the gradient. The findings in dynamic subaortic stenosis are different. The increased inotropy contributes to a real

50

increase in the degree of muscular obstruction: while the left ventricular systolic pressure and gradient rise, the aortic pressure falls. This so-called Brockenbrough sign [25] may also be seen with subaortic "muscular stenosis" at the bulboventricular foramen in patients with single ventricle and transposition of the great arteries.

Mitral Stenosis/Insufficiency

With both mitral valve obstruction and leakage, assessment of which abnormality contributes most to left atrial hypertension can be difficult. Calculation of mitral valve area, using standard formulae (see below) will give an estimate of the obstruction if one knows the regurgitant fraction. This calculation relies on a precise estimate of the transvalvar gradient during diastole alone. In combined disease, the "v" wave will be higher than usual. Since the wedge pressure phasic tracing may be delayed a variable amount of time, the "v" wave may be "displaced" from its proper position (under the left ventricle systolic curve) into ventricular diastole, creating the impression of a considerable transvalvar mitral gradient [26]. Thus, the extent to which a diastolic gradient is due to the misplaced "v" wave should be resolved by measuring left atrial pressure directly (Fig. 3-18).

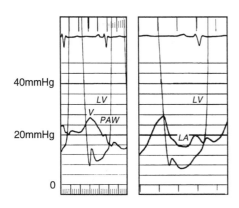

Figure 3-18: Simultaneous tracings in the same patient from the left ventricle and left atrium (right) and between left ventricle and pulmonary artery wedge (left). The wedge tracing is slightly delayed, giving the appearance of a large diastolic gradient. The paper speed is twice as fast in the righthand panel.

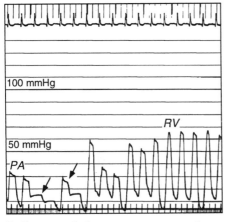

Figure 3-19: An end-hold catheter is pulled from pulmonary artery; when the catheter tip temporarily wedges in the myocardium (arrow), the tracing becomes truncated.

Trouble-Shooting Pressure Measurements

The system for recording intracardiac pressures can fail in many ways. Constant attention to the appearance of a pressure tracing is required. Each pressure must be related to the patient's clinical status, expected findings, and known or suspected anatomic and physiologic condition. A catheterization is like a puzzle: everything must fit with everything else. Unexpectedly low pressures may be due to a loose connection between the transducer and catheter tip, or a hole in the catheter. The catheter tip may be plugged or clotted or it may be wedged against a cardiac or vascular wall. Tip obstruction may be intermittent, especially when pulling from pulmonary artery to right ventricle with an end-hole catheter.

Figure 3-20: Three left ventricular pressure tracings from the same patient. On the left, there is overshoot; in the panel on the right, air in the transducer has produced considerable damping.

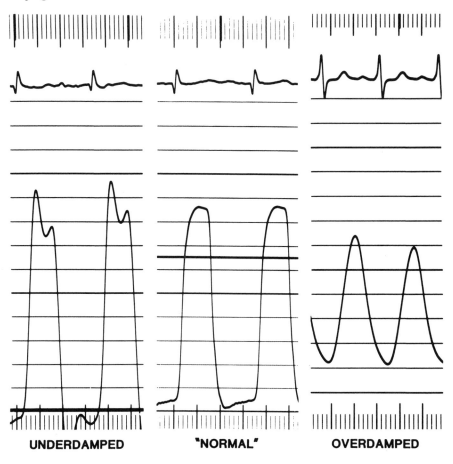

UNDERDAMPED   "NORMAL"   OVERDAMPED

If the tip becomes wedged only during systole, one may see a particularly truncated (and inaccurate) ventricular tracing (Fig. 3-19). Both atrial appendages can entrap a catheter tip: a small volume of fluid is compressed, giving the appearance of very high atrial "a" waves. Ordinarily, one never measures pressures in appendages; however it can be difficult to recognize that the catheter is wedged in an appendage with variant anatomy. Pulmonary veins contract in ventricular systole, and can cause catheter "entrapment", producing an inaccurately high "v" wave.

Partial catheter obstruction, or a compressible fluid in the system (i.e., air) will alter the frequency response of a catheter/transducer/recorder system and the measured pressure wave. If this distortion is incomplete, standing waves may be set up within the system and produce catheter "overshoot" or "fling" (Fig. 3-20). Such tracings typically drop well below baseline in early diastole and have a notched systolic peak. If the problem persists after thorough flushing of the catheter and transducer, drawing blood back into the catheter will change the viscosity of the system and may actually improve the tracing. More commonly, partial obstruction or air in the system will produce a damped tracing (Fig. 3-20). This must be corrected by flushing; if flushing doesn't work, the catheter is probably kinked and should be removed. Rarely, a pressure tracing will appear "damped" because the catheter is not where the cardiologist thinks it is. Finally, the zero and calibration settings may drift during a case. One should check the zeros and calibrations not only at the beginning and end of a catheterization but also at the time of any important numbers, or whenever the pressure measurement does not "fit" or ideally, before every tracing.

2. BLOOD OXYGEN MEASUREMENTS AND SHUNT DETECTION

The original cath lab method for measuring blood oxygen was the Van Slyke manometric method [27], which measured the total amount of oxygen in the blood (both dissolved in plasma and bound to hemoglobin). All catheterization laboratories now rely on the spectrophotometric method of determining the percentage of hemoglobin that is saturated with oxygen. Spectrophotometers measure the amount of light (optical density) transmitted through a tube (or cuvette) at a given wave length by both oxygenated and deoxygenated hemoglobin. The amount of light absorbed is proportional to the thickness of the cuvette, the concentration of the oxyhemoglobin (or deoxyhemoglobin), and the extinction coefficient of that particular wave length. Oxyhemoglobin absorbs at a wavelength = 600 nm, and deoxyhemoglobin at 506.5 nm. Their respective concentrations are calculated from Beer's law yielding the percentage of hemoglobin. This reliable method ignores the amount of dissolved oxygen in plasma, which is proportional to the oxygen tension (mmHg, or torr) The solution constant for oxygen is 0.003, i.e. 0.003 ml of oxygen is dissolved in 100 ml of plasma for every torr of oxygen tension. Thus, if the $_pO_2$ is 333, 1 ml of oxygen will be dissolved. Since the amount of oxygen carried on hemoglobin is much greater (1.36 ml O_2 per gram of Hgb), neglecting the dissolved oxygen will produce an error of 1.0-1.5% in O_2 content when the patient is breathing room air. Larger errors must be corrected for when the patients breathes more than 21% oxygen. Measuring O_2 saturation directly, rather than calculating it from the oxygen-hemoglobin dissociation curve, is independent of factors that may increase (alkalosis, hypothermia, fetal hemoglobin) or decrease (acidosis, fever) hemoglobin/oxygen affinity. Spectrophotometers are thus subject to relatively few errors. Carboxyhemoglobin absorbs light at virtually the same wave length and with the same extinction coefficient as oxyhemoglobin. As normal blood has less than 1% carboxyhemoglobin (except in heavy smokers) this error is small. Bilirubin also absorbs some light at the same wave length as oxyhemoglobin, and markedly elevated bilirubin levels may falsely raise estimated oxygen saturations.

The oxygen saturations of intracardiac blood in normal adults have, like pressures, been well studied; similar data in infants and children are hard to come by. Previous chapters in texts on pediatric cardiology [28-30] have relied largely on estimates of what are normal oxygen saturations in children. Data are, however, available from several sources, including early workers [11,31], exercise studies in normal children [13], and a large study of children with aortic or pulmonary valvar stenosis, normal cardiac outputs, and no intracardiac shunts [32]. Data from the latter study are listed in table 3-2. In most cases, abnormalities in cardiac oxygen levels will be due to left to right or right to left shunts. One non-shunt abnormality cannot be overemphasized. The first measurement made at catheterization should be a saturation from the superior vena cava. Saturations of 70 - 80% are to be expected and indicate that the patient has some hemodynamic reserve. A saturation of 30 - 60%, however, should incite concern; such patients, regardless of their anatomy, have little cardiac reserve. We immediately assess adequacy of ventilation, fluid status, acid base status and proceed with the study with a considerably heightened concern about risks and duration. Conventionally, in congenital heart disease, at least two closely spaced sets of saturations and pressures in the right heart are obtained. The first initial set, in order, consists of superior vena cava, right lateral atrial, right ventricular and pulmonary arterial and wedge values, followed by a retrograde left heart set of values to assess the "lie of the land". The second consists of this series in reverse order during oxygen consumption measurement.

Trouble-Shooting Oximetry Values

The most common problem with an oxygen saturation measurement occurs when an end-hole catheter is used to sample in the pulmonary artery. One can partially (or intermittently) "wedge" the catheter in a distal pulmonary vessel, causing the removal of a mixture of pulmonary capillary (fully saturated) and pulmonary artery blood. This can occur with free return of blood, and is prevented by sampling in central pulmonary arteries.

TABLE 3-2. Normal intracardiac oxygen saturation data in children.

Cardiac chamber	Mean value	Normal range
Superior vena cava	77.1%	66.8-87.3%
Right atrium	78.4%	69.1-87.4%
Pulmonary artery	76.7%	67.1-86.3%

The inferior vena cava (IVC) is a notoriously inconsistent site for oximetric sampling. Hepatic venous saturation is frequently quite low; and renal blood is quite high. This poor mixing is even accentuated in the fetus, where the orientations of the ductus venosus, hepatic vein and IVC have been observed to set up spiral streams that persist in the heart [33], allowing highly saturated blood to cross the foramen ovale. We only sample the IVC in cases of anomalous pulmonary venous drainage or arteriovenous malformations below the diaphragm. Rarely, one will obtain a very high (86-89%) saturation from the innominate or subclavian vein, particularly in a well-sedated older child (Table 3-2), due to return of highly oxygenated blood from the arm. Anomalous venous drainage from the lungs must be sought, but we do not perform angiography to look for systemic arteriovenous malformations in such children unless warranted by the rest of the clinical and hemodynamic picture. Finally, novice catheterizers may be shocked when deeply cyanosed blood comes from what appears (by catheter course) to be the low left atrium. The normal coronary sinus oxygen saturation is frequently 40-50% .

Shunt Detection: Oximetry
Several studies are available that define the minimum change in blood oxygen level needed to reliably demonstrate an intracardiac shunt. In adults, the studies by Barratt-Boyes and associates [34] and Dexter and associates [35] suggested that interchamber right heart oxygen saturation differences as small as 3% (right ventricle to pulmonary artery) or as large as 9% (superior vena cava to pulmonary artery) could reliably detect a left to right shunt. The most completely collected and analyzed study in children comes from Freed and colleagues [32], who reported right heart oximetries from over 1,000 children with isolated valvar (aortic and pulmonary) stenosis. A single set of blood samples was obtained, and the timing of the samples was selected to minimize sampling interval. Care was taken to use the

lateral wall of the right atrium for sampling. The minimum saturation difference to detect a shunt at the 99% confidence limit is listed in table 3-3, there being on average < 1% mean saturation difference between any of these chambers.

TABLE 3-3. Oximetric detection of shunts in children.

Chambers sampled	Minimum saturation difference (67)	Multiple samples*
Superior vena cava-right atrium	8.7%	(7%)
Right atrium-right ventricle	5.2%	(4%)
Right ventricle-pulmonary artery	5.6%	(4%)

* Early studies [35] showed that, if more than one set of samples is obtained, and if care is taken to obtain the samples as rapidly as possible (less than one minute apart), these numbers can be reduced.

Thus, each of these sites can be used to represent mixed venous blood with some accuracy. Nonetheless, the more distal site (i.e., the pulmonary artery) will have the best mixing and the smallest error. Superior vena caval blood is probably close to mixed venous blood because the contribution of inferior vena cava (high saturation) and coronary sinus blood (low saturation) tend to cancel each other. Similar data are not available for detection of right to left shunts. Ordinarily, we become suspicious of a right to left shunt if the aortic saturation is less than 95% or if there is a 2% or greater stepdown between left atrial (or left ventricular) and aortic blood.

Trouble-Shooting Shunt Detection
In the face of pulmonary disease, especially when nonuniform, detection and quantification of shunts can be difficult. Sampling all four pulmonary veins and averaging them is worth doing but cannot be considered entirely accurate: almost half of all pulmonary blood flow will ordinarily return via the right lower lobe pulmonary vein, whereas less than 15% will return from the left upper lobe. Even weighting the samples (using normal flow distributions) is hazardous, since alveolar collapse induces local pulmonary vasospasm, moving blood away from the diseased lung. The use of the SVC saturation to calculate atrial left to right shunts assumes that red blood does not regurgitate up that vessel. This may be misleading in atrial defects after pulmonary arteriography; contrast frequently refluxes up the SVC on recirculation when there is tricuspid valve regurgitation or left ventricular to right

56

atrial shunts. In such situations, mixed venous samples should include the innominate vein. Finally, the size of the shunt that can be detected will vary with the cardiac output. If the output is high, and mixed venous blood is 84% with a left atrial saturation of 95%, one will only detect shunts of 50% or more. If the output is low, and mixed venous saturations are 65%, one can reliably detect shunts as small as 15%.

3. BLOOD GAS MEASUREMENTS

A systemic arterial blood gas is required some time during catheterization: the blood gas will serve as an internal control measure of oxygen saturation measurements, it will reveal whether acidosis or respiratory depression affects the patient's clinical status, or falsely increases pulmonary vascular resistance. Blood gases may also be used to assess both intrapulmonary shunting and gross inequalities of ventilation and perfusion.

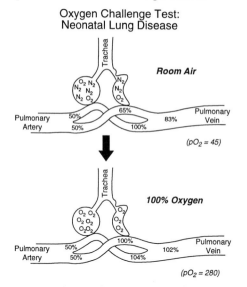

Oxygen Challenge Test:
Neonatal Lung Disease

Figure 3-21: Example of how cyanosis produced by pulmonary disease may respond to oxygen administration: partially ventilated airways will deliver much more oxygen to the pulmonary capillaries, causing arterial pO_2 to rise considerably.

Cyanosis from intracardiac right to left shunting will be largely resistant to administered oxygen; increasing the oxygen content of returning pulmonary venous blood will have little impact on the final arterial oxygen saturation. In contrast, right to left pulmonary shunting is highly dependent on inspired oxygen (Figs. 3-21 and 3-22). Carbon dioxide tension in blood can assess respiratory quotients, which are known to change with exercise in children [13]. Pulmonary vein CO_2 tensions should always be measured when gross ventilation/flow discrepancies are suspected. If congenital or post-operative abnormalities cause marked inequalities in flow distribution, both lungs will have fully saturated blood in their respective pulmonary veins. The lung receiving both flow and ventilation will have a "normal" pulmonary vein blood gas profile: the CO_2 "stepdown" will be 4-6 torr. The ventilated, but underperfused, lung will remove virtually all of the CO_2 it receives, resulting in a very low CO_2 tension in its draining pulmonary vein (Fig. 3-23). This physiology should be suspected in the postoperative patient who requires a large minute ventilation to maintain a normal arterial CO_2 [36].

Oxygen Challenge Test: Cyanotic Heart Disease

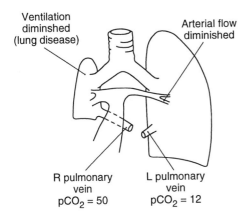

Room Air

Trachea

O₂ N₂ / N₂ N₂ / N₂ O₂   O₂ O₂ / N₂ N₂ / N₂ N₂

Right Ventricle — 50% / 50% — 100% / 100% — 100% — 83% Aorta — 50% Cardiac Shunt 50% — (pO₂ = 45)

100% Oxygen

Trachea

O₂ O₂ / O₂ O₂ / O₂ O₂   O₂ O₂ / O₂ O₂ / O₂ O₂

Right Ventricle — 50% / 50% — 104% / 104% — 86% Aorta — 50% Intracardiac Shunt 50% — (pO₂ = 49)

Figure 3-22: Cyanosis due to extra pulmonary shunting will be largely unresponsive to oxygen administration.

Ventilation diminshed (lung disease) — Arterial flow diminished

R pulmonary vein pCO₂ = 50   L pulmonary vein pCO₂ = 12

Figure 3-23: Retention of CO₂ due to a large mismatch of ventilation and perfusion. Normally, alveolar and pulmonary venous pCO₂ levels are less than 5 mmHg apart, but when a large area of the lung is ventilated but underperfused, the alveolar (and pulmonary venous pCO₂ levels) on that side will be quite low, whereas mixed arterial pCO₂ levels may be elevated.

58

4. CARDIAC OUTPUT MEASUREMENTS

Measurements of cardiac output and regional blood flows have preoccupied cardiac physiologists for decades [37, 38]. Clinical cardiologists now have a number of available accurate flow measurement techniques. In pediatric cardiology, indexed flow rather than unindexed values permit comparison between patients of different sizes.

All blood flow measurements rely on either the measurement of velocity and subsequent conversion to flow or the indicator dilution technique. The common velocity techniques employ either the Doppler shift produced by moving RBC's on an ultrasound signal [39] or the current of a moving conductor (the ions in blood) through a magnetic field [40]. Each technique uses the instantaneous cross-sectional area of the vessel and the integrated velocity of flow. The Doppler technique relies on a close relationship between peak velocity and mean velocity, and estimates mean cross-sectional area. The electromagnetic flow technique [40] requires a cannula of fixed, known diameter placed around the vessel and an externally generated magnetic field. Although rarely used for total cardiac output measurement in the intact circulation, this technique is very accurate when external flow probes are applied to single vessels (i.e. coronary arteries).

The indicator dilution principle is really quite simple and apparently was first discussed by Adolph Fick [41]. A river flows by a factory that dumps wood chips into the stream at a fixed rate. In spring, the river flows rapidly and the chips are sparsely scattered; in fall the flow slows and the chips become densely packed. In either case, the flow will be directly proportional to the amount of indicator (wood chips) added to the stream, and inversely proportional to the concentration of indicator in the stream. To calculate flow in volumes per unit time, one measures the amount of indicator (e.g. chips per hour) and the concentration of indicator in the flowing volume (e.g. chips per cubic feet). The flow (in cubic feet per hour) will be the amount of indicator divided by the concentration. The chips may be delivered to the stream as a steady stream (as oxygen is delivered), or in a bolus (as green dye or cold saline are delivered).

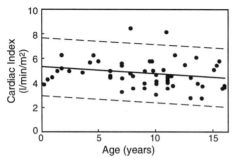

Figure 3-24: Cardiac index versus age in a group of normal children.

As with pressure measurements, normal values in children for cardiac outputs are difficult to find. From the same pooled data, in which different cardiac output measurement techniques were used, we have plotted cardiac index versus age in normal children (Fig. 3-24).

Fick Principle

If oxygen is the indicator, one measures O_2 consumption and O_2 concentrations in mixed arterial and mixed venous blood. Oxygen consumption measurements rely on the complete collection of exhaled air [42, 43]. The cooperative patient breaths through a mouthpiece, the nose gently but firmly plugged to avoid air loss. A one-way valve lets exhaled air into a Tissot spirometer that measures the volume of air without compressing it. The O_2 concentration in the spirometer is measured, subtracted from the known O_2 content of room air (20.9%), thus the oxygen consumption may be measured. This technique strains the cooperative resources of a five-year-old on the cath table, and is completely impractical under the age of three. Simplified flow-through devices obviate this problem [44]: air is withdrawn at a constant flow from a loosely fitting hood placed over the child's head . We have used such a device for many years (Waters Instruments Inc. Rochester, MN). As long as the flow rate is fast enough to bring with it all exhaled air, one can calculate the oxygen consumption. If too high a flow rate is used, the difference between room air and the collected air becomes smaller, increasing the measurement error. We have found this technique useful for measuring O_2 consumption in infants and younger children when the directions are scrupulously followed: it is particularly important that there are no hood air leaks other than the punched holes in the apron. When the digitally displayed value is unindexed, it is essential to ensure the measurement is in the correct range; knowing the body surface area is important in this regard: a crude estimate may be made by using Lowe's formula [45]:

$$BSA\ (M^2) = \sqrt[3]{WT^2(kg)} \times 0.1$$
(e.g. $8\ kg = 0.4\ M^2$; $20\ kg = 0.7\ M^2$; $32\ kg = 1.0M^2$; $60\ kg = 1.5\ M^2$)

Measurement of O2 consumption will be impossible or impractical in the intubated child or the critically ill patient studied in off hours with less than the full complement of laboratory personnel. In such cases, we rely on the formulae of LaFarge and Miettinen [46] who measured O2 consumption with spirometers in over 800 children. In children undergoing cardiac catheterization, the major determinants of O_2 consumption were age, heart rate and sex. Sedation consisted of the DPT cocktail. Their derived equations for children of varying ages and heart rates yield the results listed in table 3-4; for any given O_2 consumption listed, the 2 standard deviation range is about 45 ml o2/min-M2.

Spirometer-derived O_2 consumptions are not available for infants. Studies using the flow-through method to measure O_2 consumption in infants [47, 48] yield results that are less precise but allow for estimates of cardiac outputs. Table 3-5 lists O_2 consumption values for sedated infants from these combined studies (in ml o2/kg - min).

TABLE 3-4. Oxygen consumption in children (L/MIN-M2)

Age (yrs)	Sex	Heart rate 75	Heart rate 100	Heart rate 125	Heart rate 150
4	M	150	160	169	179
4	F	143	152	162	171
8	M	143	152	162	171
8	F	131	140	150	159
12	M	138	147	157	166
12	F	124	134	143	152
16	M	135	144	154	163
16	F	119	129	138	148

TABLE 3-5. Oxygen consumption in infants mlO_2/kg- min.

Weight	O_2 consumption
2 - 5 kg	10 - 14 ml O_2/kg
5 - 8 kg	7 - 11 ml O_2/kg

Once the oxygen consumption is known, the cardiac output may be calculated from the Fick Equation in patients without intracardiac shunts: (CO=Qp=Qs)

$$CO = \frac{VO_2}{\text{systemic artery } O_2 \text{ content - systemic vein } O_2 \text{ content}}$$

(CO = cardiac output; Qp = pulmonary flow, Qs = systemic flow, VO_2 = oxygen consumption). By convention, since hemoglobin is expressed as grams per 100 ml, O_2 content is expressed the same way:

O_2 content = (Hgb conc.)(1.36) (fractional saturation of blood)
where O_2 content is in ml of O_2 per 100 ml blood, Hgb conc. is the grams of hemoglobin per 100 ml blood, 1.36 is the number of ml of O_2 that will bind to one

gram of fully saturated hemoglobin, and the fractional saturation is determined by oximetry. The dissolved O_2 in plasma is neglected.

Although the above are expressed in volume units of 100 ml, cardiac output is expressed in liters: the denominator must therefore be multiplied by 10. Finally, since the hemoglobin concentration and maximum O_2 content are identical for arterial and venous blood, the formula may be simplified:

$$CO = \frac{VO_2}{(Ao\ sat - Pa\ sat)(Hgb\ conc.)(1.36)(10)}$$

Thermodilution

Cold saline has now replaced indocyanine green as the most commonly used indicator. A cold bolus has the distinct advantage that the cold is lost in one or two passages through a capillary bed, eliminating the recirculation curve, and simplifying the calculation of output (see below). A bucket with ice and cold water soon reaches a temperature of 0 degree C and stays there until the ice has melted. A container with sterile saline or dextrose water drawn into syringes is placed in the bucket 30 minutes prior to the study, to insure complete temperature equilibration of both fluid and syringes. A thermodilution catheter is positioned with the tip in a central PA, and the proximal port in the RA. The electrical adapter from the thermistor embedded in the catheter is connected to the computer, and the calibration factor (corrects for variabilities in catheter and thermistor) dialed in. A syringe containing 3 cc (infants 3-10 kg), 5 cc (10 - 30 kg), or 10 cc (30 + kg) of iced solution is injected rapidly into the RA via the proximal port. The first syringeful serves to cool down the catheter shaft and the output so computed is ignored. A series of three injections is made as closely together as possible (waiting for the thermistor to return to baseline between each injection) and the outputs from each recorded. The temperature at the tip should fall at least 0.5 ^{0}C (e.g., from 37.1 to 36.6) at its lowest value, and the three measurements in a clinically stable patient should be within 15% of each other. This technique is particularly useful where repeat cardiac outputs are necessary during interventional procedures such as balloon dilation of aortic stenosis. It is less useful in patients with Fontan procedures presumably because of absence of thorough mixing of the cold bolus: the initial abrupt rise in the curve is absent and the return to baseline very slow. Results in patients with significant pulmonary regurgitation can be unreliable.

Trouble-Shooting The most common problem is associated with a small temperature change. A small drop in temperature may be due to a high cardiac output but may be due to other causes. If the thermistor tip lies on, or near, the PA wall (especially if it is wedged), the wall serves as a heat sink [49], producing a falsely small area under the curve, and hence a falsely high cardiac output; the smaller the infant, the more likely the tip will be near a wall. If the injection port is not in or near the RA in freely flowing blood, the thermal bolus will lose cold before it reaches the thermistor. Respiration produces a small but measurable change in intrapulmonary arterial temperature, adding baseline noise. Finally, baseline temperature is not stable during exercise, it rises throughout the early period of body work. Despite these pitfalls, thermodilution outputs have proven relatively accurate (20%) at the time of catheterization in children [50].

Dye Curves

As the traditional gold standard for flow measurements in a biologic system, dye dilution curves have been performed using cardiogreen dye [51], Evans blue, hydrogen ions [52], freon [53], ascorbic acid [54] and radioisotopes. Although cumbersome and now rarely used, dye dilution curves are accurate, reproducible and versatile tools for analyzing cardiovascular physiology [3, 55]. Indocyanine green has become the standard: it is nontoxic, soluble, absorbs light at a wave length (800 millimicrons) unaffected by concentrations of either oxyhemoglobin or deoxyhemoglobin, and exhibits a nearly linear response to changes in light absorption with changing blood concentrations.

Cardiac Output As noted above, the cardiac output is directly proportional to the amount of the indicator delivered, and inversely proportional to the amount of indicator that is present in a syringe withdrawing blood at a constant rate. That amount could be measured directly if the indicator did not recirculate, as is done with microsphere calculations of cardiac output [56, 57]. Since green dye does recirculate, the amount of dye that would have entered the syringe without recirculation must be calculated. Constant withdrawal of blood through an optical cuvette measures the instantaneous concentration of green dye in the blood passing the catheter. A curve is generated, relating time against concentration. The initial downslope of that curve is a logarithmic decay but the tail of the downslope is distorted by recirculating blood.

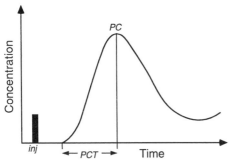

Figure 3-25: Illustration of the forward triangle method for dye curve determination of cardiac output. (Reprinted from Bloomfield, D.A. Dye Curves Baltimore:University Park Press, 1974, p.79).

To measure the cardiac output, one calculates the area under the initial, undistorted curve. In the forward triangle, a triangle is constructed from the appearance to peak concentration (Fig. 3-25), and the area of this forward triangle is assumed to be 37% of the area under of the primary curve.

The cardiac output is then

$$C.O. = \frac{\text{dye injected (mg) X 60}}{\text{(area under forward triangle)}} \quad (2.7)$$

Other more precise methods of estimating the area under the primary curve include the Stewart-Hamilton equation and the integral methods [3, 55].

Trouble-Shooting A common misconception about dye curves is the notion that they only measure the blood flow in the vessel being sampled. This is untrue. If the dye is injected in the RA and the sampling site is the RPA, blood flow measured is not RPA flow but output from the RV. In patients with intracardiac shunting, a dye curve will measure the output of the last chamber where blood is thoroughly mixed: thus, in a patient with an ASD, if one injects in the RA and samples in the PA, the curve estimates RV output. If the dye is not thoroughly mixed in a ventricular pumping chamber, output calculations will be inaccurate. In the face of a left to right shunt, recirculated blood will return earlier than usual to the downslope of the primary curve, making output calculations less accurate.

In a right to left shunt the initial portion of the curve will be distorted and no calculation of output is possible. In valvar regurgitation the regurgitant fraction will prolong the dye curve by re-mixing with the blood in the upstream chamber resulting in underestimation of cardiac output. In fact, one can estimate the degree of valvar regurgitation by applying the left to right shunt formulae.

Shunt Calculations from Dye Curves Dye curves can also be used to estimate shunt sizes, a principle which underlies the use of radionucleides to estimate left to right shunts. To some extent, the degree of distortion of the downslope (left to right shunts) or upslope (right to left shunts) is proportional to the amount of shunting. The % left to right shunt may be estimated from the following two regression curves (Fig. 3-26) [58]:

% left to right shunt = 141 C (p + Bt) - 42/Cp

and % left to right shunt = 135 C (p + 2Bt) - 14/Cp

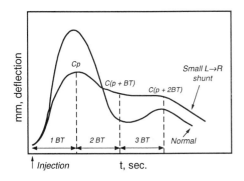

Figure 3-26: Use of a dye curve to estimate the left to right shunt when downslope of curve is smooth (usually after a superior vena cava injection site). (Reprinted from Carter, S.A., et al. J. Lab Clin Med 55:77-88, 1960.

64

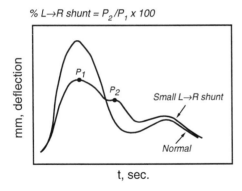

% L→R shunt = P_2/P_1 x 100

mm, deflection

P_1

P_2

Small L→R shunt

Normal

t, sec.

Figure 3-27: Use of a dye curve to estimate the left to right shunt if two distinct peaks are seen prior to recirculation. (Modified from Victoria, B.E. and Gessner, I.H.,Circulation 51:530-534, 1975).

By convention, both equations are solved and the two results averaged for the left to right shunt.

The Carter formulae are most accurate when the downslope is smooth. If two distinct peaks (the primary and the recirculation peaks) are seen, one should use a different formula [59]: % left to right shunt = (P2/P1) (100) (Fig. 3-27).

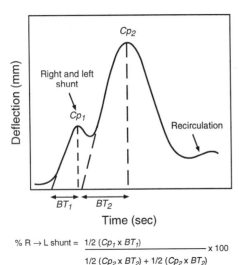

Deflection (mm)

Cp_2

Right and left shunt

Cp_1

Recirculation

BT_1 BT_2

Time (sec)

% R → L shunt = $\dfrac{1/2\,(Cp_1 \times BT_1)}{1/2\,(Cp_2 \times BT_2) + 1/2\,(Cp_2 \times BT_2)}$ x 100

Figure 3-28: Use of a dye curve to estimate the right to left shunt from a modification of the forward triangle method. (Reprinted from Carter, S.A. et al. J Lab Clin Med 55:77-88, 1960).

With right to left shunts, the upstroke of the curve is distorted. The early peak represents the dye injected into the venous site which has passed right to left through the intracardiac defect and reaches the arterial sampling site without crossing a capillary bed. The amount of right to left shunt can be calculated by a modification of the forward triangle method [60]; Fig. 3-28):

Detection of right to left shunts appears reliable, with shunts as small as 5% accurately detected. Detection of left to right shunts is not so precise, with the threshold being a shunt of about 30%.

% R to L shunt $= \dfrac{(0.5)\,(Cp1)\,(Bt1)}{(0.5)\,(Cp1)\,(Bt1) + (0.5)\,(Cp2)\,(Bt2)}$

5. SHUNTS, RESISTANCE AND VALVE AREA MEASUREMENTS.

Shunts. When there are no shunts, systemic (Qs) and pulmonary (Qp) blood flows are equal. In the presence of shunts, the Fick equation is applied to the systemic and pulmonary vascular beds separately, assuming that O_2 uptake (in the lungs) and O_2 consumption (in the rest of the body) are equal. Thus,

$$Qp = \frac{VO_2}{(PV\ sat\ -\ PA\ sat)\ (Hgb)\ (1.36)\ (10)}$$

and for the systemic circulation

$$Qs = \frac{VO_2}{(Ao\ sat\ -\ SVC\ sat)\ (Hgb)\ (1.36)\ (10)}$$

Most shunts are expressed as the absolute volume of the left to right or right to left shunt (in L/min -M2), or as the ratio of pulmonary to systemic blood flow (Qp/Qs), or the percentage of blood being shunted.

Absolute Shunt Volumes. The amount of already oxygenated blood that returns to the lungs will be inversely proportional to the oxygen saturation difference between the PA and SVC. Thus,

$$Q\ L\ to\ R = \frac{VO_2}{(PA\ sat\ -\ SVC\ sat)\ (Hgb)\ (1.36)\ (10)}$$

and

$$Q\ R\ to\ L = \frac{VO_2}{(PV\ sat\ -\ Ao\ sat)\ (Hgb)\ (1.36)\ (10)}$$

The ratio of pulmonary blood flow to systemic blood flow is perhaps the most useful shunt calculation, providing an estimate of volume loads on various cardiac chambers. Since most of the variables cancel out, and since flow is inversely proportional to saturation differences, Qp/Qs = Ao sat - SVC sat/PV sat - PA sat.

Shunt Percentages. In the presence of intracardiac shunts, "effective pulmonary blood flow" (Qep) is a useful notion. Qep is the amount of desaturated systemic venous blood flow that crosses the pulmonary vascular bed and picks up O_2. The effective pulmonary blood flow and effective systemic blood flow are equal. The "ineffective" pulmonary blood flow would be fully oxygenated blood that goes to the lungs for a redundant trip; ineffective systemic blood flow is the portion of desaturated blood that returns to the body.

$$Qep = Qes = \frac{VO2}{(PV\ sat - SVC\ sat)\ (Hgb)\ (1.36)\ (10)}$$

The absolute left to right shunt is Qp - Qep; and the percent of total pulmonary blood flow that is shunted blood is: Qp - Qep/Qp=(PA - SVC)/(PV - SVC).

Similarly, the absolute right to left shunt is Qs- Qes: and the percent of total systemic blood flow that is shunted blood is: Qs - Qes/Qs = (PV - Ao)/(PV - SVC).

Resistances. In an attempt to estimate the force that "resists" blood flow through a vascular bed, physiologists have calculated vascular resistances by dividing the pressure drop across the vascular bed by the indexed flow; the higher the resistance, the more pressure that will be needed to maintain a constant flow. Calculations of vascular resistances may be in Woods units (mmHg X min/L) derived by dividing the mean pressure by the flow, or in dyne sec cm -5. The latter unit, less commonly used, is merely the resistance in Woods units multiplied by 80. Systemic vascular resistance is therefore: SVR = (mean Ao pressure - mean RA pressure)/Qs. Since RA pressure contributes so little to the total pressure in the aorta, many cardiologists omit it from the resistance calculation.

Two different pulmonary resistances may be calculated; (a) the resistance across the vascular bed (called "arteriolar" resistance) and (b) the total resistance.

(a) PAR = (mean PA pressure - LA pressure)/Qp

(b) Total PVR = (mean PA pressure)/Qp.

In adults, body size is less variable than in children, and resistances are often uncorrected for body surface area. In children, resistances are calculated using the cardiac index (cardiac output/body surface area): the raw resistance is divided by the body surface area to get the corrected resistance. One must be careful in comparing calculated resistance values between pediatric and adult patients (especially with different publications and centers) to note whether the resistances have been indexed. Although useful, resistance alone is an inadequate method to gauge the anatomic or physiologic state of a vascular bed. For example, if the cardiac output across any vascular bed is increased, the bed will partially and passively "stretch" to accommodate the higher flow: calculated resistance will fall. No vascular bed is rigid; each is compliant to one degree or another. A "normal" resistance at normal flow is more normal than a "normal" resistance at high flow. Several methodologies have been designed to overcome this interdependence in the pulmonary vascular bed [61].

Valve Areas. Several formulae were derived by Gorlin and Gorlin [62] to estimate the area across a stenotic valve. These formulae assert that the valve area is directly related to the flow across the valve and inversely related to the square root of the pressure drop. They use the total flow across the valve when the valve is open. One needs a measured cardiac output, a mean heart rate and superimposed pressure tracings from the cardiac chambers above and below the valve in question. If one does not obtain the two pressures simultaneously (with two catheters or a single catheter with two pressure sampling sites) a pullback tracing can be used, but the two tracings must be carefully matched at the same heart rate.

For semilunar (aortic and pulmonary) valves,

$$\text{valve area} = \frac{\text{systolic flow (ml/sec)}}{(44.5)(\text{square root of mean gradient})}$$

$$\text{indexed valve area} = \frac{\text{systolic flow (ml/sec - M2)}}{(44.5)(\text{square root of mean gradient})}$$

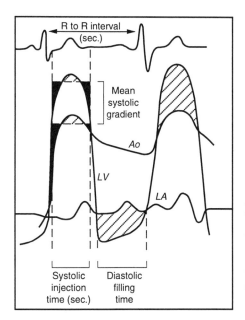

Figure 3-29: Calculation of valve areas depends on estimation of the mean gradient across either the aortic or mitral valve and the time that the valve is open.

To determine systolic flow, (in ml/sec), the time that the aortic (or pulmonary) valve is open (systolic ejection time) is measured directly from the combined great vessel/ventricular pressure tracing: the places where the two lines cross (Fig. 3-29) marks opening and closure. When the total cardiac output is divided by the percent of the cardiac cycle during which the valve is open, one obtains systolic flow:

$$\text{systolic flow (ml/sec)} = \frac{(C.O.)(\text{R to R interval})}{(60)(\text{systolic ejection time})}$$

Thus, for a child with a cardiac index of 3,000 ml/min, a heart rate of 100 (i.e., an R to R interval of 0.6 sec), a systolic ejection time of 0.24 sec, and a mean aortic gradient of 49 mmHg, the indexed aortic valve area will be:
systolic flow = (3,000) (0.6)/(60) (0.24) = 125 ml/sec/M2, and
A.V.A./M2 = 125/(44.5)(7)=0.40 cm$_2$ M2.

68

The mean systolic gradient may be obtained in two ways: vertical lines are drawn through the places where the aortic and ventricular tracings intersect, and horizontal lines are visually estimated to get average aortic and ventricular systolic pressure (Fig. 3-29). The difference between the two lines is the mean gradient. A more accurate method uses planimetry. Planimeters determine the surface area of an irregular area; if the area between the systolic tracings (Fig. 3-29) is known in cm_2 it is divided by the distance (on the paper) between valve opening and closure, to get the average distance between the systolic lines. Computer programs now solve for these variables.

Bache and associates [63] modified the Gorlin formula for semilunar valves to use the peak to peak systolic gradient,

A.V.A. = systolic flow/(37.8) (square root of peak gradient + 10).

The measurements of mitral or tricuspid valve areas are identical in principle to those of semilunar valves, substituting the diastolic flow from the diastolic filling time, the mean diastolic pressure, and a different constant:

$$\text{mitral valve area} = \frac{\text{diastolic flow (ml/sec)}}{(31.5)(\text{square root of mean diastolic gradient})}$$

diastolic flow = (C.O.) (R - R interval)/(60) (diastolic filling time)

Trouble-Shooting Valve Area. As noted above, if wedge pressure is used instead of atrial pressure, the time delay between the two tracings may cause one to estimate filling times incorrectly and (especially with associated mitral regurgitation) mean diastolic gradient. Similarly, if a peripheral artery is used instead of the central aorta, the gradient and timing will be off. More importantly, if there is significant valvar regurgitation, most estimates of cardiac output will only estimate the flow across the valve that stays across the valve; the regurgitant fraction must cross the valve with each heart beat, but will not be measured by Fick, indocyanine green dye, or thermodilution outputs. If regurgitation is ignored, the calculated valve area will be smaller than the real valve area.

REFERENCES

1. Baim, DS, Grossman, W. Cardiac Catheterization, Angiography and Intervention. Baltimore: Williams & Wilkins, 1996.
2. Zimmerman, H.A., Intravascular Catheterization. Springfield, IL: Charles C. Thomas, 1966.

3. Yang, S.S., Bentivoglio, L.G., Maranhao, V. and Goldberg, H. From Cardiac Catheterization to Hemodynamic Parameters. Philadelphia: F.A. Davis Co., 1978.

4. Hale, S. Statical Essays. Vegetable Staticks, Vol. ll (3rd ed.) London: W. Inrys and R. Maonday, 1738.

5. Adams, F.H. and Lind, J. Physiologic studies on the cardiovascular status of normal newborn infants. Pediatrics 19:431-37, 1957.

6. Emmanoulides, G.C., Moss, A.J., Duffie, E.R., Jr. and Adams, F.H. Pulmonary arterial pressure changes in human newborn infants from birth to 3 days of age. J. Pediatr. 65:327-33, 1964.

7. Sproul, A. and Simpson, E. Stroke volume and related hemodynamic data in normal children. Pediatr. 33:912-18, 1964.

8. James, L.S. and Rowe, R.D. The pattern of response of pulmonary and systemic arterial pressures in newborn and older infants to short periods of hypoxia. J. Pediatr. 51:5-11, 1957.

9. Lucas, R.V., Jr., St. Geme, J.W., Jr., Anderson, R.C., Adams, P. and Ferguson, D.J. Maturation of the pulmonary vascular bed. Am. J. Dis. Child. 101:467-75, 1961.

10. Rowe, R.D., and James, L.S. The normal pulmonary arterial pressure during the first year of life. J. Pediatr. 51:1-4, 1957.

11. Kjellberg, S.R., Mannheimer, E., Rudhe, U. and Jonsson, B. Diagnosis of Congenital Heart Disease. Chicago: Year Book Publishers, 1955.

12. Cummings, G.R., Hemodynamics of supine bicycle exercise in "normal" children. Am. Heart J. 93:617-22, 1977.

13. Lock, J.E., Einzig, S.A., and Moller, J.H. Hemodynamic responses to exercise in normal children. Am. J. Cardiol. 41:1278-84, 1978.

14. Paton, A., Reynolds, T.B. and Sherlock, S. Assessment of portal venous hypertension by catheterization of hepatic vein. Lancet 1:918-21, 1953.

15. Wagenvoort, CA., Heath, D. and Edwards, J.E. The pathology of the Pulmonary Vasculature. Springfield IL: Charles C. Thomas, 3-35, 1964.

16. Connolly, D.C., Kirklin, J.W. and Wood, E.H. The relationship between pulmonary artery wedge pressure and left atrial pressure in man. Circ. Res. 2:434-440, 1954.

17. Hellens, H.K., Haynes, F.W. and Dexter, L. Pulmonary "capillary" pressure in man. J. Appl. Physiol. 2:24-29, 1949.

18. Werko, L., Varnaskas, E., Eliasch, H., Lagerlof, H., Senning, A. and Thomasson, B. Further evidence that the pulmonary capillary venous pressure pulse in man reflects cyclic pressure changes in the left atrium. Circ. Res. 1:337-39, 1953.

19. Hawker, R.E. and Celermajer, J.M. Comparison of pulmonary artery and pulmonary venous wedge pressure in congenital heart disease. Br. Heart J. 35:386-91, 1973.

70

20. Adatia, I., Moore, P., Jonas R.A., Colan, S.D., Lock, J.E., Keane, J.F. Clinical course and hemodynamic observations after supra-annular mitral valve replacement in infants and children. J.Am. Coll. Cardiol. 29:1089-94, 1997.

21. Levin, A.R., Spach, M.S., Boineau, J.P., Canent, R.V., Jr., Capp, M.P. and Jewett, P.H. Atrial pressure-flow dynamics in atrial septal defects (secundum type). Circulation 37:476-88, 1968.

22. Shabetai, R., Fowler, N.O., and Guntheroth, W.G. The hemodynamics of cardiac tamponade and constrictive pericarditis. Am. J. Cardiol. 26:480-89, 1970.

23. Meany, E., Shabetai, R., Bhargave, V., Shearer, M., Weider, C., Mangiardi, L.M., Smalling, R. and Peterson, K. Cardiac amyloidosis, constrictive pericarditis, and restrictive cardiomyopathy. Am. J. Cardiol. 38: 547-66, 1976.

24. Bush, C.A., Stang, J.M., Wooley, C.F. and Kilman, J.W. Occult constrictive pericardial disease. Diagnosis by rapid volume expansion and correction by pericardiectomy. Circulation 56:924-30, 1977.

25. Brockenbrough, E.C., Braunwald, E., Morrow, A.G.: A hemodynamic technique for the detection of hypertrophic subaortic stenosis. Circulation 23:189-94, 1961.

26. Schoenfeld, M.H., Palacios, I.F., Hutter, A.M., Jacoby, S.S., and Block, P.C. Underestimation of prosthetic mitral valve area: Role of transseptal catheterization in avoiding unnecessary repeat mitral valve surgery. J. Am. Coll. Cardiol. 5:1387-92, 1985.

27. Van Slyke, D.D. and Neill, J.M. Blood gasses I. J. Biol. Chem. 61:524-84, 1942.

28. Rudolph, A.M. Cardiac catheterization and angiography. In Congenital Diseases of the Heart. Chicago: Year Book, 1974.

29. Jarmakani, J.M. Catheterization and Angiocardiography, and Heart Disease in Infants, Children, and Adolescents. Baltimore: Williams & Wilkins, 1983.

30. Rowe, R.D. Cardiac catheterization. In Heart Disease in Infancy and Childhood. New York: Macmillan, 1978.

31. Rudolph, A.M., and Cayler, G.C. Cardiac catheterization in infants and children. Pediatr. Clin. North Am. 5:907-43, 1958.

32. Freed, M.D., Miettinen, O., Nadas, A.S. Oximetric detection of intracardiac left-to-right shunts. Br. Heart J. 42:690-94, 1979.

33. Rudolph, A.M. Distribution and regulation of blood flow in the fetal and neonatal lamb. Circ. Res. 57:811-21, 1985.

34. Barratt-Boyes, B.G. and Wood, E.H. The oxygen saturation of blood in the venae cavae, right-heart chambers, and pulmonary vessels of healthy subjects. J. Lab. Clin. Med. 50:93-06, 1057.

35. Dexter, L., Haynes, F.W., Burwell, L.S., Eppinger, E.C., Sagerson, R.P. and Evans, J.M. Studies of congenital heart disease II. The pressure and oxygen content of blood in the right auricle, right ventricle, and pulmonary artery in control patients, with observations on the oxygen saturation and source of pulmonary "capillary" blood. J. Clin. Invest. 26:554-60, 1947.

36. Fuhrman, B.P., Pokora, T.J., Bessinger, F.B., Jr. and Lucas, R.V., Jr. Hypercarbia in the infant with congenital cardiac disease. Pediatr. Cardiol. 2:245-50, 1982.

37. Stewart, G.N. Researches on the circulation time and on the influences which affect it. IV: The output of the heart. J. Physiol.22:159-83, 1987.

38. Kinsman, J.M., Moore, J.W., Hamilton, W.F. Studies on the circulation. I: Injection method. Physical and mathematical considerations. Am. J. Physiol. 89:322-39, 1929.

39. Hatle, L. and Angelson, B., Doppler Ultrasound in Cardiology. Philadelphia: Lea & Febiger, 1985.

40. Kolin, A. A new approach to electromagnetic blood flow determination by means of catheter in an external magnetic field. Proc. Soc. Nat. Acad. Sci. 65:521-27, 1970.

41. Fick, A. Uber die Messung des Blutquantums in den Herzventrikeln. Sits der Physik-Med ges Wurtzberg, 1870, p.16.

42. Van Slyke, D.D. and Neill, J.M. The determination of gases in blood and other solutions by vacuum extraction and manometric measurement. J. Biol. Chem. 61:523-84, 1924.

43. Scholander, P.F. Analyzer for accurate estimation of respiratory gases in one half cubic centimeter samples. J. Biol. Chem. 167: 235-50, 1947.

44. Lister, G., Hoffman, J.I.E. and Rudolph, A.M. Oxygen uptake in infants and children: A simple method for measurement. Pediatrics 53: 656-62, 1974.

45. Vaughan III, V.C.: Growth and Development in Nelson, Textbook of Pediatrics: Philadelphia W.B. Saunders pg. 37, 1975.

46. LaFarge, C.G. and Miettinen, O.S. The estimation of oxygen consumption. Cardiovasc. Res. 4:23-30, 1970.

47. Kappagoda, C.T., Greenwood, P., Macartney, F.J. and Linden, R.J. Oxygen consumption in children with congenital disease of the heart. Clin. Sci. Mol. Med. 45:107-14, 1973.

48. Baum, D., Brown, A.C., Church, S.C. Effect of sedation on oxygen consumption of children undergoing cardiac catheterization. Pediatrics 39: 891-95, 1967.

49. Wessel, H.U., Paul, M.H., James, G.W. and Grahn, A.R. Limitations of thermal dilution curves for cardiac output determinations. J. Appl. Physiol. 30:643-52, 1971.

50. Freed, M.D. and Keane, J.F. Cardiac output measured by thermodilution in infants and children. J. Pediatr. 92:39-42, 1978.

51. Fox, I.J. and Wood, E.H. Indocyanine green: Physical and physiological properties. Proc. Mayo Clin. 35:732-44, 1960.

52. Vogel, J.H.K., Grover, R.F. and Blount, S.G. Jr. Detection of the small intracardiac shunt with the hydrogen electrode. A highly sensitive and simple technique. Am. Heart J. 64:13-21, 1962.

53. Amplatz, K., Jeffrey, R.E., Gobel, F.L., Wang, Y., Gathman, G.E., Moller, J.H. and Lucas, R.V. Jr. The freon test: A new sensitive test for the detection of small cardiac shunts. Circulation 39:551-56, 1969.

54. Frommer, P.L., Pfaff, W.W. and Braunwald, E. The use of ascorbate dilution curves in cardiovascular diagnosis. Application of a technique for direct intravascular detection of indicator. Circulation 24: 1227-34, 1961.

55. Bloomfield, D.A. Dye Curves. Baltimore: University Park Press, 1974.

56. Heymann, M.D., Payne, B.D., Hoffman, J.I.E. and Rudolph, A.M. Blood flow measurements with radionuclide-labelled particles. Prog. Cardiovasc. Dis. 20:55-79, 1977.

57. Einzig. S., Nicoloff, D.M. and Lucas, R.V., Jr. Myocardial perfusion abnormalities in carbon monoxide poisoned dog. Can. J. Physiol. Pharmacol. 58:396-405, 1980.

58. Carter, S.A., Bajec, S.F., Yannicelli, E. and Wood, E.H. Estimation of left to right shunts from arterial dilution curves. J. Lab. Clin. Med. 55:77-88, 1960.

59. Victoria, B.E. and Gessner, I.H. A simplified method for quantitating left to right shunts from arterial dilution curves. Circulation 51:530-34, 1975.

60. Thorburn, G.D. Estimates of cardiac output from forward part of indicator dilution curves. J. Appl. Physiol. 16:891-95, 1961.

61. Kulik, T.J. and Lock, J.E. The assessment of pulmonary vascular tone: A review of experimental methodologies. Pediatr. Pharmacol. 4:73-83, 1984.

62. Gorlin, R. and Gorlin, G. Hydraulic formula for calculation of area of stenotic mitral valves, other valves, and central circulatory shunts. Am. Heart J. 41:1-29, 1951.

63. Bache, R.J., Wang, Y. and Jorgeson, C.R. Hemodynamic effects of exercise in isolated valvular aortic stenosis. Circulation 44: 1003-13, 1971.

4. ANGIOGRAPHY OF CONGENITAL HEART DISEASE

Taylor Chung, M.D.
Patricia E. Burrows, M.D.

BASIC ROENTGENOLOGY
Comprehensive review of physical principles of roentgenology is beyond the scope
of this chapter [1-3]. The following is a brief introduction to the basic principles on
roentgenology for the cardiologists who perform catheterizations and
interventional procedures.
X-ray in the Catheterization Lab
Basic physics and fundamental x-ray image characteristics
X-ray photons are generated from an x-ray tube (Fig. 4-1), a glass vacuum tube
containing a cathode (negative terminal) and an anode (positive terminal). An
electric current passes through a tungsten filament coil (cathode) and heats it, such
that electrons are 'boiled off' the filament (thermionic emission). These electrons
are accelerated towards the anode within the tube by the application of a large
electrical voltage, measured in kilo-volts peak (kVp), across the cathode and the
anode. This stream of electrons is the tube current, measured in milliAmperes
(mA). The kinetic energy of these high-velocity electrons, after striking the
spinning tungsten disc (anode), are transformed mostly to heat energy and a few x-
ray photons. The actual area of electron impact on the tungsten target is called the
focal spot of the x-ray tube (Fig. 4-1). This anode disc spins, yielding a greater
surface area and allows x-rays to be generated more rapidly without damage to the
surface of the disc from excessive temperature.

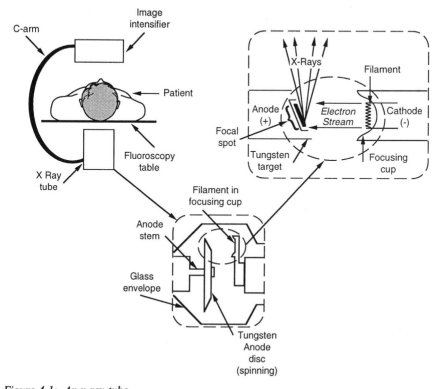

Figure 4-1: An x-ray tube.

74

The energy carried by each x-ray photon depends on the applied voltage (kVp) while the rate of x-ray production depends on the tube current (mA). The total number of x-rays per pulse of radiation (mAs) is the product of the current (mA) and the duration of the pulse of x-ray in seconds(s). Since an angiogram of the thoracic aorta, for example, is effectively a 'map' of the varying degrees of attenuation of the x-ray photons by the different tissues of the chest (skin, fat, muscle, bone, lung tissue with air, etc.) and the iodine of the contrast agent in the aorta, the quality of the image is directly related to the mAs and the kVp settings of the x-ray tube, and the size of the focal spot. The ability of each constituent of the body part to attenuate the x-ray photons is a function of its atomic number, density, and thickness, and the energy of the x-ray photons.

Density, contrast, noise, quantum mottle, temporal and spatial resolution (blurring) are the terms that describe image quality. Density is the degree of blackening of the cine image on film; the analogy on the fluoroscopy monitor is the brightness. For a given kVp, density or brightness is determined by the mAs used per pulse of radiation to form the image. Contrast refers to the variation of density between different tissue constituents within the image. In general, contrast is improved by reducing the kVp and increasing the mAs; this reduces the energy carried by each x-ray photon and increases the radiation dose to the patient.

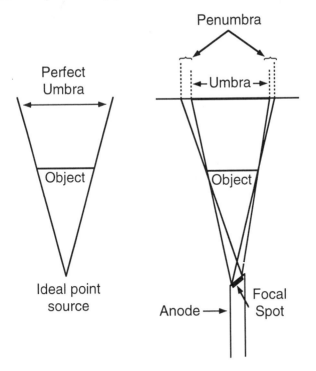

Figure 4-2: Geometric blurring from a finite size focal spot. Umbra = shadow. Penumbra = region of partial illumination surrounding the umbra or the geometric unsharpness.

Quantum mottle (sometimes referred to as noise) is the point-to-point random variation in density or brightness oF the image due to the limited number of photons exiting the patient to form the image. Quantum mottle can only be reduced by increasing the mAs to the patient. Temporal resolution refers to the blurring in the image due to motion of objects during the exposure pulse. Spatial resolution refers to the degree of unsharpness in the edges of stationary objects due to the finite size of the focal spot (Fig. 4-2). Thus, blurring can be minimized by smaller focal spots and shorter exposure pulses.

Image quality can, therefore, be manipulated by varying the technical parameters: kVp, mAs, and focal spot size of the x-ray tube. For different patient size and different projections through the same patient, the thickness and the types of tissue the x-ray photons need to penetrate will be different (e.g. lateral view of the upper mediastinum will require the photons to penetrate much more bony tissue than a frontal view given the location of the humeri). These parameters need to be adjusted to obtain the optimal image quality.

The interplay between image quality parameters and technical parameters for cineangiography is discussed in great detail by Moore [3]. For example, compare a frontal projection with no angulation to a double-oblique 4-chamber projection. To obtain similar density, the 4-chamber view will require more energetic photons in order to penetrate the thicker body part. Therefore, higher kVp is needed. However, as the more energetic photons can penetrate thicker body part, the difference in density between various portions of the image is less and the overall image contrast suffers. As an alternative to increasing the kVp, the mAs could be increased which will create more photons per pulse of radiation due to higher tube current and/or longer exposure pulse. This will result in more darkening of the image even though the penetrating power of each of the photons remains unchanged (the kVp is constant). Hence, one can balance the increase of kVp and mAs to achieve optimal density and maintain adequate image contrast in the 4-chamber view <u>assuming the object can be stationary during the exposure</u>.

Now consider blurring and focal spot size. As discussed, blurring can come from gross object motion (such as the normal physiologic motion of the cardiac chambers and vessels) or from magnification secondary to a finite focal spot source of x-ray photons rather than a true point source (Fig. 4-2). To decrease geometric blurring, one would always want to use the smallest focal spot size. However, due to thermal limits on the tungsten anode of the x-ray tube, a small focal spot cannot generate as many photons per unit time as a large focal spot. Thus, for a given density and contrast requirement, it takes a longer exposure time to obtain an image such that physiologic motion causes unsharpness. Hence, a trade-off between temporal and spatial resolution always exists due to the choice of focal spot size when imaging objects that are not stationary.

Consider again the previous example of the 4-chamber view. In order to retain tissue contrast, one should increase the mAs rather than the kVp. However, because of physiologic motion blurring as discussed above, there is a limit to the duration of the exposure pulse and there is always a maximum mA for a certain focal spot size. We may need to switch to a larger focal spot which will decrease the spatial sharpness of the resultant image as the lack of temporal sharpness is dominating overall image quality. As one can see, optimization of various technical parameters and the trade-offs is essential to acquiring a high quality, diagnostic cineangiogram.

Hardware

Most modern labs have the x-ray tube mounted on a single plane C-arm or 2 C-arms in a bi-plane design. For a frontal (PA) projection, the x-ray tube mounted on one end of a C-arm is positioned below the table with the x-ray beam traversing a supine patient from posterior to anterior and collected by the image intensifier (II) tube mounted on the opposite end of the C-arm (Fig. 4-1).

76

The II tube (Fig. 4-3) captures the x-ray pattern in space exiting from the patient and converts it into a light pattern. This light pattern is amplified within the II resulting in a bright enough image to be seen by human photopic (daylight) vision with reasonable radiation doses to the patient. This amplified light output can be directed through an optic lens to a television camera for fluoroscopic monitoring or to a cine camera for cineangiography (recording onto 35 mm cine film) (Fig. 4-3). During a "cine run", 10 to 20% of the II output is directed through the image distributor to the TV port allowing for simultaneous monitoring of the cine run. In a "filmless cine" system, the light output of the II tube is coupled to a high-quality video display unit (VDU). The analog video output of the VDU is then amplified and converted to a digital signal through an analog-to-digital (A/D) converter. This is the fluoroscopic image to be recorded in a digital format that can be stored, and replayed with or without image-enhancing post-processing.

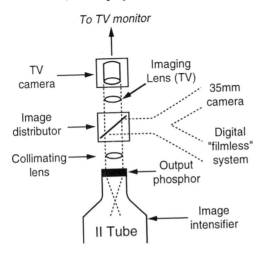

Figure 4-3: The image intensifier tube captures the x-rays that passed through the patient, converts and amplifies them to light which is then directed to TV monitors and camera for 35mm cine film recording, or coupled to video display unit (VDU) for digital filmless system.

Performing cardiac angiography without cine film had been equated to erecting a "tower of Babel" in the cardiac catheterization laboratory [4]. However, with advancement in technology, the "filmless" catheterization laboratory is now a reality. Although digital angiography systems in diagnostic radiology departments have been the norm for many years, the requirements for a digital cineangiographic system have only been developed in recent years.

In 1994, an ad hoc committee, with representation from the American College of Cardiology (ACC), the American College of Radiology (ACR), and the National Electrical Manufacturers Association (NEMA), defined the requirements for Basic Cardiac X-ray Angiographic Studies. This work was built on existing standards of digital imaging and communications in medicine (DICOM) by ACR-NEMA known in the industry as DICOM version 3.0. Each frame of a cineangiogram study requires a 512 x 512 spatial resolution. The gray-scale of each element (pixel) of this 512 x 512 matrix is represented by 8 bits (1 byte) allowing for $2^8 = 256$ steps of gray-scale. Thus, each frame requires 262,144 bytes or a quarter of 1 Megabyte (MB). The Ad hoc committee determined that the maximum number of frames per study is slightly below 4,800 (99 th percentile) with an average of 2,200 frames. Digital storage medium needs a capacity of 1,200 MB or 1.2 Gigabytes (GB) without the aid of data compression. This is roughly equivalent to storing 5 months of a daily newspaper [5].

Data transmission is a significant issue. As an aside, a potentially confusing technical aspect for the readers is the units used for data transmission rate. Megabits per second (Mbps) is used in reference to transmission rate across a network. Megabytes per second (MBps) is used in reference to data transfer rate within a computer system. The standard 30 frames per second (fps) of conventional cineangiograms translates to data rate of 7.5 MBps or 60 Mbps. Due to overhead, actual network rates never achieve the specified rate so that real-time streaming rates of 100 Mbps without data compression are estimated [6]. For comparison, commercially available modem on an analog telephone line in 1998 has a data rate of 0.0288 Mbps. With high-speed wide bandwidth network, streaming rates of up to 45 Mbps can be achieved on point-to-point digital service lines (DS-3 lines) [6]. Data compression, either reversible (lossless) or nonreversible (lossy), is needed. Currently, 2:1 lossless compression is possible and accepted within the DICOM 3.0 standard. The standards for clinically acceptable maximal compression rate has yet to be determined.

The Basic Cardiac X-ray Angiographic Studies currently accept a minimum data rate of 1 MBps or 8 Mbps which is approximately a quarter of the real-time acquisition rate of 30 fps with 2:1 compression. Although real-time transmission of cine runs is not yet practical, the cineangiograms can be stored into an on-line digital storage system, RAID (Redundant Array of Independent Discs), capable of handling 100 - 200 studies (with reversible compression algorithm) without manual intervention by a human operator. A study can be retrieved from the RAID in seconds onto a display monitor system (workstation), allowing the cineangiograms to be viewed in 'real-time' speed. In addition, another digital storage device called a jukebox which contains multiple optical discs or magnetic tapes, can be used for long-term archive. Typically, each study stored on the RAID is also simultaneously stored in the jukebox in the background. These jukeboxes are capable of storing 1,500 to 2,000 studies (with reversible compression algorithm) without manual intervention by a human operator. When all the discs in the jukebox are full, they will need to be manually stored and replaced with blank discs. In order to review an old study on the jukebox but not on the RAID, it typically takes 10 to 20 minutes to transfer an average length study from the jukebox to the RAID. Most advanced systems also have databases, departmental information systems, and even hospital information systems linked with the display system thus allowing comprehensive review of all forms of data on each patient and reporting of the cineangiogram.

The standard exchange medium for 30 years has been the 35-mm cineangiographic film. The chosen medium for the Basic Cardiac X-ray Angiographic Studies application is the compact disk recordable (CD-R). This medium, demonstrated at the 1995 ACC conference, showed that studies can be successfully retrieved by systems from different vendors for display. Current CD-R technology can allow storage of 650 MB per disk. This capacity can accommodate the requirement of single storage unit per patient-study similar to cineangiogram films. It is estimated that 35 mm film (including processing and storage) costs approximately $100 per patient-study compared with $12 for CD-R [5].

Radiation Safety

The radiation exposure to both patient and personnel from diagnostic and interventional procedures in a cardiac catheterization laboratory exceeds the exposure of all other forms of diagnostic imaging. It is, therefore, of utmost importance for all personnel involved, especially the cardiologist performing the catheterization, to understand the risk of radiation and to limit the radiation level to as low as reasonably achievable (ALARA concept) [7, 8].

There are three radiation units commonly used: the Roentgen (R), the radiation absorbed dose (rad), and the "rad equivalent man" (rem). By definition, the Roentgen is a unit of exposure, quantifying the amount of energy of the x-ray produced by measuring the amount of ionization of air caused by the x-ray. One R is defined as the amount of x-ray needed to ionize a cubic centimeter of air (pressure = 1 atmosphere, temperature = 0^0C) into 2.08 billion ion pairs or 2.58 x 10^{-14} coulombs/kg of air. The rad and the rem are measurements of the amount of energy absorbed or the dose, not exposure. When an x-ray photon is attenuated or absorbed in the patient's tissue, some or all of the energy is 'unloaded' into the tissue. For x-ray radiation, a rad is equivalent to a rem which is not the case for other types of radiation. The rem is used in many state and federal radiation control regulations to specify the maximum permissible doses (MPD) for radiation workers. Table 4-1 lists the current MPDs summarized from the recommendation by the National Council on Radiation protection and Measurement (NCRP) [9]. Cardiologists and cath lab personnel including anesthesiologists, nurses, and technologists are all radiation workers. Radiation workers must be monitored by film badges which are calibrated to estimate the occupational radiation dose received by the worker from the degree of blackening on the piece film in the worker's film badge.

TABLE 4-1

Summary of Recommendations for Annual Maximum Permissible Dose*

| | Dose | |
	mSv	Rem
Total body	50	5
Lens of eye	150	15
All other individual organs (e.g., red marrow, breast, lung, gonads, skin, extremities)	500	50
Embryo-fetus exposure	5	0.5

*Modified from ref [9].

The relationship between R and rad (f factor), depends on the previously discussed characteristics of the tissue irradiated, i.e. atomic number, thickness, density, and on the energy of the x-ray photons. For example, soft tissue has an f factor between exposure in R to absorbed dose in rad of 0.9 compared with bone having an f factor of 4.0. In 1985, new international, SI, units were developed to replace the rad and rem as follows: 100 rad = 1 Gray (Gy); 100 rem = 1 Sievert (Sv).

Radiation injuries can be either deterministic or stochastic in nature. Deterministic radiation injuries (tissue injury, cataract production) occur when a number of cells are involved; a threshold dose is required and the severity of the injury is proportional to the dose above the threshold. Stochastic radiation injuries (genetic effects and carcinogenesis) are believed to be caused by injury to a single cell. Typically, a threshold dose is not required. The probability of an injury is proportional to the dose, but the severity is independent of the dose.

For cataract induction, a threshold of about 250 rem has been defined as the dose at which diffuse lens opacities begin to form [10]. If radiation workers adhere to ALARA guidelines which require occupational dose to be below the MPD values whenever possible and one assumes cardiologists receive 5 rem per year over their professional career, it would take a minimum of 50 years to reach the threshold dose. With protective lead glasses and appropriate side shields, the dose to the lens can be further reduced.

For genetic effects, the estimated doubling dose for radiation-induced mutations is approximately 100 rem [8]. The protective lead apron (a minimum of 0.5 mm lead equivalent) which must be worn by all personnel in the cath lab attenuates at least 90% of the potential occupational exposure due to stray radiation. Since the MPD for the whole body including the gonads is 5 rem per year, all personnel should receive less than 0.5 rem of occupational dose annually to his/her gonads underneath the protective apron. Thus, the genetic risk, especially during the child bearing years, is quite low.

For carcinogenesis, the estimate for cancer deaths in low exposure (tens of rad) has to be extrapolated from high-exposure data (hundreds of rad). There is no direct evidence that low-dose background radiation, which everyone is subjected to, causes malignant diseases. In the United States, the average natural background radiation at sea level is equivalent to a whole-body dose of about 0.3 rem per year. Thus, a radiation worker in the cath lab would need to receive 2 to 3 rem on their film badges worn outside of the protective apron to result in an whole-body occupational dose equivalent to background radiation. If one assumes that naturally occurring low-dose radiation causes death by cancer with a risk of 1 in 10 million, this has been estimated to be equivalent to the risk of death by riding an automobile for 1,000 miles, or smoking 30 cigarettes, or 3 cross-country return flights on a commercial airline [3].

Nonetheless, a cineangiography study easily delivers the highest radiation exposure to the patient amongst various diagnostic studies [7, 8, 10, 11]. It has been estimated from dose measurement and calculations performed in the department of Radiology and at the cardiac catheterization lab at Children's Hospital, Boston, that 10 minutes of continuous fluoroscopy and 1 minute of cine run time at 30 fps is equivalent to approximately 1000 frontal and lateral chest films! With the advent of complex interventional procedures which may involve over 100 minutes of fluoroscopy and multiple minutes of cineangiogram, patient entrance skin doses in hundreds of rads are not uncommon. This problem is compounded if the x-ray unit produces excessive rates of radiation exposure [12]. In addition to the stochastic risks discussed above, deterministic skin damage must be monitored and avoided. Transient skin erythema, and permanent skin erythema have threshold doses as little as 2 and 6 Gy [13]. Temporary and permanent epilation has been reported at 3 to 7 Gy [13]. More serious skin damage such as dry or moist desquamation, dermal necrosis, or atrophy occur at threshold doses starting at 10 Gy [13]. Hence, the cardiologist must protect the patient and all the personnel in the lab. The following is a list of highly recommended methods to reduce radiation risk for both patient and lab personnel according to the ALARA concept.

1. Keep fluoroscopic and cineangiographic times as short as possible. Do not activate fluoroscopy unless full attention is devoted to the fluoroscopy monitor. The II tubes and collimator blades should be positioned while fluoroscopy is off and only turned on when necessary to check position. Biplane fluoroscopy is seldom needed. With current fluoroscopic technology, one can make use of last-image-hold to check catheter position with short burst of fluoroscopy time. The angiographer's hands should never be within the primary x-ray beam.

2. Use the smallest possible radiation dose to achieve adequate image contrast and spatial resolution needed during fluoroscopy. The x-ray tube parameters need to be matched by technologists to the size of the patient and the projection. The image intensifier should always be as close to the patient as possible to minimize scattered radiation and dose. Collimators should be used at all times, in both fluoroscopy and cineangiography, to minimize the volume of tissue irradiated. Also, variable-rate pulsed-fluoroscopy as opposed to continuous fluoroscopy is now widely available through many manufacturers. A reduction of the pulse rate from 30 frames per second to 7.5 frames per second can be accompanied by a reduction of patient entrance exposure by a factor of 2 with no difference in the noise perceived in the image [14, 15]. In addition, radiation dose to the lab personnel is reduced by 35% [16].

3. Plan ahead and acquire the least numbers of cine runs to obtain the maximum amount of information. Remember that one minute of cine run is equivalent to 10 minutes of continuous fluoroscopy in terms of radiation exposure for the patient and cath lab personnel.

4. During a cine run, all personnel, if possible, should leave the laboratory area; all remaining personnel should be behind leaded shields and away from the table. Radiation obeys the "inverse-square law": the radiation dose decreases as a square of the distance from the source.

5. All personnel must wear lead aprons in the cath lab. Wrap-around aprons are preferred. Leaded thyroid shields and eyeglasses are highly recommended. An x-ray shield made of leaded glass or acrylic should be available suspended from the ceiling to protect the angiographer's head and neck. It is the responsibility of the cardiologist performing the catheterization to confirm that all personnel have protective aprons on prior to the start of the study.

6. It is mandatory that all personnel wear their film badges properly near the level of the thyroid gland, outside the apron at all times while in the cath lab and keep a monthly record of their cumulative doses. There needs to be a radiation safety officer in the department/institution to oversee the periodic monitoring of all radiation workers' doses. Also, refresher radiation safety courses on an annual basis are recommended. An active maintenance program must be in place for all x-ray equipment to insure optimum image quality at the least possible radiation dose to patient and cath lab personnel [7].

Contrast Agents

This discussion is limited to iodine-based intravascular contrast material. All currently available water soluble contrast agents are based on a tri-iodinated benzoic acid derivatives [17] (Fig. 4-4).

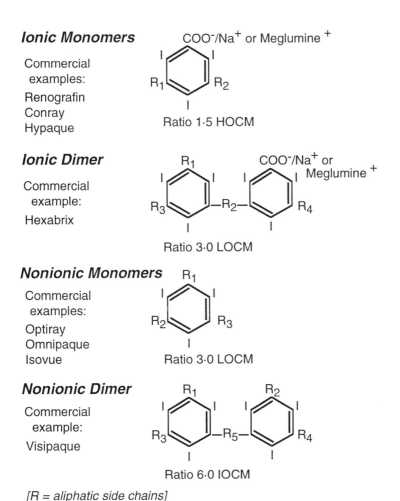

Ionic Monomers

Commercial examples:
Renografin
Conray
Hypaque

Ionic Dimer

Commercial example:
Hexabrix

Nonionic Monomers

Commercial examples:
Optiray
Omnipaque
Isovue

Nonionic Dimer

Commercial example:
Visipaque

[R = aliphatic side chains]

Figure 4-4: Basic chemical structures of water soluble iodinated contrast agents. HOCM = high osmolality contrast medium; LOCM = low osmolality contrast medium; IOCM = isotonic contrast medium; ratio = number of iodine atoms on one contrast molecule : number of particles in solution from one contrast molecule. R = aliphatic side chains. I = iodine.

Their basic chemical structure is that of a benzene ring with 3 iodine atoms in the 1, 3, 5-positions. Single ring structures are called monomers; double ring structures are dimers. They can be classified as high-osmolality contrast media (HOCM), low-osmolality contrast media (LOCM), and most recently, isotonic contrast media (IOCM) [18, 19]; or ionic versus nonionic contrast media. Most LOCM are nonionic compounds with the exception of Ioxaglate (Table 4-2).

82

TABLE 4-2   Comparison of Conventional Contrast Agents[a]

Generic Name	Trade Name	Iodine (mg/ml)	Osmolality (mOsm/kg)	Viscosity (cp) 25⁰C	37⁰C
Ionic Monomers (HOCM[b])					
Diatrizoate Sodium 8% Meglumine 52%	Renografin-60	292.5	1420	5.9	4.0
Diatrizote meglumine	Reno-M-60	282	1500	4.6	4.0
Diatrizote sodium	Hypague 50%	300	1550	3.43	2.43
Diatrizote meglumine	Hypague 60%	282	1415	6.16	4.10
Diatrizote Sodium 10% Meglumine 66%	Renografin-76	370	1940	13.8	8.4
Diatrizote Sodium 25% Meglumine 50%	Hypague-M 75%	385	2108	12.69	7.99
Iothalamate sodium	Conray-400	400	2300	7.0	4.5
Ionic Dimer (LOCM[c])					
Ioxaglate Sodium 19.6% Meglumine 39.3%	Hexabrix	320	600	15.7	7.5
Nonionic Monomers (LOCM[c])					
Ioversol	Optiray 350	350	792	14.3	9.0
	Optiray 320	320	702	9.9	5.8
	Optiray 240	240	502	4.6	3.0
Iopamidol	Isovue 370	370	796	20.9	9.4
	Isovue 300	300	616	8.8	4.7
	Isovue 200	200	413	2.0	3.3
Iohexol	Omnipaque	350	862	18.5	11.15
	Omnipaque	300	709	10.35	6.77
	Omnipaque	240	504	4.43	3.08
Nonionic Dimers (IOCM[d])					
Iodixanol	Visipague	320	290	26.6	11.8

a   Modified from H.W. Fischer [20].
b   HOCM is High Osmolality Contrast Media.
c   LOCM is Low Osmolality Contrast Media.
d   IOCM is Isotonic Contrast Media.

All HOCM are ionic compounds which are either sodium or meglumine salts of diatrozoic acid. They disassociate in solution to two particles, a cation and an anion. Therefore, for every three iodine atoms, there are 2 particles in solution representing a ratio 1.5 contrast media [20]. Since osmolality is defined as the concentration of dissolved solute per unit of solvent, these agents are significantly hyperosmolar, 5 to 8 times higher, with respect to serum osmolality (280 mOsm/kg). The osmolality is important as many of the adverse effects from iodinated contrast agents are thought to be secondary to hyperosmolality. The iodine to particle ratio for ionic dimer, Ioxaglate, and the nonionic monomers are 3.0 [20] and therefore are lower in osmolality, although still higher than serum osmolality. The newest class of contrast agents, non-ionic dimers, is slightly hypotonic to the serum with an iodine to particle ratio of 6. The commercial product of non-ionic dimer, iodixanol, is isotonic to blood with the addition of sodium chloride and calcium chloride [21]. The viscosity is high (Table 2) such that iodixanol has been used in adult cardioangiography studies only in 320 mg of Iodine/ml concentration and warmed to 37°C for the ease of injection through catheters [21].

Reactions to contrast media can be classified as nonidiosyncratic or idiosyncratic [22]. Nonidiosyncratic reactions are related to the physical and chemical properties of the media such as hyperosmolality and chemtoxicity of the molecule. Hemodynamic effects such as vasodilation resulting in flushing and hypotension, cardiac arrythymias and bradycardia, cardiac ischemia, negative inotropic effect, pulmonary hypertension with vasospasm, pulmonary edema, acute renal dysfunction, nausea and vomiting are all examples of nonidiosyncratic reactions.

Idiosyncratic reactions are "anaphylactoid" or "allergic-like" reactions, but not true hypersensitivity reactions. These reactions do not uniformly recur and antibodies to contrast agent are not well characterized [22]. The exact mechanism of these reactions is not yet understood and may be multifactorial involving nonimmunological release of vasoactive substances, activation of complement system, activation of contact system with release of kelikrein and other kinins, or a central nervous system reaction. Hives, urticaria, itching, laryngeal edema, bronchospasm, and circulatory collapse are all examples of idiosyncratic reactions [17]. In acute clinical settings, differentiation between the two classes of reaction may not be possible.

Besides the cardiovascular and pulmonary systems, contrast agents can have an adverse effect on renal function. Adult patients at higher risk are those with underlying renal insufficiency and diabetes mellitus [23]. There are, however, limited data on the effects of iodinated contrast agents on the pediatric kidney [24]. Hypoperfusion states would likely be an additional risk factor for contrast-induced renal failure in pediatric patients with congenital heart diseases. Contrast is eliminated primarily by glomerular filtration. With contrast induced renal failure, clearance of the iodinated contrast will be markedly delayed such that nephrograms will persist at 24-hour follow-up and vicarious excretion of contrast through the biliary system will occur.

At our institution, nonionic contrast agents have been in routine use since the late 1980's. Although there are no large studies comparing the use of HOCM vs LOCM in pediatric cardiac catheterizations, many studies in the adult literature documented fewer hemodynamic and electrophysiologic changes with LOCM [25, 26]. Adverse reactions, including idiosyncratic reactions from the use of LOCM both at cardiac catheterization and with intravenous administration, are fewer than with HOCM in both adult [27] and pediatric patients [24]. In two of the largest comparison studies [28, 29], the overall adverse reaction rates for HOCM ranged from 3.8 to 12.8%, and severe reaction rates of 0.09 to 0.22% compared to rates for LOCM of 1.2 to 3.1% and 0.02 to 0.04% respectively. In Palmer's study, two deaths occurred in the ionic group (79,278 patients). In Katayama's study, there was one death in each group (169,284 patients in ionic group vs. 168,363 patients in the nonionic group). Although there are no similiar large comparison studies available for children, the frequency of serious reactions is likely no higher. Initial clinical results in adult patients with the use of IOCM have been encouraging [19, 21], although there are limited data published with pediatric patients. The high viscosity of IOCM may be an issue with smaller catheter sizes used in pediatric cases.

In the cardiac catheterization lab at Children's Hospital, Boston, LOCM with concentration of 350 mg of iodine per milliliter is used in conventional cineangiograms. The concentration can decrease to 240 mg of iodine per milliliter if digital subtraction technique is used. The contrast media ought to be kept in a warmer close to body temperature prior to injection in order to decrease its viscosity and improve the flow rate through catheters. Although the upper limits for contrast toxicity have not, to our knowledge, been established, our upper limits when using LOCM with 320 mg to 350 mg of iodine per milliliter is 4 to 6 milliliter/kilogram body weight. However, if the patient has normal renal function, with stable hemodynamics, and has good urine output, in a long catheterization case, higher amounts of contrast have been used without adverse outcome.

GENERAL ANGIOGRAPHY GUIDELINES IN CONGENITAL HEART DISEASE

The role of angiocardiography has evolved significantly in recent decades, influenced by advances in noninvasive imaging, such as echocardiography, radionuclide angiocardiography and magnetic resonance imaging and magnetic resonance angiography (Chapter 1). In order to minimize radiation exposure and contrast load, each cardiac catheterization should be carefully planned in advance, utilizing appropriate catheter selection, catheter placement, quantity and rate of contrast injection and angiographic projection.

Important characteristics to consider prior to catheter selection include French size and length, catheter composition, position and number of injection holes, shape, and presence or absence of balloon tip. Catheter selection is also influenced by the route and degree of difficulty of catheter placement into the site to be injected, the size of the patient, and the flow rate required. Torque catheters tend to be shaped, thick-walled catheters which incorporate a stainless steel braided layer. The wall stiffness imparts torquability. Some uses of these catheters are transvenous placement into the pulmonary artery, across ventricular septal defects, and retrogradely into coronary arteries. Disadvantages include stiffness, which can result in an increased incidence of cardiac perforation or stain, and small internal diameter, which limits contrast flow rates. Thin-walled catheters have less torquability, but are more flexible, track along guidewires more readily, and deliver high contrast flow rates. Endhole catheters are useful for selective, relatively small volume injections by hand, such as into coronary arteries, aortopulmonary collaterals, and other small or medium-sized arteries. Rapid, high volume injection through endhole catheters is undesirable, as associated catheter whip often results in displacement of the catheter tip, and wedging into the myocardium or an arterial branch, possibly resulting in perforation or stain. Contrast injections into cardiac chambers, main pulmonary trunk or aorta should be made through a multi-side-hole catheter. Multiple side holes facilitate high contrast flow rates, high velocity of injection and minimal catheter whip.

Catheter Selection

Characteristics of catheters commonly used in pediatric angiocardiography are described in Table 4-3.

When choosing a pigtail catheter, the position of the side holes should be noted. The side holes may be placed either within the loop of the pigtail, or in the straight shaft of the catheter just proximal to beyond the pigtail loop. Side holes within the catheter loop allow precise contrast placement in small infants. Double lumen balloon-tipped catheters when the balloon is inflated with carbon dioxide allow for flow directed catheter placement, such as for ventriculography or pulmonary angiography.

They are also useful for balloon occlusion angiography, to elucidate systemic venous anatomy or, with balloon occlusion of the neonatal aorta, to evaluate anatomy of the coronary arteries or aortopulmonary collaterals. End-hole balloon-tipped catheters can be used for wedge angiography, forcing contrast through a capillary bed to opacify the vessel on the other side.

Taper of the catheter tip is important. Catheters inserted into the femoral artery or vein directly over a guidewire (rather than through an introducer sheath) must be tapered to the size of the guidewire, in order to minimize vascular trauma.
Maximum contrast flow rates are related to catheter internal diameter, the number and size of side holes, and catheter length, as well as the viscosity of the contrast medium. As a general rule, in order to minimize access vessel trauma, the smallest French size which will accomplish the necessary contrast flow rate should be selected for small patients. In order to maximize contrast flow rate, the shortest useful catheter length should be chosen. For example, left ventriculography and aortography can be performed in neonates using a 3 French, 40 cm long pigtail catheter introduced into the femoral artery over a guidewire.
The use of cut-off pigtail catheters with intraluminal guidewires during interventional procedures is an innovative technique which facilitates acquisition of hemodynamic and angiographic data without the risk of losing catheter position or extending vascular tears after balloon dilation angioplasty [30]. In this technique, the looped portion of a pigtail catheter is cut off and advanced over a guide wire. The side holes are placed across the area of interest. A Y-connector is attached to the catheter, the valve is closed tightly over the wire, and the side arm is connected to the high pressure tubing of an injector pump. The side arm can also be used for obtaining hemodynamic measurements.

86

TABLE 4-3 Catheter Flow Rates and Volumes

Catheter diameter, length	Flow, volumes at rupture
PIGTAILS, CORDIS	
6F, 100 cm long	24 cc @ 24 cc/sec
7F, 100 cm long	31 cc @ 31 cc/sec
PIGTAILS, U.M.I. (Thinwall)	
3F, 40 cm long	8 cc @ 15 cc/sec; 10 cc @ 13 cc/sec
3F, 50 cm long	6 cc @ 15 cc/sec; 10 cc @ 10 cc/sec
4F, 50 cm long	10 cc@ 20 cc/sec; 15 cc @ 15 cc/sec
4F, 80 cm long	14 cc @ 10 cc/sec
5F, 80 cm long	10cc @ 24 cc/sec; 20 cc @ 20 cc/sec
5F, 100 cm long	18 cc @ 18 cc/sec
6F, 80 cm long	35 cc @ 35 cc/sec
6F, 100 cm long	30 cc @ 30 cc/sec
7F, 100 cm long	40 cc @ 40 cc/sec
PIGTAILS, U.M.I. (Thinwall-Cutoff, with Guidewire in situ)	
5F, 80 cm long, with 0.025 wire	10 ml @ 10 ml/sec
6F	
7F, 100 cm long with 0.035 wire	18 ml @ 20 ml/sec
BERMAN BALLOON ANGIOGRAPHICS, CRITIKON	
4F, 50 cm long	5 cc @ 5 cc/sec
5F, 50 cm long	15 cc @ 15 cc/sec
5F, 80 cm long	12 cc @ 12 cc/sec
6F, 60 cm long	20 cc @ 20 cc/sec
6F, 90 cm long	17 cc @ 17 cc/sec
7F, 60 cm long	22 cc @ 22 cc/sec

Catheter Position
The choice of catheter position must be guided by the type of information desired. The anatomy of any chamber is best delineated when the chamber is filled directly. For example, ventricular septal defects are best evaluated angiographically by left ventricular injection, even if the left ventricle is the lower pressure chamber, because of the smoother surface of the left ventricular side of the septum. Atrioventricular and semilunar valves are best evaluated by echocardiography. Using angiocardiography, the morphology of the cardiac valves is best assessed by upstream contrast injection and appropriate projections. The assessment of atrioventricular valve regurgitation is often imprecise due to the presence of the catheter across the valve, and injection or catheter induced cardiac arrhythmias. Aortic valve insufficiency should be evaluated by retrograde aortic injection, with careful positioning of a multi-side-hole catheter well above the valve commissures.

Imaging of the central pulmonary arteries is best accomplished by injecting in the main pulmonary artery, while intrapulmonary branches should be studied by separate injections in the ipsilateral central pulmonary artery branch. This way, the individual segmental branches are profiled with a combination of frontal and lateral projections.

Balloon occlusion techniques are useful in certain situations. Balloon occlusion to arrest flow during contrast injection permits dense opacification of the desired structures, with a minimal amount of contrast medium [31, 32]. Upstream balloon occlusion is useful for opacification of the peripheral pulmonary arteries and pulmonary veins, as well as to study systemic venous anatomy, such as persistent left superior vena cava, inferior vena caval anomalies and venous collaterals. Downstream balloon occlusion is used, in neonates, to produce dense opacification of coronary arteries, patent ductus arteriosus, aortic arch or aortopulmonary collaterals.

Some catheter positions are known to have a high rate of complications and should be avoided. For example, one can cross the ventricular septum through a septal defect from the right ventricle, and be tempted to perform left ventriculography. The catheter will frequently be directed posteriorly, behind a papillary muscle of the mitral valve, and be partially entrapped. A brisk contrast injection in this position will commonly stain the left ventricle.

After catheter placement, and prior to power injection, it is important to assess the catheter tip position. This can be done by fluoroscopy and a small test injection of contrast medium. The catheter tip should move freely in the cardiac chamber, away from papillary muscles, trabeculations or valve apparatus. Pigtail catheters in the aorta or pulmonary artery should be positioned with the pigtail fully looped, to avoid direct injection into a coronary artery or other small branch.

Contrast Delivery

General guidelines for the quantity and rate of contrast delivery are listed in Table 4-4. In general, for anatomic definition, contrast should be delivered through the catheter as rapidly as possible, generally in one second or less. Normal blood and cardiac volumes are relatively higher in infants than in older children, so angiography in infants requires larger volumes (ml per kg) of contrast medium. The volume of contrast medium injected should be modified according to the size and flow rate of the chamber or vessel being studied. For example, higher volumes and flow rates are required to opacify aortic branches in patients with large aortopulmonary communications than in those without shunts. Likewise, greater intracardiac contrast injections are required in patients with large intracardiac shunts than in patients with ventricular outflow tract obstructions. Smaller injections are sufficient in patients with decreased cardiac output.
Selective contrast injections into peripheral arteries or veins require variable contrast volumes and rates, depending upon the flow characteristics of the vessel.

88

TABLE 4-4

General Guidelines for Contrast Injections in Congenital Heart Disease

Chamber Vessel	Normal Size	Increased Volume normal flow	Marked Increase volume & flow
Aorta	1.0 cc/kg	1.0 cc/kg	1.5 cc/kg
LV	1.0 cc/kg	1.0 cc/kg	1.5 cc/kg
LA	1.0 cc/kg	1.0 cc/kg	1.5 cc/kg
MPA	1.0 cc/kg	1.2 cc/kg	1.5 cc/kg
RV	1.0 cc/kg	1.0 cc/kg	1.5 cc/kg
RA	1.0 cc/kg	1.0 cc/kg	1.5 cc/kg
R, LPA	0.5 cc/kg	1.0 cc/kg	1.0 cc

A high flow rate is much more important than volume.

Selection of Appropriate Angiocardiographic Projections

The septal contours and connections between chambers and great vessels are variable and complex. For optimal angiocardiographic imaging, a thorough

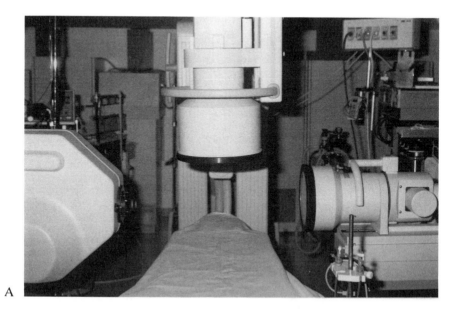

A

Figure 4-5: Image intensifier position for standard projections.
A) frontal and lateral; B) 30º RAO and long-axial oblique; C) 30º RAO and 4-chamber view (hepatoclavicular); D) cranial-angulated frontal (sitting-up) and lateral; E) Caudal-angulated frontal (laid-back aortogram for TGA) and lateral.

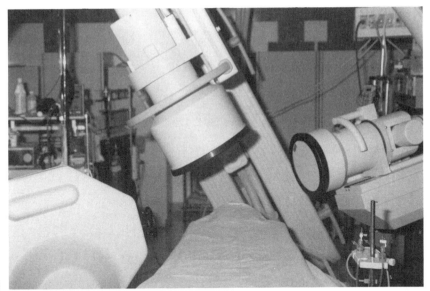

B

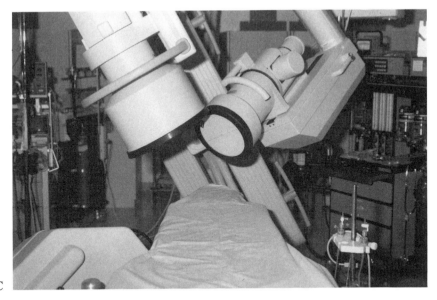

C

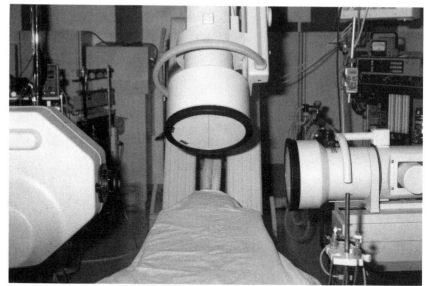

D

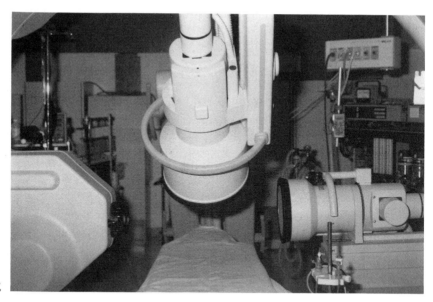

E

knowledge of normal cardiac anatomy, and anatomy of complex congenital cardiac anomalies is necessary. Angiocardiography produces a two-dimensional projection of a three dimensional structure. Ideally, the anatomic structure being evaluated should be profiled by the selected projection. Projections used for angiocardiography include frontal, lateral and right and left oblique projections, without or with the addition of axial (craniocaudal or caudocranial) angulation (Fig. 4-5).

In the past, the use of fixed vertical and horizontal x-ray systems required that oblique and angled projections were achieved by changing the position of the patient on the angiography table, with the risk of awakening the sedated child. Modern cardiac catheterization labs are equipped with biplane C-arms, which facilitate the acquisition of complex projections without changing the position of the patient on the table [33-37]. In general, the child is positioned supine, with the arms extended above the head.

Table 4-5 lists the projections most commonly used to image congenital cardiac defects, with a brief description of the structures profiled and chambers or vessels routinely studied with each view. The following are some generalizations.

TABLE 4-5 Angiographic Projections

Projection	Degrees	Chamber/Vessel	Lesions
Frontal	0^0	RV	TGA, DORV
		PA Branch	PA Stenosis
			Pulmonary Vein Stenosis
			Anomalous Pulmonary Veins
Cranial Frontal;	30^0 Cranial	RV	PS, TOF, DORV
	30^0 Cranial, 15^0 LAO	MPA	PA Stenosis, ASD
Caudal Frontal	450 Caudal	Ascending Aorta	TGA, DORV
RAO	300 RAO	LA	Mitral Stenosis
		LV	Mitral Valve Abnormality Anterior VSD
LAO	60-700 LAO	Aorta	Aortic Valve Abnormality Coarctation PDA
Long Axial Olique	700 LAO	LV	Membranous VSD
	300 Cranial		Outlet VSD, Midrabecular VSD LVOT Obstruction
Four Chamber Projection	450 LAO	LV	AV Septal Defect
	450 Cranial		Midrabecular VSD
		RVPV	ASD
		PA	ASD
		RA, LV	Complex AV Connections
Lateral	900	RV	PS, TGA, DORV, Coarctation, PDA

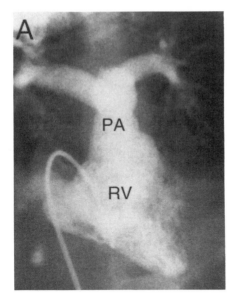

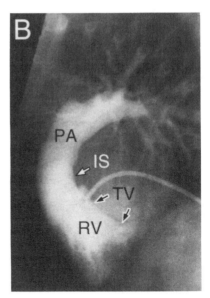

Figure 4-6:A & B. Normal right ventriculogram, cranially angled frontal (A) and lateral (B) projections. Note the superimposition of the heart on the abdominal contents, elongation of the RVOT and central pulmonary arteries. The infundibular septum (IS) is seen separating the pulmonary and tricuspid valves (TV). To profile the origin of the left pulmonary artery, additional left anterior obliquity could be added to the frontal projection. (PA = pulmonary artery, RV = right ventricle)

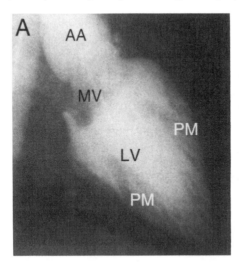

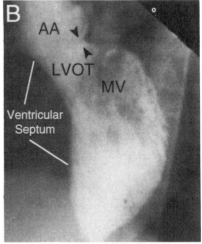

Figure 4-7:Retrograde left ventriculogram, long axial oblique projection (LAO 70°, craniocaudal angulation 30°), and RAO (30°) projection.A. The RAO projection provides a profiled view of the mitral valve annulus and the two papillary muscles. (AA = ascending aorta, lvot = left ventricular outflow tract, LV = left ventricle, MV = mitral valve, pm = papillary muscle). B. The long axial oblique projection demonstrates the normal sigmoid

shape of the left ventricular surface of the interventricular septum. The left ventricular outflow tract is profiled. Arrowheads indicate the aortic and anterior mitral valve leaflets.

Standard frontal and lateral projections are useful for systemic venous anatomy, peripheral pulmonary arterial anatomy, and RV anatomy, in selected complex anomalies. Cranial angulation elongates the right ventricular outflow tract and central pulmonary arteries (Fig. 4-6).

The right anterior oblique projection (Fig. 4-7A) profiles the normally positioned atrioventricular valve annuli, the left ventricular papillary muscles, the infundibular septum, defects in the anterior interventricular septum, the left main coronary artery and its bifurcation, the anterior and posterior descending coronary arteries and the right coronary artery. In the lateral projection, the infundibular septum and pulmonary valve are profiled in hearts with normal relations. The cranially angled steep left anterior oblique projection (30 degrees cranial, 70 degrees LAO) (Fig. 4-7B) normally elongates and profiles the midtrabecular and membranous ventricular septum, the left ventricular outflow tract, the left ventriculoinfundibular fold (distance between the posterior aortic valve and anterior mitral valve leaflets), the bifurcation of the left coronary artery, the distal branches of the right coronary artery, and the origin of the left pulmonary artery. The cranially angled shallow left anterior oblique projection (hepatoclavicular view, 45 degrees cranial and 45 degrees LAO) elongates and profiles the atrioventricular connections, the inlet or posterior interventricular septum, the pulmonary outflow tract and the pulmonary venous connections. The left anterior oblique projection (70 degrees LAO) optimally images the aortic arch. Caudal angulation (barrel, laid back projection) is used with downstream balloon occlusion to define the origins, branching pattern and epicardial course of the coronary arteries in patients with transposition of the great arteries, prior to arterial switch procedure [31, 38, 39]. In complex congenital heart disease, innovation is frequently helpful in producing optimal results.

Angiographic Techniques in Specific Lesions:
Recommended angiographic technique for a selection of common lesions is described below. While these are techniques to optimally image the most important anatomic aspects of these lesions, each study should be tailored according to the clinical needs of individual patients.

Membranous (Paramembranous) Ventricular Septal Defect

Left ventriculogram;
        Catheter position: apex of ventricle, away from mitral valve
        Catheter: balloon angio catheter across the foramen ovale and
             mitral valve, or retrograde pigtail catheter
        Contrast: 1 - 1.5 cc/kilogram, delivered as rapidly as possible
             (1 second or less)
        Projection: Long axial oblique (70 degree LAO, 30 degree
             cranial angulation) and orthogonal RAO (Fig. 4-8)

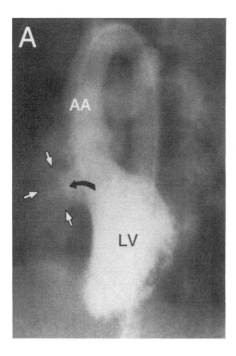 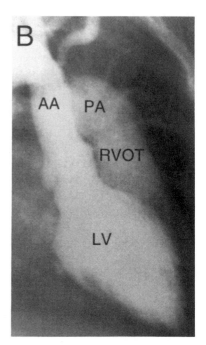

Figure 4-8:   *Membranous (paramembranous) ventricular septal defect*
A. Retrograde left ventriculogram, long axial oblique projection. The VSD is seen as a break (black arrow) in the profiled interventricular septum, beneath the aortic valve. Linear radiolucencies (arrowheads) represent the tricuspid valve tissue which is adjacent to the VSD.
B. Right anterior oblique projection. The right ventricular outflow tract and pulmonary artery are opacified indicating an interventricular shunt. The membranous VSD is not profiled in this projection but occasionally is seen "end on" (AA = ascending aorta, LV = left ventricle, PA = pulmonary artery, RV = right ventricle, RVOT = right ventricular outflow tract)

Comment: The long axial oblique projection profiles the membranous septum and the smooth midtrabecular septum and elongates the LVOT. The membranous or paramembranous VSD is seen as an extension of the contrast column across the interventricular septum, below the commissure between the right and noncoronary cusps of the aortic valve, and behind the septal leaflet of the tricuspid valve. With a membranous VSD, contrast collects under or around the tricuspid valve leaflets before opacifying the right ventricular outflow tract.   Long axial oblique projection also evaluates the left   ventricular outflow tract, permitting identification or exclusion of associated subaortic obstructions, and abnormal (prolapsing) aortic valve. The RAO projection sometimes permits visualization of the VSD "on end", especially if small, evaluation of the right ventricular outflow tract, and exclusion or identification of associated RVOT obstructions.   Associated LV-RA shunt can be diagnosed by identification of the contrast jet opacifying the right atrium in both projections.

Aortogram:
>Catheter position: ascending aorta
>Catheter: retrograde pigtail catheter
>Contrast: 1 cc per kilogram over 1 second or less
>Projection: LAO/RAO
>Comment: Aortography is useful for evaluation of the aortic valve and arch, especially for exclusion of aortic valve prolapse and regurgitation, and patent ductus arteriosus. It also adds information regarding the coronary artery anatomy.

Muscular Ventricular Septal Defect

Left ventriculogram
>Catheter position: apex of left ventricle
>Contrast: 1 – 1.5 cc per kilogram, delivered as rapidly as possible (1 second or less)
>Projections: four chamber projection (Fig. 4-9), long axial oblique/RAO (Fig. 4-10)
>Comment: Patients with trabecular VSD frequently have more than one defect, so that multiple projections are useful to evaluate the entire septum.

The RAO projection is useful in profiling the infundibular septum, and defects in the anterior conal septum (anterior to the septal band) (Fig. 4-10). As described above, the long axial oblique projection profiles defects in the midtrabecular septum. The four chamber projection, or cranially angled shallow LAO projection is useful to evaluate defects in the posterior trabecular septum, and around the atrioventricular valve.

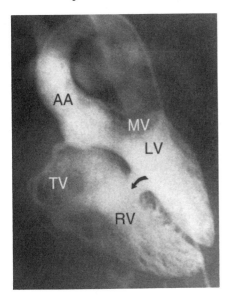

Figure 4-9: Multiple trabecular ventricular septal defects. Retrograde left ventriculogram, four chamber projection, profiles the mitral and tricuspid valves, and the midtrabecular VSD (arrow). Additional VSDs located closer to the apex are more anterior in location and are not profiled in this projection. (AA = ascending aorta, LV = left ventricle, MV = mitral valve, RV = right ventricle, TV = tricuspid valve)

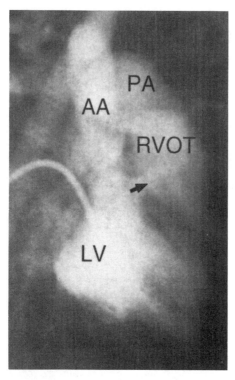

Figure 4-10:   Anterior   trabecular (conal) ventricular septal defect.
Transvenous left ventriculogram, right anterior oblique projection, profiles the anterior trabecular or conal VSD (arrow).
(AA = ascending aorta, LV = left ventricle, PA = pulmonary artery, RVOT = right ventricular outflow tract)

Defects In The Atrioventricular Septum

Left ventriculogram

> Catheter position: apex of left ventricle, antegrade across mitral valve or retrograde across the aortic valve
> Catheter: pigtail or balloon tipped catheter
> Contrast: 1 – 1.5 cc per kilogram over 1 second (or more with severe mitral regurgitation)
> Projection: four chamber projection (45 degree LAO, 45 degree cranial) (Fig. 4-11) and reciprocal cranially angled RAO
> Comment: The four chamber projection is the optimal view to evaluate the atrioventricular valves and inlet or posterior interventricular septum. Abnormal position of the atrioventricular valve attachments, common or partitioned atrioventricular valve, the presence and/or extent of ventricular septal defect, size of the ventricles, and type and severity of atrioventricular valve regurgitation are clearly demonstrated. The reciprocal cranially angled RAO projection is useful to evaluate the infundibular septum, the possibility of confluent conoventricular-inlet VSD and right ventricular outflow tract obstruction.

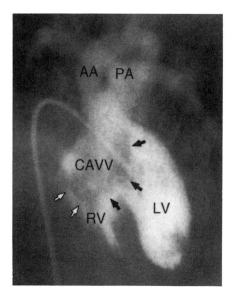

Figure 4-11: Complete atrioventricular septal defect (atrioventricular conal defect) Transvenous left ventriculogram, four chamber projection demonstrates the common atrioventricular valve (arrows) and a VSD around the valve.
(AA = ascending aorta, CAVV = common atrioventricular valve, LV = left ventricle, PA = pulmonary artery, RV = right ventricle)

Right ventriculogram
        Catheter position: RV apex
        Catheter: balloon tipped multi-side hole catheter
        Contrast: 1 - 1.5 cc per kilogram over 1 second
        Projection: cranially angled RAO/lateral
        Comment: Right ventriculography is indicated to evaluate associated RVOT obstruction. These projections will evaluate the RV outflow tract, infundibular septum, pulmonary valve and the pulmonary arteries.

Atrial Septal Defect

Left atrial injection
        Catheter position: right upper pulmonary vein
        Catheter: balloon-tipped angiocatheter
        Projection: Four chamber projection (45 degree LAO, 45 degree cranial) (Fig. 4-12)
        Comment: Although no longer needed for diagnosis, left atrial angiography is frequently used during device closure of atrioseptal defects. Transesophageal echocardiography is often used in conjunction with angiography to determine the relationship between the margins of the ASD, and adjacent tricuspid, mitral and aortic valves.

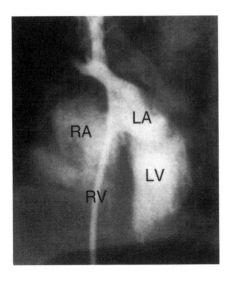

Figure 4-12:Secundum type atrial septal defect
Transvenous right upper pulmonary vein injection, four chamber projection, profiles the defect in the mid-atrial septum, with a rim of atrial septal tissue above (posterior) and below (anterior), between the defect and the atrioventicular valves.
(LA = left atrium, LV = left ventricle, RA = right atrium, RV = right ventricle)

Left ventriculogram
    Catheter position: Left ventricular apex
    Catheter: Balloon tipped angiocatheter antegrade, pigtail retrograde
    Contrast: 1 - 1.5 cc/kg in one second
    Projections: Four chamber projection (Fig. 4-13), right anterior oblique
    Comment: For primum ASD, LV angiography is useful to assess LV size, atrioventricular valve function, integrity of ventricular septum.

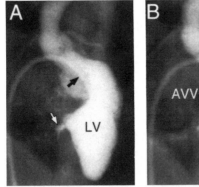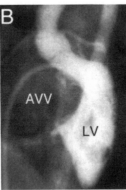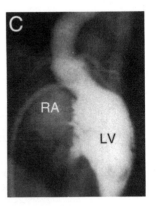

Figure 4-13:Primum atrial septal defect
A, B, & C. Transvenous left ventriculogram, four chamber projection, in diastole, (A&B) and systole (C) demonstrates the abnormal attachments of the cleft anterior mitral valve leaflets (arrowheads) to the intraventricular septum. The gap between the leaflets represents the "cleft". During systole (C) there is contrast regurgitation through a jet between the leaflets of the cleft mitral valve, into right atrium.
(AVV = atrioventricular valve, LV = left ventricle, RA = right atrium)

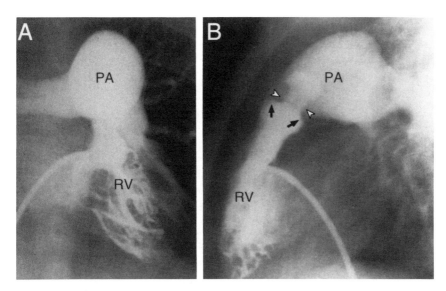

Figure 4-14:Usual pulmonary valve stenosis. A. Transvenous right ventriculogram, frontal projection demonstrates right ventricular hypertrophy and marked post-stenotic dilatation of the main and left pulmonary arteries. B. Lateral projection demonstrates an obstructed infundibulum, thickened and doming pulmonary valve leaflets (arrows), contrast jet (arrowheads) and post-stenotic dilatation of the main pulmonary artery. (PA = pulmonary artery, RV = right ventricle)

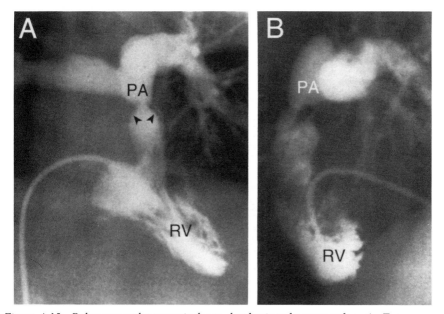

Figure 4-15: Pulmonary valve stenosis due to dysplastic pulmonary valve. A. Transvenous ventriculogram, cranially angled frontal projection demonstrates thickening and doming of a pulmonary valve (arrowheads) with a small annulus.

100

B. Lateral projection emphasizes thickening of the valve margins. Note the lack of post-stenotic dilatation of the main pulmonary artery.
(PA = pulmonary artery, RV = right ventricle)

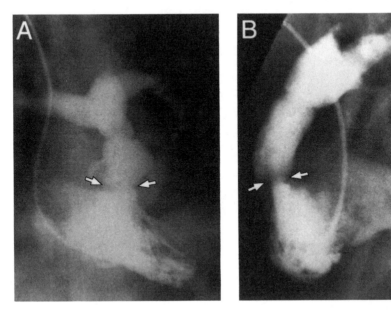

Figure 4-16: Subpulmonary stenosis (double chambered right ventricle)
A & B. Transvenous right ventriculogram, cranially angled frontal projection (A) and lateral projection (B) demonstrate focal obstructing muscle bundle (arrows) at the level of os infundibulum.

Pulmonary Stenosis

Right ventriculogram
>Catheter position: apex of right ventricle
>Catheter: balloon angiocatheter
>Contrast: 1 cc per kilogram over 1 second
>Projection: Cranially angled frontal and lateral (Figs. 4-14,4-15 & 4-16)
>Comment: In the presence of severe right ventricular hypertrophy, the catheter tip can become entrapped and produce myocardial staining during the injection. The balloon of an angiographic catheter should be inflated in the right atrium prior to crossing the tricuspid valve. The lateral projection is usually the best for demonstrating the nature of pulmonary valve stenosis and associated subpulmonary fixed or dynamic narrowing.

Left Ventricular Outflow Tract Obstructions

Left ventriculogram
      Catheter position: midportion left ventricle
      Catheter: pigtail, balloon angiocatheter
      Contrast: 1 cc per kilogram over 1 second
      Projection: long axial oblique (Figs. 4-17 & 4-18) /RAO
      Comment: Left ventriculography is used, not only to evaluate the aortic valve, but also the subaortic outflow tract (which is elongated in the long axial oblique projection), the midtrabecular septum (which may have anomalous muscle bundles), and the anterior leaflet of the mitral valve. Left ventriculography optimally demonstrates subaortic membranes, hypoplasia of the aortic valve annulus, and thickening of the aortic valve leaflets.

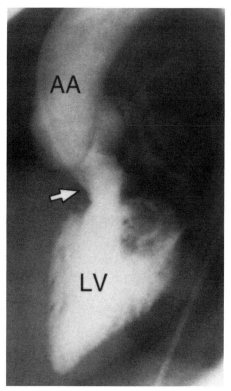

Figure 4-17: Discrete fibromuscular subaortic stenosis.
Left ventriculogram, long axial oblique projection, demonstrates a focal subaortic indentation (arrow).
(LV = left ventricle, AA = ascending aorta).

102

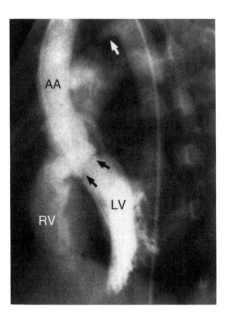

Figure 4-18: Discrete subaortic stenosis, subaortic membrane with membranous VSD.
Retrograde left ventriculogram, long axial oblique projection, demonstrates a membranous VSD, and obstructing subaortic membrane (arrows). Note also the PDA (white arrow).
(AA=ascending Aorta, LV=left ventricle, RV=right ventricle)

Aortogram
Catheter position: ascending aorta
Catheter: pigtail
Contrast: 1 cc per kilogram as rapidly as possible
Projections: RAO, LAO, Lat (Figs. 4-19, 4-20 & 4-21)
Comment: The catheter should be positioned close to the aortic valve for optimal imaging of the valve leaflets, but above the valve commissures, in order to assess aortic valve regurgitation. The field of view should include the left ventricle, in order to accurately assess the severity of the aortic regurgitation. In the presence of supravalvar aortic stenosis, additional injections may be necessary to profile the coronary ostia.

103

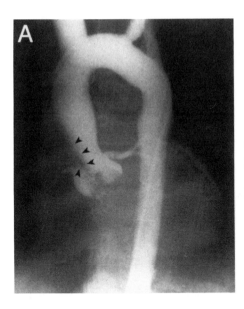 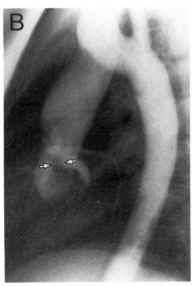

Figure 4-19: Aortic valve stenosis with absence of non-right coronary commissure
A. Retrograde ascending aortogram, frontal projection, demonstrates systolic doming of the aortic valve leaflets and an eccentric radiolucent jet (arrowsheads).
B. Retrograde aortogram, lateral projection, demonstrates the typical doming of the aortic valve leaflets, with a radiolucent jet (arrows) outlining the orifice, and post-stenotic dilatation of the ascending aorta.

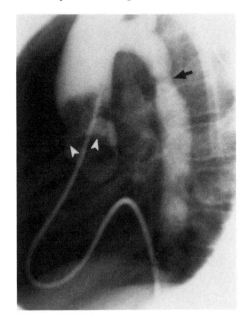

Figure 4-20: Bicuspid aortic valve with coarctation of the descending aorta. Transvenous ascending aortogram demonstrates two symmetric aortic valve cusps with absence of intercoronary commissure (arrowheads), with a discrete coarctation of the descending aorta (arrow) note mild hypoplasia of the aortic isthmus.

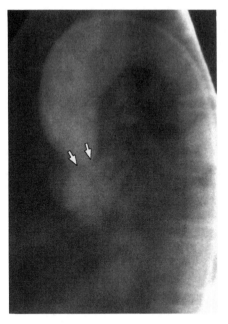

Figure 4-21: Discrete supravalvar aortic stenosis.
Retrograde aortogram, left anterior oblique projection, demonstrates discrete obstruction (arrows) above the aortic valve, and just above the origins of the coronary arteries.

Coarctation

Aortogram
    Catheter position: ascending aorta or aortic arch
    Catheter: pigtail, balloon angiocatheter
    Contrast: 1 cc per kilogram as rapidly as possible
    Projection: RAO/LAO, Lateral (Fig. 4-22)
    Comment: Isolated coarctation of the descending aorta is accurately diagnosed by echocardiography or magnetic resonance imaging, so angiography is generally carried out only in the presence of associated complex congenital heart disease, or simultaneously with catheter intervention. In neonates with patent ductus arteriosus and transverse aortic arch hypoplasia with coarctation of the isthmus, the arch and isthmus may be best imaged by catheterization of the descending aorta via the patent ductus arteriosus, and descending aortic balloon occlusion angiography.

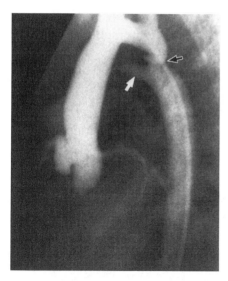

Figure 4-22: Juxtaductal coarctation of the descending aorta.
Retrograde aortogram, lateral projection demonstrates discrete posterior lateral indentation in the descending aorta (black arrow) opposite a small patent ductus arteriosus (white arrow).

Transposition Of The Great Arteries, Preoperative

Left ventriculogram
        Catheter position: apex of left ventricle, antegrade across the
            foramen ovale
        Catheter: balloon tipped angiocatheter
        Contrast: 1 cc per kilogram as rapidly as possible
        Projection: long axial oblique (Fig. 4-23 A & B & Fig. 4-24)/RAO

106

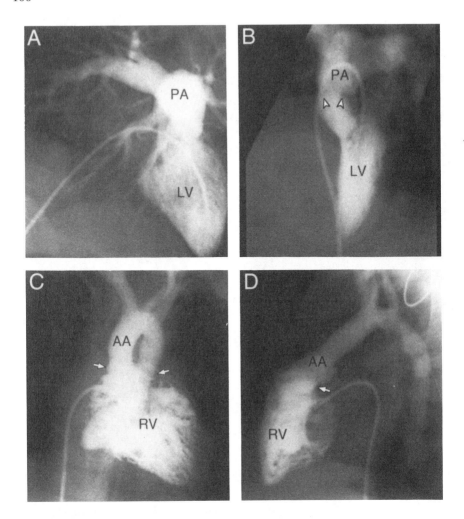

Figure 4-23: Transposition of the great arteries (SDD) with pulmonary valve stenosis.
A & B. Transvenous left ventriculogram, right anterior oblique (A) and long axial oblique
(B) projections. The pulmonary artery (PA) is situated above the morphologic left ventricle
(LV), with no infundibulum between the pulmonary valve and the mitral valve. The long
axial oblique projection (B) profiles the LV outflow tract and demonstrates pulmonary valve
stenosis (arrowheads).
C & D. Transvenous right ventriculogram, (RV) frontal (C) and lateral (D) projections. The
aortic valve is positioned rightward and anterior, separated from the tricuspid valve by the
infundibulum (arrows).
(AA = ascending aorta).

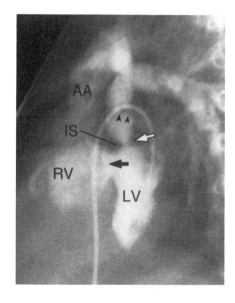

Figure 4-24: Transposition of the great arteries (SDD) with VSD and pulmonary stenosis.
Transvenous left ventriculogram, long axial oblique projection, demonstrates the aorta (AA) rising above the morphologic right ventricle RV), and the pulmonary artery rising above the morphologic left ventricle (LV), with a membranous VSD, (black arrow). Unlike Fig. 4-23, this heart demonstrates conus (white arrow) beneath the pulmonary artery. Posterior deviation of the infundibular septum (IS) with prominence of the left ventriculo-infundibular fold results in subpulmonary stenosis. There is also pulmonary valve stenosis (arrowheads).

Comment: The LAO projection is important to assess the size of the left ventricle, status of the intraventricular septum, and the left ventricular outflow tract. Elongation of the LVOT is necessary to exclude a variety of potential causes of LVOT obstruction which occur in transposition of the great arteries. This projection also evaluates the origin of the left pulmonary artery (Fig. 4-24). The RAO projection is useful in assessing the anterior interventricular septum, and the mitral valve.

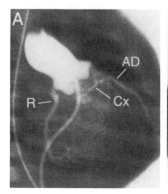
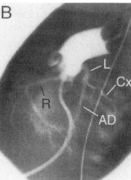
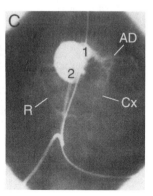

Figure 4-25: Balloon occlusion antegrade aortography in a neonate with transposition of the great arteries (SDD) and normal coronary arteries.
A & B. Standard right anterior oblique (A) and long axial oblique (B) projections with balloon occlusion of the distal ascending aorta produce excellent opacification of the coronary arteries, which are seen to arise normally from the facing sinuses of valsalva.
C. Caudal or barrel projection further defines the spatial relationship of the coronary arteries. The facing sinuses are labelled 1 and 2.
(AD=anterior descending, CX=circumflex, L= left coronary artery, R=right coronary artery).

Right ventriculogram (optional)
    Catheter position: antegrade or retrograde in the body of the right
    ventricle
    Catheter: balloon angiocthater (antegrade) or pigtail (retrograde)
    Contrast: 1 cc per kilogram over 1 to 1.5 seconds
    Projection: frontal and lateral (Fig. 4-23 B & C)
    Comment: These projections are useful in defining the size and
    function of the morphologically right ventricle, status of
    the infundibular septum, aortic valve and aortic arch.

Ascending aortogram
    Catheter position: distal ascending aorta (antegrade), proximal
    ascending aorta (retrograde)
    Catheter: balloon angiocatheter (antegrade), pigtail (retrograde)
    Contrast: 1 cc per kilogram over a second or less
    Projections: caudally angled frontal and lateral, RAO/LAO (Fig. 4-26).

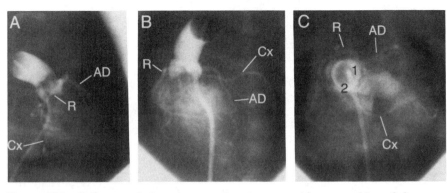

*Figure 4-26: Balloon occlusion aortogram in a neonate with transposition of the great
arteries (SDD) and, origin of the right and left coronary arteries from the number one
facing sinus.*
*A&B. Balloon occlusion antegrade aortogram in right anterior oblique (A) and long axial
oblique (B) projections demonstrate the right coronary artery and left anterior descending
arteries to arise from a common trunk. The right coronary artery passes anterior to the RV
outflow tract to reach the right atrial-ventricular groove. The circumflex artery rises
separately from the number two facing sinus.*
*C. Caudal or barrel projection confirms the spatial orientation of the coronary artery
branches as described above. (AD=anterior descending, CX=circumflex, L= left coronary
artery, R=right coronary artery).*

Comment: Ascending aortography is useful prior to arterial switch
surgery, to definite the origins, branching pattern and epicardial course of
the coronary arteries. The caudally angled frontal projection is best for
profiling the origins of the coronary arteries, but must be performed with
distal flow arrest, using antegrade positioning of a balloon tipped multi-
side-hole catheter. The balloon is inflated in the distal ascending aorta,
resulting in dense opacification of the coronary arteries. Incomplete flow
arrest will lead to suboptimal imaging, so, if the aorta cannot be
occluded, standard RAO/LAO projections should be obtained for better
image quality.

L-Transposition Of The Great Arteries

Left ventriculogram
>Catheter position: apex of morphologic left ventricle, antegrade
>Catheter: balloon angiocatheter or pigtail
>Contrast: 1 cc per kilogram as rapidly as possible
>Projections: cranially angled RAO/LAO (Fig. 4-27 A & B)
>Comment: These projections are used to image the intraventricular septum, subpulmonary LVOT, and the pulmonary arteries. The cranially angled LAO projection is also used when evaluating the pulmonary veins and intra-atrial septum.

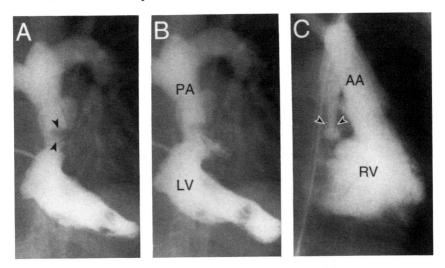

Figure 4-27: Corrected transposition of the great arteries (SLL) with VSD and pulmonary stenosis.
A & B transvenous injection in the left ventricle (LV), cranially angled frontal projection shows that the pulmonary artery (PA) arises above the morphologic left ventricle. There is subvalvar pulmonary stenosis caused by prolapse of tricuspid valve tissue (arrowheads) through the ventricular septal defect.
C.. Retrograde injection into the morphologic right ventricle (RV), frontal projection, shows the aorta (AA) arising, to the left of the pulmonary artery, above the right ventricular infundibulum. The left ventricular outflow tract and pulmonary artery fill via the VSD.

Right ventriculogram
>Catheter position: apex of morphological right ventricle.
>Catheter: pigtail (retrograde) or balloon angiocatheter (antegrade).
>Contrast: 1 cc per kilogram over 1 second.
>Projections: frontal and lateral (Fig. 4-27 C & D).
>Comment: Retrograde catheterization of the right ventricle is preferred, for optimal evaluation of the tricuspid valve, which is often abnormal and regurgitant in this condition. In the absence of a ventricular septal defect, slower injection may help to reduce ventricular ectopic beats.

Double Outlet Right Ventricle

Left ventriculogram

        Catheter position: apex of left ventricle, antegrade via foramen
ovale, or retrograde, via aortic valve and VSD
Catheter: balloon angio (antegrade) or pigtail (retrograde)
Contrast: 1 – 1.5 cc per kilogram as rapidly as possible
Projection: long axial oblique/RAO
Comment: These projections are used for evaluation of the left
ventricular size, mitral valve, ventricular septum (VSD), the relationship
between the great vessels and the VSD, and the status of the aortic-mitral
continuity. In the presence of atrioventricular valve anomalies, inlet VSD
or multiple VSD's, the four chamber projection (45 degree LAO, 45
degree cranial) should be added.

Right ventriculogram

        Catheter position: antegrade or retrograde in apex of right ventricle
Catheter: balloon angiocatheter or pigtail
Contrast: 1.5 cc per kilogram over 1 second or less
Projection: frontal and lateral (Figs. 4-28 & 4-29). Additional cranially
angled frontal projection may be necessary for pulmonary arterial
anatomy.
Comment: The anatomy of the infundibulum and ventriculo-
arterial relations is variable in double outlet right
ventricle. The right ventriculogram is used to evaluate
the position and orientation of the infundibular septum,
presence of subarterial obstruction, the relationship
between great arteries and ventricular septal defect, as
well as anomalies of the great arteries. The field of view,
especially in the lateral projection should include the
aortic arch.

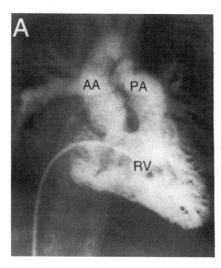 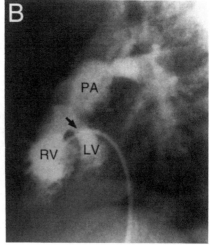

Figure 4-28: Double outlet right ventricle (SDD)
A. Right ventriculogram, frontal projection, shows both great arteries rising above the infundibulum of the right ventricle, with their outflow tracts separated by the infundibular septum. A pulmonary artery band is present.
B. Lateral projection confirms the "side by side" relationship of the great arteries and the outlet VSD (arrow). (AA=ascending aorta, LV=left ventricle, PA= pulmonary artery, RV=right ventricle). (see previous page)

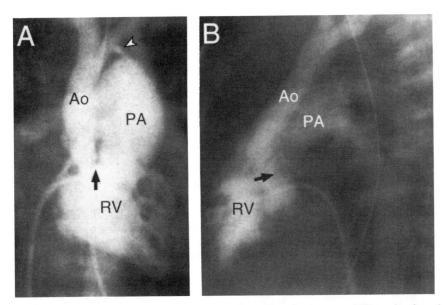

Figure 4-29: Double outlet right ventricle (SDD) with subpulmonary VSD and subaortic stenosis and coarctation of the aorta.
A & B Transvenous right ventriculogram, frontal, (A) and lateral (B) projections demonstrates both great arteries rising above the right ventricular infundibulum, separated by the infundibular septum (arrow), which is displaced toward the right. The subaortic stenosis is associated with the small ascending aorta and severe coarctation of the descending aorta (arrowhead). The lateral projection confirms the subpulmonary location of the VSD (arrow).

Aortogram, for coronary artery anatomy, and arch anomalies.
(see Transposition of the Great Arteries)

Total Anomalous Pulmonary Venous Connection

Pulmonary arteriogram
Catheter position: global injections in the main, and individual injections in the right and left pulmonary arteries
Catheter: balloon angiocatheter
Contrast: 1 – 1.5 cc per kilogram, depending on the presence of obstruction of pulmonary veins
Projection: frontal and lateral
Comment: Injection in the main pulmonary artery is useful, especially if combined with digital subtraction imaging, in opacifying the entire pulmonary venous system simultaneously. This technique may cause

reactive pulmonary vasospasm in infants with pulmonary venous hypertension. Separate injection of 1 cc per kilogram per lung should be made in each pulmonary artery, in the presence of high flow. In addition, retrograde transvenous catheterization of the anomalous pulmonary vein is frequently possible and informative. Balloon occlusion of patent ductus arteriosus may be useful, in the presence of severely obstructed veins, to reduce the right to left shunting into the aorta.

Left ventriculogram
      Catheter position: apex of left ventricle
      Catheter: balloon angiocatheter (antegrade) pigtail (retrograde)
      Contrast: 1 cc per kilogram over 1 second or less
      Projection: long axial oblique and RAO
      Comment: left ventriculography is performed in TAPVC, in order to evaluate left ventricular size and the ventricular septum. It may be omitted if these anomalies are not suspected after echocardiography.

Tricuspid Atresia

Left ventriculogram
      Catheter position: apex of left ventricle
      Catheter: balloon angiocatheter or pigtail
      Contrast: 1 cc per kilogram as rapidly as possible
      Projection: Four chamber projection or long axial oblique and RAO (Fig. 4-30) is used to assess size and function of the left ventricle, number and position of ventricular septal defects, ventriculoatrial relations and anomalies of the pulmonary arteries and aorta.

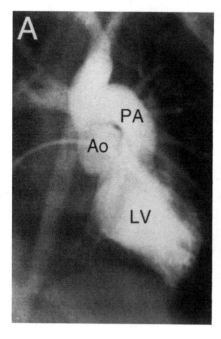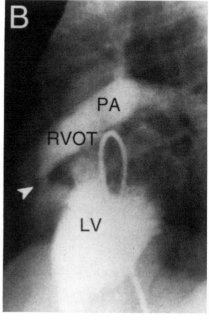

Figure 4-30: Tricuspid atresia with ventricular septal defect.
A. Transvenous left ventriculogram, right anterior oblique projection. The aorta (A_O) rises above the left ventricle (LV). The pulmonary artery (PA) is opacified.
B. Long axial oblique projection demonstrate the opacification of the right ventricular outflow (RVOT) tract through a VSD (not profiled). Note the subpulmonary stenosis (arrowhead). (see previous page)

Superior Vena Cavagram
  Catheter position: Left innominate vein
  Catheter: balloon angiocatheter, balloon inflated
  Contrast: 0.5 - 1 cc per kilogram, as rapidly as possible
  Projection: frontal and lateral projections
  Comment: Venous angiography is performed to define the upper body systemic venous return, in preparation for a Glenn shunt or Fontan procedure. In particular, the presence or absence of a left superior vena cava is important to determine.

Special Angiographic Studies

Digital Angiography:

Digital subtraction angiography is a computer enhanced imaging system which subtracts the background structures from the contrast injection, permitting excellent contrast resolution. For best results, 1024 matrix and excellent patient motion control are necessary. Digital subtraction angiography is ideal for imaging structures which do not require a high frame rate, such as the pulmonary circulation, thoracic aorta and systemic branches. Because of the high contrast resolution, structures which are only faintly opacified with conventional radiography can be clearly imaged.
Digital angiography without subtraction also has advantages over conventional radiographic imaging. The digital nature of the acquired image permits post acquisition manipulation of density and contrast levels, image zoom or magnification, and measurement techniques. Modern archival techniques result in reduced cost of production and storage of angiographic studies in comparison with conventional cineangiography. The disadvantages include slightly reduced geometric definition, and the need for specialized work stations for viewing.

Pulmonary Venous Wedge Angiography

Wedged injection into the pulmonary veins is useful to produce retrograde opacification of small or proximally obstructed central pulmonary arteries, in conditions such as pulmonary atresia and ventricular septal defect with small central pulmonary arteries (Fig. 4-31), absent central pulmonary artery, or postoperative central pulmonary arterial occlusion. Contrast staining of the pulmonary parenchyma and extravasation into the adjacent bronchus may occur, but is usually well tolerated [40].

114

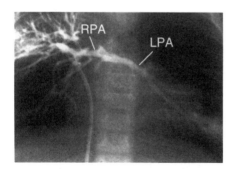

Figure 4-31: Wedge pulmonary vein injection in pulmonary atresia with VSD. A balloon tipped catheter is wedged in the right upper pulmonary vein. contrast injection refluxes into the right pulmonary (RPA) artery, outlining a confluence as well as the left pulmonary artery (LPA).

Technique
1. Advance balloon tip end-hole catheter across the atrial septum into right or left pulmonary veins. If necessary, transeptal needle technique should be employed. With the tip free in a fairly large vein, inflate the balloon so that the catheter tip is wedged. Confirm the wedged position with a small contrast injection.
2. Deflate the balloon, taking care to keep position stable. Attach to the hub of the catheter a 10 or 20 cc syringe in which contrast (0.3 cc per kilogram) and 5 to 15 cc of saline have been carefully layered, the saline being drawn up first and the contrast second. Keep the syringe tip down.
3. Inflate the balloon again, and hand inject the contrast/saline contents of the syringe fully, forcing the contrast through the capillary bed with the saline, as fast as is manually possible.
    Comment: Serious complications from this technique have been reported with the use of non-balloon end-hole catheters.

Selective Coronary Arteriography

In general, ventriculography and aortography, using appropriate projections, are sufficient to identify anomalies of origin and distribution of coronary arteries associated with complex congenital heart diseases such as tetralogy of Fallot, transposition of the great arteries, double outlet right ventricle and other lesions. Indications for selective coronary arteriography in children include Kawasaki's disease, coronary artery fistulae, anomalous left coronary artery from the pulmonary artery, pulmonary atresia with intact ventricular septum, and patients who have undergone cardiac transplantation.
Right and left coronary artery curves are currently available in 4.5 French sizes (Judkin's, Cook), 5 French (Amplatz Cook), 6.5 French (Cook), and 7.3 French. Since considerable catheter manipulation is often necessary, it is best to introduce these catheters through a femoral arterial sheath [41].
When the catheter is free in the ascending aorta, it is attached to a manifold that allows easy switching between saline flushing, pressure monitoring and contrast injection. The catheter is filled with contrast, and pressure and the EKG are continuously recorded. In children as in adults, the right coronary artery arises from the right cusp in a nearly straight anterior direction, and the left coronary artery arises in the postero leftward direction. The right coronary curve can often be manipulated into both orifices. Once either orifice is engaged by the free catheter tip (as determined by a good arterial pressure wave and frequent small test injections), biplane coronary arteriography is obtained in the long axial oblique, frontal, lateral, LAO and RAO views.

Balloon Occlusion Aortography

Balloon occlusion is useful in neonates or infants to stop flow, resulting in superior opacification of the desired structures [31, 38, 39]. The aorta is catheterized antegradely with a balloon-tipped angiocatheter. The balloon is inflated immediately prior to contrast injection, and then deflated.

Catheter position: Ascending aorta (for coronaries) (Fig. 4-26). Descending aorta (for aortopulmonary collaterals) (Fig. 4-32)
Catheter: Balloon tipped angiocatheter
Contrast: 1 cc per kilogram as quickly as possible
Projections: Frontal and lateral for descending aortography, oblique and barrel (caudal) for coronaries

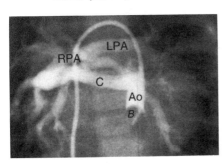

Figure 4-32: Balloon occlusion descending aortogram for a demonstration of aortopulmonary collaterals. The balloon tipped angiographic catheter has been advanced from the right ventricle into the ascending and then the descending aorta. Contrast injected behind the inflated balloon (B) produces dense opacification of the aortopulmonary collateral (C) which then refluxes into the right and left pulmonary arteries. (AO= aorta, C= aortopulmonary collateral, LPA=left pulmonary artery, RPA= right pulmonary artery).

REFERENCES

1. Curry TS, Dowdey JE, Murry RC. Christensen's introduction to the physics of diagnostic radiology. In: 4th ed. Philadelphia, PA: Lea and Febiger, 1990
2. Sprawls P. The physical principles of diagnostic radiology. In: Rockville, MD: Aspen, 1977
3. Moore RJ. Imaging principles of cardiac angiography. In: Rockville, MD: Aspen, 1990
4. Nissen SE, Pepine CJ, Bashore TM. Cardiac angiography without cine film: erecting a "tower of Babel" in the cardiac catheterization laboratory. J Am Coll Cardiol 1994;24:834-837
5. Stewart BK. Exchange media and networks for digital fluoroscopy and cineangiography. In: Syllabus: categorical course in physics. Oak Brook, IL: Radiological Society of North America, 1995:153-165
6. Holmes Jr. DJ. To compress or not, that is the question. Catheterization and Cardiovascular Diagnosis 1995;36:382
7. Balter S. Guidelines for personnel radiation monitoring in the cardiac catheterization laboratory. Cathet Cardiovasc Diagn 1993;30:277-279
8. Johnson LW, Moore RJ, Balter S. Review of radiation safety in the cardiac catheterization laboratory. Cathet Cardiovasc Diagn 1992;25:186-194
9. Recommendations on limits for exposure to ionizing radiation. NCRP Report 91. In: National Council on Radiation Protection and Measurements, 1987
10. Merriam GR, Focht EF. A clinical study of radiation cataracts and the relationship to dose. Am J Roentgenol 1957;77:759-785

116

11. Schueler BA, Julsrud PR, Gray JE, et al. Radiation exposure and efficiency of exposure-reduction techniques during cardiac catheterization in children. Am J Roentgenol 1994;162:173-177
12. Cagnon CH, Benedict SH, Mankovic NJ, et al. Exposure rates in high-level-control fluoroscopy for image enhancement. Radiology 1991;178:643-646
13. Wagner LK, Eifel PJ, Geise RA. Potential biological effects following high x-ray dose interventional prodcedure. JVIR 1994;5:71-84
14. Aufrichtig R, Xue P, Thomas CW, et al. Perceptual comparison of pulse and continuous fluoroscopy. Med Phys 1994;21:245-256
15. Hernandez RJ, Goodsitt MM. Reduction of radiation dose in pediatric patients using pulsed fluoroscopy. Am J Roentgenol 1996;67:1247-1253
16. Holmes Jr. DR, Wondrow MA, Gray JE, et al. Effect of pulsed progressive fluoroscopy on reduction of radiation dose in the cardiac catheterization laboratory. J Am Coll Cardiol 1990;15:150-162
17. Parker JE, Bettmann MA. Angiographic contrast media. In: Taveras J, Ferrucci J, eds. Radiology: Diagnosis-Imaging-Intervention. Vol 2. Philadelphia: J. B. Lippincott Company, 1992:Ch 135A, pp 1-10.(Yucel K, ed. Vascular Radiology).
18. Dawson P, Howell M. The non-ionic dimers: a new class of contrast agents. Br J Radiology 1986;59:987-991
19. Tveit K, Bolstad KD, Haugland T, et al. Iodixanol in cardioangiography. Acta Radiologica 1994;35:614-618
20. Fischer HW. Catalog of intravascular contrast media. Radiology 1986;159:561-563
21. Klow NE, Levorstad K, Berg KJ, et al. Iodixanol in cardioangiography in patients with coronary artery disease. Acta Radiologica 1993;34:72-77
22. Cohan RH, Dunnick NR. Intravascular contrast media: adverse reaction. Am J Roentgenol 1987;149:665-670
23. Parfrey PS, Griffiths SM, Barrett BJ, et al. Contrast material-induced renal failure in patients with diabetes mellitus, renal insufficiency, or both: a prospective controlled study. NEJM 1989;320:143-149
24. Cohen MD. A review of the toxicity of nonionic contrast agent in children. Invest Radiol 1993;28:S87-S93
25. Bettmann MA, Bourdillon PD, Gopalan R, et al. Contrast agents for cardiac angiography: effects of a nonionic agent vs a standard ionic agent. Radiology 1984;153:583-587
26. Barrett BJ, Parfrey PS, Vavasour HM, et al. A comparison of nonionic, low-osmolality radiocontrast agents with ionic, high-osmolality agents during cardiac catheterization. NEJM 1992;326:431-436
27. Siegle RL. Rates of idiosyncratic reactions: Ionic versus nonionic contrast media. Invest Radiol 1993;28:S95-S98
28. Palmer FJ. The RACR survey of intravenous contrast media reactions: final report. Australas Radiol 1988;32:426-248
29. Katayama H, Yamaguchi K, Kozuka T, et al. Adverse reactions to ionic and nonionic contrast media: the report from the Japanese Committee on the safety of contrast media. Radiology 1990;175:621-628
30. Verma R, Keane JF. Use of cutoff pigtail catheters with intraluminal guidewires in interventional procedures in congenital heart disease. Cathet Cardiovasc Diagn 1994;33:85-88
31. Keane JF, McFaul R, Fellows K, et al. Balloon occlusion angiography in infancy: methodology, uses and limitations. Am J Cardiol 1985;56:495-497
32. Fiddler GI, Partridge JB. Balloon occlusion angiography in critically ill neonates. Cath Cardiovasc Diagn 1983;9:309-312

33. Culham JAG. Physical principles of image formation and projections in angiocardiography. In: Freedom RM, Mawson JB, Yoo SJ, Benson LN, eds. Congenital Heart Disease. Vol 1. Armonk: Futura Publishing Company, 1997:39-93

34. Bargeron LM, Jr, Elliot LP, Soto B, et al. Axial cineangiography in congenital heart disease. Section I: Technical and anatomical considerations. Circulation 1977;56:1975-1083

35. Elliot LP, Bargeron LM, Jr, Bream PR, et al. Axial cineangiography in congenital heart disease. Section II: Specific lesions. Circulation 1977;56:1084-1093

36. Fellows KE, Keane JF, Freed MD. Angled views in congenital heart disease. Circulation 1977;56:485-490

37. Freedom RM, Mawson JB, Yoo SJ, et al. Congenital Heart Disease. In: Armonk, NY: Futura Publishing Company, Inc., 1997: 1-662. vol 1).

38. Mandell VS, Lock JE, E MJ, et al. The "laidback" aortogram: an improved angiographic view for demonstration of coronary arteries in transposition of the great arteries. Am J Cardiol 1990;65:1379-1383

39. Yoo SJ, Burrows PE, Moes CAF, et al. Evaluation of cornary arterial patterns in complete transposition by laid-back aortography. Cardiol Young 1996;6:149-155

40. Alpert BS, Culham JAG. A severe complication of pulmonary vein angiography. Brit Heart J 1979;41:727-729

41. Formanek A, Nath PH, Zollikofer C, et al. Selective coronary arteriography in children. Circulation 1980;61:84-94

5. CATHETER INTERVENTION: BALLOON ANGIOPLASTY:
Experimental Studies, Technology and Methodology.

Phillip Moore, M.D.
James E. Lock, M.D.

HISTORY

Dotter and Judkins first described transluminal angioplasty in 1964 [1]. Using a surgical cutdown, they introduced solid cylindrical dilators of sequentially increasing diameters to enlarge the vessel lumen of iliac and femoral arteries. Ten years later Gruentzig [2] successfully applied Dotter's concept to a percutaneously placed inflatable noncompliant balloon, demonstrating effective dilation of iliac and femoral arteries. In 1975 the technique was applied to the coronary arteries [3]. At that time, the prevailing hypothesis of the mechanism of vessel enlargement was redistribution of soft atheromatous plaque. Pediatric cardiologists were therefore slow to apply the technique to congenital vessel stenoses. Animal studies in the early 80s [4, 5, 6] showed the mechanism of vessel enlargement by angioplasty to be intimal and medial injury with presumed healing in an open position; the door opened to the rapid application of balloon angioplasty to a variety of congenital vascular stenoses. In a trio of case reports in 1982, Singer et al. reported angioplasty of a coarctation in an infant [7], Driscoll et al. unsuccessfully dilated pulmonary vein stenosis [8], and Rocchini et al. treated SVC obstruction [9]. By 1983 the technique had been successfully applied by Lock and colleagues to series of patients with pulmonary artery stenosis, coarctation, and venous stenosis including atrial baffle obstruction [10,11,12].

The late 80s witnessed an exponential increase in clinical experience with angioplasty for congenital stenoses. Advances in methods and technology led to smaller, more effective balloon catheters and guidewires, which improved success rates and minimized complications, even in small neonates. A voluntary collaborative registry of 27 institutions, the Valvuloplasty and Angioplasty of Congenital Anomalies Registry (VACA) assessed angioplasty procedures performed from 1981 through 1986; the results were published in 1990 [13,14,15]. Angioplasty became a routine treatment for a variety of native and postoperative lesions. The development of high pressure balloons [16,17] and endovascular stenting [18] in the late 80s further improved the success rates with angioplasty, increasing its already prominent role in the treatment of congenital and acquired vascular stenosis.

PRINCIPLES OF ANGIOPLASTY

Physical Principles
The dilating force on a stenotic lesion, the radial or outward force a balloon exerts, is dependent on balloon diameter, balloon inflation pressure, balloon compliance, balloon length, lesion severity, lesion compliance, lesion length [19, 20],

120

and other factors. According to the law of Laplace, the circumferential force or tension (T) exerted on the wall of an inflated balloon is directly proportional to the pressure (P) within the balloon and the radius (R) of the balloon (T= PxR). Therefore, larger balloons will require less pressure than smaller balloons to generate the same dilating force. Consequently, larger vessels will require less pressure to dilate and rupture than smaller vessels. To be an effective dilator a balloon should be as non-compliant as possible. The diameter of a compliant balloon, when placed across a stenotic vessel where the narrowing and the surrounding vessel have the same compliance, will enlarge preferentially under the normal vessel (because of its increased diameter) without increasing the diameter of the stenotic segment. Eventually the balloon ruptures under the normal segment and little is accomplished. A totally non-compliant balloon will increase its diameter equally across the lesion at increasing inflation pressures.

Figure 5-1: Subtle waist seen in a balloon produced by a stenotic aortic valve. Note the waist is seen on both sides of the balloon. A subtle waist generates a limited dilating force that may be adequate for dilation of a valve but not a stenotic vessel.

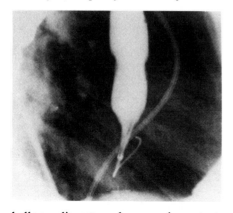

The length of the balloon also plays an important role. Compliant balloons will deform longitudinally as they increase their diameter with increasing inflation pressures so a shorter compliant balloon will exert a more concentrated dilating force on the lesion than a longer compliant balloon. In contrast, length has little effect if the balloon is totally noncompliant because no deformation will occur.

Lesion diameter in relation to the balloon diameter plays an important role in determining the dilating forces, making the choice of the balloon diameter critical for each lesion. The dilating radial force vector is greater in a tight high-grade stenosis than in a shallow stenosis (Fig. 5-1).

This dilating force decreases as the waist on the balloon is eliminated. If the balloon is relatively small compared to the lesion, the waist produced will be subtle (Fig 5-1) and the vector of the dilating force small. This force can be increased by increasing inflation pressure, putting the balloon at risk for rupture. If the balloon is large for the stenosis and the waist is quite tight (Fig 5-2), the dilating force will be large and effective, however the larger balloon may put the normal vessel, proximal and distal to the stenosis, at greater risk of injury.

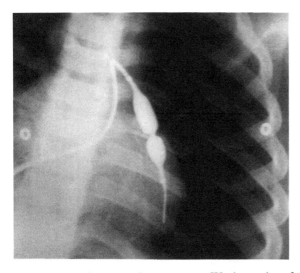

Figure 5-2: Marked waist produced by a severe stenosis in a left pulmonary artery. The large size of the balloon on either side of the waist may injure the normal vessel.

In addition, once the vessel begins to tear, it will rapidly tear all the way to the full balloon diameter. If the vessel wall is not thick at the narrowed site, there will be insufficient adventitia to maintain vascular integrity, causing vascular rupture. We have therefore found that "intermediate" waists are the most effective and safest for dilation of nearly all lesions (Fig 5-3).

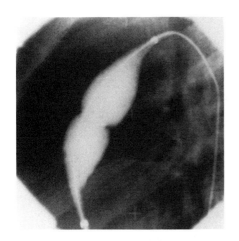

Figure 5-3: Moderate waist produced by a stenotic pulmonary valve. Elimination of such a waist at higher pressures optimizes obstruction relief with minimal risk for normal vessel injury.

EXPERIMENTAL STUDIES

The mechanism of vessel enlargement from balloon dilation of congenital or post-operative lesions has been proven by experimental studies [4, 5, 6, 21, 22], intravascular ultrasound [23 - 25], and post surgical/autopsy series [26 - 29] to be tearing of the intima, media, and rarely adventitia with subsequent healing and scarring. There is no clinical or experimental evidence to suggest that "stretching" a lesion without at least partial wall disruption leads to any permanent improvement. Tears can occur along the length of the vessel or across its diameter and may be superficial (into the intima) or deep, extending through the media into the adventitia. Balloon dilation always causes some endothelial injury but the most common and effective injury is a deep medial tear [25]. Dissection of the intima and/or media may occur when the tear extends circumferentially > 25% of the vascular circumference and results in an intraluminal flap (Fig. 5-4).

Figure 5-4: Angiographic and intravascular ultrasound (IVUS) images of a coarctation before and after balloon dilation. Despite no obvious angiographic appearance of wall injury, a medial tear with intimal flap (arrow) is easily seen on IVUS

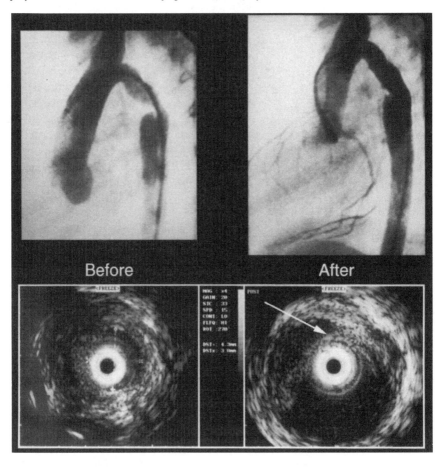

This has been reported in up to 15% of procedures when evaluated with intravascular ultrasound. Lesions are nearly always in the area of the obstruction itself but can extend above or below the lesion, particularly if a large balloon (> 150% diameter of the native vessel) or a long balloon is used in a tortuous vessel. Our understanding of the vascular response to balloon dilation remains incomplete. Once the media has been torn, blood dissects below the medial layers. The endothelial damage in the intima promotes platelet adherence to exposed subendothelium. This initiates interactions between cellular matrix proteins in the adventitia, smooth muscle cells in the media and endothelial cells in the intima which lead to healing/scar formation.

Local release of compounds such as vascular endothelial growth factor, basic fibroblast growth factor, and nitric oxide appear to play a role in balancing the inverse relationship between re-endothelialization and smooth muscle proliferation [30-32]. There can be loss and disarray of smooth muscle cells in some areas, resulting in marked thinning of the media with excessive proliferation of smooth muscle cells or neointimal hyperplasia, a potential cause of restenosis.

ANGIOPLASTY CATHETER CHARACTERISTICS

The variety of balloon and catheter configurations available for angioplasty of congenital stenosis is extensive although few have actually been approved by the FDA for the treatment of congenital heart disease in children. Most have been approved for use for peripheral vessels, coronary arteries, or valvuloplasty in adults. FDA approval does not seem to identify balloon catheters that are inherently superior for the management of congenital lesions. It is crucial to consider properties of both the catheter and balloon when selecting an angioplasty catheter for a particular congenital lesion [18,19] (Fig. 5-5).

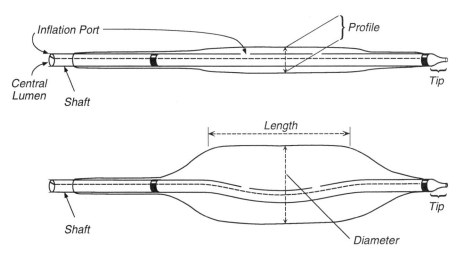

Figure 5-5: Anatomy of an angioplasty catheter in inflated and deflated states. The French size refers to the shaft of the catheter but the profile refers to the diameter of the deflated balloon, which dictates the sheath requirements.

Guidewire Lumen

All current angioplasty catheters currently used for congenital heart disease are delivered to the stenosis over a guidewire. Guidewire lumen diameters range from .014" to .038". Most smaller balloons (< 5-6 mm) used for congenital stenosis have an .018" lumen and most large balloons a .035" lumen. The stiffer the guidewire, the more likely a catheter will be able to follow the wire. There should be a close fit between the lumen and the wire; if the lumen is larger than the wire the gap at the tip can snag on tissue as the balloon moves through the skin, vessels, or heart causing vascular or catheter tip damage and catheter immobilization.

Tip Design

The longer the catheter tip, the smoother the taper of the distal balloon, lowering the catheter's profile and improving its ability to track over a wire. However, a longer catheter tip may prevent reaching a stenosis if it is near an acute angulation in a vessel or bifurcation. In addition, a short catheter tip and balloon taper minimize the trauma to adjacent normal vessels during dilation. For congenital stenosis, especially those in the distal pulmonary artery bed or around vascular curves, a short distal tip is generally preferable.

Shaft Design

Balloons are mounted on catheter shafts ranging in diameter from 3 Fr. to 9 Fr. Most are a true double lumen design with the shaft composed of a polyester, polyethelene, nylon or polyamide derivative. The balloon is attached to the end of the shaft by adhesive and/or thermal bonding. The outer, smaller lumen that is connected to the side port inflates the balloon and may be round, crescent, or a semi circle. It is the area of this second lumen and the length of the catheter which determine the inflation/deflation time of the balloon. The larger this lumen and shorter the catheter the faster the inflation/deflation time. Shaft stiffness is determined by diameter, material and construction design. A rigid shaft will allow easy passage through the inguinal fascia and vessel wall if no sheath is used. A softer more flexible shaft will follow a tortuous guidewire course more easily with less potential trauma to vessels and the heart. Since angioplasty of congenital lesions rarely occurs at the end of a straight line, soft flexible shafts are generally preferable. Obviously, the smaller the shaft diameter the less the vascular trauma from angioplasty, but the longer the inflation/deflation times. In general, the smaller the shaft size the better. The one exception is when considering using an angioplasty balloon for placement of a balloon expandable stent: larger stents may not crimp tightly to an angioplasty catheter with an extremely small shaft.

BALLOON CHARACTERISTICS

Balloon Profile

The balloon profile is the diameter of the catheter over the balloon when it is deflated. This profile determines the French size of the sheath required for passage. With current technology, the balloon profile for larger balloons (≥ 16 mm diameter) is typically 2 or more French sizes larger than the catheter shaft, while for smaller diameter balloons it is 1-2 French sizes larger. There are no advantages to a larger balloon profile. For many balloons, the deflated profile after full inflation is 1-2 French sizes larger than prior to inflation. Thus, many balloons won't come out through the same sheath they went in through. One manufacturer (Olbert) has developed ingenious, double shaft designs that stretch the balloon's length as it passes through the skin or an obstruction to minimize the balloon profile.

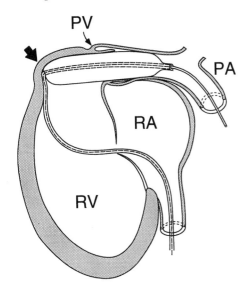

Figure 5-6: Long balloons straighten curved cardiovascular structures during inflation and may cause damage at their proximal or distal ends. This is the probable mechanism of right ventricular free wall injury after pulmonary valve dilation. (Reprinted with permission from Am J Cardiol 55:210, 1985.)

Balloon Length

By convention, manufacturers list as the balloon length the "flat" part of the balloon, often the site of balloon length markers on the shaft.

The shoulder leading up to the balloon is not counted and may be either steep or shallow; on newer balloons they may be mixed with a steep distal shoulder and a shallow proximal shoulder. Shallow shoulders allow for a better balloon taper and lower overall profile but significantly add to the total balloon length. Very long balloons improve stability during inflation if properly positioned. However, since a long balloon will straighten a curved cardiovascular structure at full inflation (and thus may cause injury at the tips of the balloon), shorter balloons (2-3 cm) are preferred for most congenital lesions (Fig 5-6). The exception is aortic stenosis in the older child in whom a 4-6 cm long balloon significantly improves stability for valve dilation.

Balloon Shape

Virtually all balloons have a circular cross-section: wall stress is distributed equally around the circumference and thus will predictably tear the valve or vessel at its weakest point, and they fold to a relatively small profile. Their disadvantage is that during inflation, blood flow across the balloon filled obstruction is abolished. The use of two or three separate balloons, or trefoil balloons mounted on the same shaft will allow blood through interstices during full inflation. Simultaneous double balloon dilation has the advantage of smaller profiles that minimize sheath requirements and potential vascular injury, although they require multiple sites of vascular entry. There are limited data evaluating the unequal distribution of wall stresses that may occur with this technique although no untoward clinical effects have been reported [33].

Balloon Strength, Rupture Characteristics

Most current balloons are made from one of five basic classes of plastic polymers: polyvinyl chloride, polyethylene, polyethylene teraphthalate, nylon, or reinforced polyurethane. Important characteristics of balloon material include compliance (degree of stretch at low pressure), yield strength (pressure at which permanent deformation of the balloon material occurs), ultimate tensile strength (pressure at which balloon rupture occurs), and scratch resistance (ease of perforation). The optimal balloon is extremely scratch resistant and non-compliant, with a very high yield strength equal to the ultimate tensile strength. This maximizes the dilating forces at the lesion and minimizes the chances of balloon rupture or normal vessel injury. This is particularly important in congenital lesions such as branch pulmonary artery stenosis, recoarctation or homograft stenosis, which often require very high dilating pressures for success. Finally, should balloon rupture occur, no plastic should fragment off and the balloon should tear longitudinally. Balloons that are torn circumferentially are very unpleasant: they may umbrella open upon removal from the skin, cause vessel injury, and may be unremovable without an extensive surgical dissection.

Balloon Diameter

In our opinion diameter is the most important variable in choosing a balloon. The proper balloon diameter for a given lesion is based both on experimental studies [5,6] and accumulated clinical experience [13,14]. Both the diameter of the stenosis and the diameter of the surrounding normal vessel must be considered when choosing the balloon diameter. Too small a balloon will be ineffective; too large will result in vessel injury and possibly rupture. Often balloon diameter must be adjusted based on the appearance of a balloon inflated to low pressure. Care must be taken when evaluating the appearance and disappearance of balloon waists. A partially inflated balloon may fold giving the false impression of a waist on one side only. Furthermore, a bona fide waist may disappear not only because of successful dilation but also because of a small shift in position of the balloon or lesion.

SPECIFIC LESIONS

Native Aortic Coarctation

Coarctation is usually due to discrete posterior infolding of the aorta near the ductus arteriosus. The abnormality may extend distally or be associated with hypoplasia of the transverse arch. Histology shows predominantly intimal, but some medial, thickening which protrudes into the vessel lumen. Depletion and disarray of the medial elastic tissue, known as cystic medial necrosis, commonly occurs adjacent to the area of coarctation. Distal to the coarctation intimal proliferation and disruption of the elastic tissue may occur due to high velocity flow through the coarctation.

Despite the extensive clinical information that has accrued since the initial description in 1982, balloon dilation of native coarctation remains controversial. Most centers prefer surgery to angioplasty for infants < 6 months of age because of the unacceptable restenosis rate of 55% at short term follow up [34 - 36].

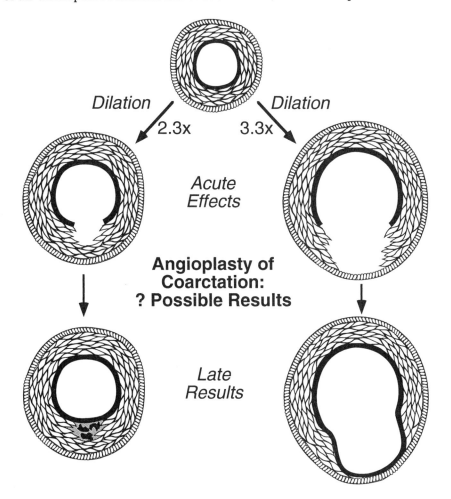

Figure 5-7: Probable mechanism of aneurysm formation after angioplasty. Over-distention may cause a complete transmedial tear resulting in loss and disarray of supporting smooth muscle cells causing a weakening in the vessel wall.

There is currently no consensus on the optimal treatment of native coarctation in older children: the only randomized trial comparing surgery to balloon dilation[36] reported similar immediate results with a higher rate of aneurysm formation and restenosis with angioplasty. Restenosis occurs more often with young age and a hypoplastic transverse arch. Aneurysms following dilation occur in 2 to 5% of patients and appears related to the degree of anatomic enlargement (Fig. 5-7). Progression of aneurysms at intermediate follow up are uncommon but their long term fate remains a major concern. As expected, hospital charges and length of stay are considerably shorter with dilation than with surgery [37].

Based on the clinical data currently available, we do not recommend balloon dilation of native coarctation in infants or children less than 2 years of age unless at increased risk from the standard operative approach (Table 5-1). Long term results of surgery may outweigh the immediate benefits of balloon dilation, especially if the long-term adverse effects of relatively small coarctation gradients are worse than previously suspected. In high-risk surgical patients, balloon dilation has proven to be a very useful procedure. For older children with favorable anatomy, primary balloon dilation can and should be offered as an alternative treatment to surgery. Whether the reduction in acute morbidity and medical costs associated with balloon dilation outweigh the increased need for late repeat intervention and unknown risks of aneurysm formation remain to be seen.

Table 5-1. Probable indications for balloon angioplasty of native aortic coarctation.

---

1. Severe left ventricular dysfunction.
2. Severe pulmonary hypertension or other pulmonary diseases that would raise the risks of thoracotomy.
3. Recent intracranial hemorrhage (berry aneurysm).
4. Other major systemic illnesses.

Procedure

Patients are seen the day before the procedure for a screening physical examination, standard routine lab tests, and type and cross for a unit of blood. Four extremity blood pressure measurements are recorded as a baseline. On the morning of the procedure, a peripheral intravenous line is placed for standard sedation. A femoral venous catheter permits right heart hemodynamic measurements, cardiac output determination, and rapid venous access if needed later in the procedure. We take considerable pains to enter only the anterior femoral arterial wall for any retrograde dilation procedure to minimize bleeding and vessel injury. The puncture site is placed relatively proximally to enter the largest bore femoral vessel possible, heparin is administered intravenously (100 units / kg) intravenously and activated clotted times (ACT) are monitored at 45 to 60 minute intervals. Repeat doses of 50 units / kg of heparin maintain an ACT > 200 seconds. A 4-7 F pigtail catheter is used to complete the left heart hemodynamic study. For larger patients, a 6 or 7 F marker pigtail catheter improves measurement on the angiogram. The coarctation anatomy and transverse arch are precisely defined by angiography, including definition of the narrowest part of the obstruction in two views. The first balloon is chosen using the criteria listed in Table 5-2

With the patient on supplemental oxygen, the pigtail is positioned in the left ventricle. A guidewire, chosen to fit the angioplasty balloon, is curved by hand or a ventricular apex wire used so it will curl in the left ventricle without causing significant ectopy. Recently, we have begun "parking" the wire in the right subclavian artery to reduce ectopy and the risk of emboli. Extra lidocaine is given locally and analgesic given systemically. After enlarging the skin incision, the angioplasty balloon can be prepared on the table or in the descending aorta by initially inflating with CO_2 to remove air and then filling with a dilute (4 to 1) contrast/saline solution. We take considerable care to keep the balloon wetted, turning it so it remains folded as it enters the sheath (usually counterclockwise), and to keep the wire taut to facilitate passage and minimize ectopy. We take pains to leave these large bore catheters and sheaths in the artery for as short a time as possible. The balloon is centered under the obstruction and inflated to low pressure to evaluate the waist. Recording the inflation so replay is available is advantageous. If no waist is seen the balloon is repositioned until one is certain the balloon is centered on the lesion. If still no significant waist is seen, then the catheter is replaced by the next largest size (remaining within the maximal parameters set in Table 5-2). If a very tight waist is seen (Fig. 5-2), we do not inflate to high pressure; we remove the balloon and put in a smaller size. This process may need to be repeated several times to optimize dilation and minimize complications.

After choosing the correct balloon, it is inflated with a pressure gauge until either the waist disappears or the maximal safe inflation pressure is reached. Inflation times need not be longer than 30 seconds. One should only exceed the recommended burst pressure of the balloon with caution: balloon rupture can lead to aneurysm formation as well as other vascular injury. One should always know the actual (not the manufacturer's) maximum inflation pressure maximum for the balloons in use in one's laboratory. The actual burst pressures for commonly used balloons are listed in Table 5-3.

TABLE 5-2. Coarctation angioplasty balloon size

a. > 2.5 but no greater than 5 times the coarctation diameter
b. 100% but no greater than 110 % the diameter of the aorta above or below the coarctation
c. the shortest balloon possible, 2 cm for infants and children, 3 or 4 cm for adolescents and adults
d. smallest possible shaft and balloon profile to minimize arterial sheath size

TABLE 5-3. Recommended and rupture inflation pressures for selected balloon catheters

Balloon name (Manufacturer)	Balloon Diameter (mm)	Max Inflation Pressure (ATM) Manufacturer	Actual
LOWER PRESSURE			
Schwarten (Mallinkrodt)	4	5	8
Proflex 5 (Mallinkrodt)	6	6	8
Tyshak (Braun)	8	5	6
Accent (Cook)	8	8	10
Accent (Cook)	12	5	8
XXL (Meditech)	12	8	16
Tyshak (Braun)	16	2	4
HIGHER PRESSURE			
Sub four (Meditech)	4	10	14
Ranger (Scimed)	4	12	20
Ultrathin Diamond(Meditech)	6	15	18
Z-med (Braun)	12	7	12
Blue max (Meditech)	12	17	> 20
Z med (Braun)	16	5	8
XXL (Meditech)	16	5	14

Tearing of the coarctation site almost always causes chest pain or, less commonly, throat, arm or ear pain. The pain usually subsides within a minute or so after balloon deflation: persistent severe pain can herald an extensive aortic tear. During the procedure, experienced nursing personnel monitor blood pressure from an arm cuff, manage the airway, and administer extra analgesia/sedation as needed. We routinely inspect fluoroscopically the mediastinum before and after dilation of the aorta or pulmonary arteries and have blood available in the room at the time of dilation. Acute hypertension, which fortunately occurs rarely following balloon angioplasty, should be treated aggressively to prevent extension of an aortic tear. Adequacy of analgesia should be assessed but if hypertension persists, or if the aortic tear appears larger than desired, we treat with intravenous beta-blockers.

Once the vessel has been dilated, leave the guidewire in position, remove the angioplasty catheter, rotating counterclockwise through the sheath, and replace it with a Gensini or cut pigtail. (If one uses a pigtail catheter without a wire after successful dilation, the tip of the pigtail may snag on the intimal tear during pullback and cause considerable trauma). A repeat angiogram and gradient are obtained, in that order. If there is concern of residual stenosis on the angiogram then the pullback should be obtained over the wire. When recrossing a recently (< 2 month) dilated vessel, very soft wires, preferably looped, will reduce the risk of vascular injury.

Finally, the sheath is removed and pressure is applied to the arterial entry site. It is quite important to perform this task correctly: the hole in the artery is proximal to the hole in the skin, and applying pressure on the latter site may result in visual hemostasis, but a subinguinal hematoma. Further, if too much pressure is applied for too long (> 30 minutes) one can propagate clots above and below the bleeding site, promoting sustained vascular thrombosis. After 5-10 minutes of heavy pressure, one should attempt to gently reduce pressure to allow blood flow through the vessel (palpable pedal pulse) but not through the hole in the artery. In general, pressure application will be needed 10 to 20 minutes after arterial angioplasty. We never rely on sandbags or mechanical devices to achieve hemostasis.

Complications

Balloon angioplasty of native coarctation is a safe procedure, even for patients with substantial associated diseases. Death has been reported in less than 1% of patients in the largest multicenter series [38] and appears related to the patient's pre-morbid condition at the time of the procedure. Aortic rupture has been reported but is extremely rare and has mostly been related to balloons with very tight waists. Aortic aneurysms, usually small, have been reported in 2 to 7% of patients. The incidence is partly dependent on definition and technique used for detection. Progression of aneurysms at intermediate follow up is rare, but does occur. Neurologic events have occurred in less than 1 % of patients and have been associated with inadequate anticoagulation or prolonged positioning of a deflated balloon around the arch. Because of the reports of rare but significant late complications, we monitor patients for at least 12 hours after the procedure

132

with a reliable I.V. in place. Trauma to the femoral artery is the only real morbidity we have encountered with the incidence of clinically detectable injury at discharge below 5% with our current practice of low profile balloons, heparinization during the case and aggressive treatment with streptokinase later if a palpable pulse is absent. Of more concern, however, is the 40% incidence of significant iliofemoral artery stenosis noted at follow up when evaluated with non invasive studies such as Doppler or MRI [39]. Risk factors for vessel injury include larger catheter / sheath size and small patient size.

Results
Immediate success, if defined as an increase in coarctation diameter with residual gradient less than 20 mmHg, occurs in 80-90 % of patients dilated with an average gradient reduction of 75% (Fig 5-8).

Figure 5-8: Successful balloon angioplasty of a coarctation in a child with associated mitral stenosis.

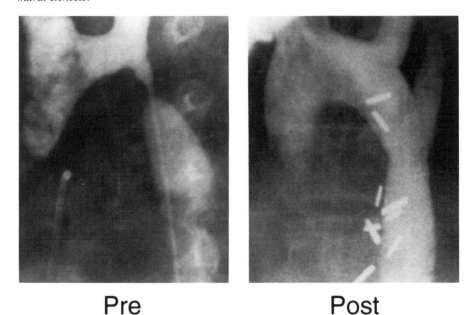

Pre   Post

In general, gradient relief after angioplasty of native coarctation has been less complete than that seen after surgical repair. Restenosis rates at intermediate follow up are directly related to age at dilation: 85% for neonates, 35% for infants, and 10% for children over 2 years. Long term follow up remains limited but for children older than 1 month at dilation freedom from restenosis at 10 years is approximately 65% [34]. Repeat dilation of restenosis has immediate results similar to initial dilation [40] however follow up data is currently unavailable.

Recurrent Aortic Coarctation

Operative management of recurrent coarctation can be difficult. Operative mortality has been reported in 0 to 15%. Significant morbidity, including paraplegia and late aneurysm formation have been reported in up to 6% [41]. These risks are particularly concerning for those patients with recoarctation following arch reconstruction for single ventricle physiology, who will need additional surgeries to achieve complete palliation. For these reasons we consider balloon angioplasty the treatment of choice for recurrent coarctation, including patients who have had complex repair of interrupted arch or aortic atresia.

Procedure
The technique is virtually the same as noted above for native coarctation. Recurrent coarctations are, however, somewhat less compliant lesions and often require higher inflation pressures with high pressure balloons. Occasionally, long periods (2-4 minutes) of high pressure inflation will eliminate a waist when more conventional periods of inflation (e.g. 15-30 seconds) fail. As in native coarctation dilation, patients are monitored in hospital for 12 to 24 hours after the procedure with a reliable intravenous line in place. Patients who have recurrent coarctation following complex arch reconstruction for interruption, aortic atresia, or hypoplastic left heart syndrome often have associated hemodynamic lesions (single ventricle physiology, VSD, PA band, sub AS, etc).

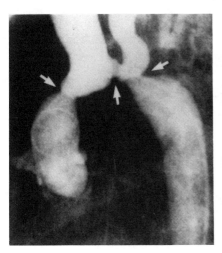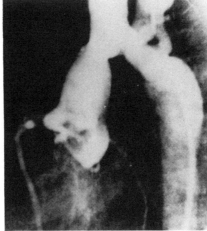

Figure 5-9:   Successful dilation angioplasty of several aortic obstructions (arrows) following repair of an interrupted aortic arch.

We therefore often intubate and ventilate these patients to optimize stability. The aortic obstructions following arch interruption repair are unpredictable, occurring in the ascending, transverse, or descending aorta and may be multiple (Fig 5-9).

Several aortograms are often necessary to adequately define the obstructions.

Recoarctation following arch reconstruction for aortic atresia or hypoplastic left ventricle is almost always at the distal end of the anastomosis in the proximal descending aorta.   Angiographic definition is best obtained with a balloon occlusion descending aortogram using a balloon tipped catheter passed antegrade from the right ventricle (Fig 5-10).   The technique for dilation in these patients differs from that described above.   A 5-7 F balloon tipped end-hole catheter is passed from the right ventricle through the pulmonary valve across the anastomosis to the descending aorta.   Often the area of coarctation is quite narrow and tortuous so a torque wire is used to advance into the descending aorta.   These patients are often unstable with poor ventricular function so it is imperative to perform the dilation as rapidly as possible

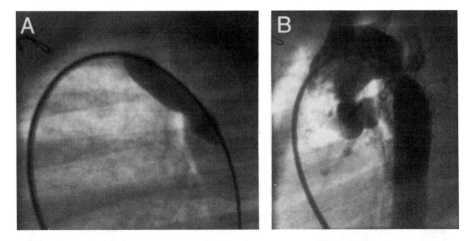

Figure 5-10:   Antegrade balloon dilation of a recoarctation (A) in a patient with hypoplastic left heart syndrome 4 months after stage 1 Norwood palliation (B) = post dilation cine.

Occasionally, the wire or catheter will prop open the tricuspid valve and induce cardiac arrest even prior to dilation.   Cardiopulmonary resuscitation is often required.   Because of the tortuous catheter course through the heart a short (2 cm long) balloon catheter with a flexible shaft is used.

Complications

Mortality associated with balloon dilation of recoarctation is 0.7% [38] and appears, in part, due to the pre-morbid state of the patient. Aortic rupture has been reported but is extremely rare and, as in native coarctation, appears often related to oversized balloons. Neurologic complications occur in less than 1% and aneurysm formation at late follow up occurs in less than 2% [42]. Complications do not seem to correlate with the type of initial surgical repair although some have raised concerns regarding the lack of scar tissue that forms following Gore-Tex patch repair. The most significant complication remains femoral artery injury with pulse loss reported in 4 to 22 % of patients, up to 16% of whom require treatment with either heparin, thrombolytic therapy, or rarely, surgery.

Results

A successful acute result, if defined as a residual gradient < 20 mmHg, occurs in 74 to 88 % of patients dilated with an average gradient reduction of 75%. The more severe the obstruction the more likely a sub-optimal result. Long term follow up data are limited but 3 year median freedom from reintervention is 72% for those patients who have successful dilation. As expected, hypoplastic transverse arch is a risk factor for repeat intervention. Repeat angioplasty can be successfully performed; however, there is a 60% failure rate at 2 year follow up [42].

Hypoplastic / Stenotic Branch Pulmonary Arteries

The pathology of branch pulmonary artery stenosis ranges from isolated discrete central stenosis to multiple segmental stenoses associated with syndromes such as Williams' or Alagille's to diffusely "hypoplastic" arteries associated with complex intracardiac abnormalities such as pulmonary atresia with VSD. In discrete central or segmental lesions, histology most often shows medial hypertrophy with a decrease in elastic fibers and disorganization of smooth muscle cells. In addition there is usually marked intimal hyperplasia. In diffusely "hypoplastic" arteries the intima, media and adventitia may appear normal but small.

Balloon dilation or stenting of stenotic pulmonary arteries has the narrowest therapeutic window of any of the interventional procedures commonly performed in children with congenital heart disease. The mortality rate associated with the procedure has been reported as high as 3% [14] with a clinical (as opposed to angiographic or hemodynamic) benefit noted in as few as 35 % of patients in early reports [43]. Thus, patients selected for dilation should have significant cardiac disease: significantly elevated right ventricular pressures, marked inequality of pulmonary blood flow, or symptoms. Despite these facts, transcatheter dilation or stenting remains the first line treatment in most patients with pulmonary artery stenosis because of limited success with surgical repair.

136

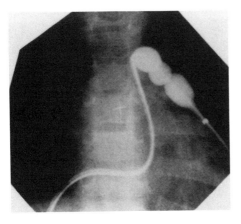

Figure 5-11: Balloon inflated across a "hypoplastic" left pulmonary artery. Note the multiple areas of stenoses demonstrated by the multiple waists.

Nearly all types of pulmonary anatomy can be successfully dilated to one degree or another. Exceptions are very rare cases of diffuse hypoplasia of the pulmonary bed extending out past the 3rd or 4th branch, and native stenoses of collateral vessels in patients with pulmonary atresia with VSD. Even in difficult patients, however, we are currently unable to predict how an individual stenotic lesion will respond to balloon dilation. Often, hypoplastic central vessels are simply vessels with serial obstructions: when one inflates a long balloon across the diffusely narrowed vessel, one sees multiple waists, as if there were 2 or 3 stenoses in a row with a relatively normal vessel in between (Fig 5-11).

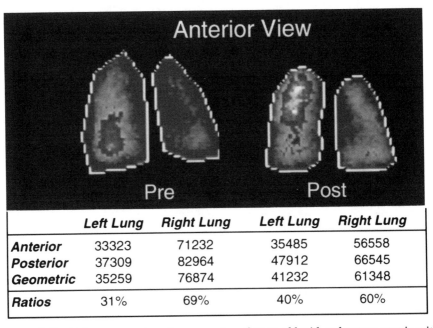

	Pre		Post	
	Left Lung	*Right Lung*	*Left Lung*	*Right Lung*
Anterior	33323	71232	35485	56558
Posterior	37309	82964	47912	66545
Geometric	35259	76874	41232	61348
Ratios	31%	69%	40%	60%

Figure 5-12: Pulmonary nuclear flow scans in a 2 year old with pulmonary atresia with ventricular septal defect who is status post surgical unifocalization before and after balloon dilation of a right lower pulmonary artery stenosis. Note the marked discrepant flow that increases significantly to the right lower lobe after dilation.

Relief of multiple stenosis can markedly enlarge a hypoplastic vessel. With the use of high pressure balloons, (> 20 atmospheres) even difficult collateral stenosis can sometimes be dilated or stretched making the lesions amenable to stent therapy. Most who recommend this are primarily dilating older patients with central stenoses; we reserve primary stenting for older patients with central obstructions.

If right ventricular hypertension is suspected to be $\geq$ systemic levels, general anesthesia is used. Femoral arterial and venous cannulation permits hemodynamic assessments and rapid arterial pressure monitoring. The patient is heparinized and activated clotting times are monitored. Because of the risk of pulmonary artery dilation, we always have blood available in the cath lab during the procedure.

Selective biplane right and left pulmonary angiograms are performed using either a cut pigtail or Gensini catheter over a guidewire. The detailed pulmonary artery anatomy defined by angiography is correlated with the information from the pre-catheterization nuclear flow scan to develop a plan for dilation. The most severe lesion is dilated first: since the balloon will be occluding the smallest amount of flow it will be the safest hemodynamic lesion to dilate. Multiple lesions may be dilated during the procedure but extreme care must be taken not to cross recently dilated lesions with anything other than a very floppy guidewire.
After angiography the end-hole catheter is placed across the lesion into the distal pulmonary artery tree. For central lesions, placement into a posterior lower lobe segment, to the level of the diaphragm in the AP view, gives the most stable position. For lesions requiring dilating balloons $\geq$ 6mm in diameter, a .035 or .038" exchange guidewire is placed distally. For lesions requiring smaller balloons, either a .014 or .018" guidewire is used. We take considerable care, including small hand injections of contrast and repositioning with a torque wire if necessary, to insure the catheter and guidewire are in the largest lobar artery available distal to the stenosis. If the exchange wire passes into a small distal vessel, balloon dilation can cause a tubular aneurysm distal to the lesion (Fig 5-13).
With the guidewire in proper distal position, the end-hole catheter removed, and a sheath that will accommodate the appropriate sized balloon catheter, a balloon is advanced to straddle the lesion. The balloon should be short with a minimal tip length, and a diameter 3 to 4 times the lesion diameter but no larger than 2 times the diameter of the normal distal pulmonary artery. Because pulmonary artery lesions are often difficult to dilate we routinely start with a high-pressure balloon [16].

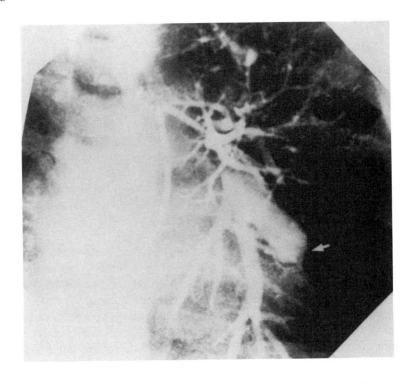

Figure 5-13: Aneurysm (arrow) produced in the distal pulmonary artery after attempted balloon angioplasty. Inflating the balloon when the distal tip is positioned in a small vessel distal to the stenosis most likely causes the aneurysm.

If the balloon is prepared outside the body as described for coarctation dilation, one must take care to recompress the balloon before using since it can be very difficult to get the balloon to cross these peripheral stenoses. As with coarctation, pulmonary artery dilation causes pain, so adequate analgesia should be given prior to inflation.

The balloon is advanced over the wire using the straightest possible wire course through the heart and pulmonary arteries. Occasionally, the formation of a large right atrial loop will contain the catheter course and force a recalcitrant catheter to follow the wire. During this maneuver, pressure on the SA or AV node may result in bradycardia or heart block. Very short, brisk, vibrating, thrusts over a tautly held wire or the use of a buttressing long sheath positioned in the main pulmonary artery may get a catheter to follow the wire when all else fails. If a standard wire keeps pulling back when the balloon is advanced into the lesion, we remove the angioplasty catheter and advance a guiding catheter past the lesion to the distal bed. The standard wire is then either exchanged for a stiff wire (such as a "Rosen" or "Amplatz extra stiff"), or rarely the stiff end of the wire (hand formed to match the curve of the pulmonary artery). With care taken to avoid perforation, this technique has proven safe and effective. If multiple lesions in series are present, the most distal lesion should be dilated first. Once the balloon is distal to that lesion, it is brought back over the wire and centered. It is better to have the balloon a bit too distal rather than too proximal. It allows for better control and will prevent the balloon from being pushed centrally out of the lesion as the proximal end of the balloon inflates. When inflated to low pressure the waist should be obvious but not marked (Fig 5-2:). If the waist is too subtle or too marked the balloon size is adjusted. Once adequate position and balloon size are established, the balloon is inflated until the waist completely disappears or the maximum inflation pressure is reached (Table 3). Because we use high-pressure balloons, this often requires an insuflator to achieve adequate inflation pressures. Inflation times are generally kept short but inflations may be repeated several times to assure a centered inflation is achieved. Rarely, prolonged inflation will succeed when standard inflation times do not. Dilation of proximal lesions may result in complete obstruction of right ventricular outflow and associated hypotension, making quick deflation and adequate recovery between inflations essential.

The balloon catheter is removed and a cut pigtail or Gensini catheter is advanced over the wire for repeat hemodynamic measurements and angiography. Once a satisfactory result has been achieved or the largest appropriate balloon has been used, the catheter and wire are removed and attention is turned to any additional lesions. Extreme care must be taken to keep catheters and wires away from the newly dilated vessel when crossing an additional lesion. Additional lesions are crossed using only a high torque floppy wire. We have successfully dilated as many as 8-10 lesions in both lungs at one procedure by dilating distal lesions first and taking extreme care to avoid previously dilated areas when crossing additional lesions.

Efficacy of balloon dilation can and should be assessed in several ways. An increase in pulsatility and mean pressure distal to the dilation as well as angiographic diameter increase suggest a beneficial effect, as does a significant fall in RV pressure. A nuclear pulmonary flow scan should be obtained after the procedure to assess redistribution of flow (Fig 5-12). Patients are monitored carefully after the procedure for at least 12 hours. If we are concerned about an aneurysm on angiogram or the development of segmental pulmonary edema (an acute increase in mean pressure to > 30 mmHg in dilated segments) we observe the patient in the ICU. Any respiratory symptoms or complaints of chest pain are evaluated immediately.

Complications

This is a hazardous interventional procedure in children, with complications quite dependent on procedural technique. Procedural related death has been reported in 3% of patients, although recent results from Boston suggest a mortality rate less than 1% in the most recent 400 cases [44]. Death has been attributed to vessel rupture due either to balloon or wire perforation, bradycardic arrest associated with supra-systemic RV pressure or severe hypoxia during dilation, and in one case, neurologic due to a paradoxical embolus. Aneurysm formation occurs in 5% [44] with one case report of late rupture causing death, occurring two weeks after dilation in a patient with Williams syndrome [45]. Transient pulmonary edema has occurred in 3% which is easily managed with supportive care, diuretics + positive pressure ventilation, without late sequelae. The most common cause of death has been pulmonary arterial rupture, usually in an artery distal to the narrowing. When a tear producing an extravascular collection of contrast is demonstrated, we watch to be certain that the hemorrhage is confined and non-progressive. If bleeding into the chest or airway is progressive, most patients will die unless the bleeding is physically corrected. Recently, we have reduced the mortalities in pulmonary artery dilation by routinely coil occluding the vessels producing unconfined pulmonary hemorrhage [44]. Similarly, death due to unmanageable hemodynamic instability in patients with William syndrome and severe bilateral outflow tract obstruction can be avoided by creating a decompressing atrial communication at the very beginning of the case.

As noted above, meticulous attention to detail is mandatory. Positioning the guidewire in the largest possible distal vessel and carefully monitoring the distal portion of the balloon during inflation will minimize distal vessel aneurysm formation. Limiting the balloon diameter to no greater than 2.5 times the normal surrounding pulmonary artery diameter will reduce vessel rupture. Aggressive support with general anesthesia, 100% O_2, and a decompressing atrial septostomy during dilation in patients with supra-systemic RV pressures will reduce the risk of bradycardic arrest.

Results
Acute success, if defined as either an increase of $\geq$ 50% of predilation diameter, an increase of > 20% of flow to the affected lung, or a decrease of > 20% in systolic right ventricular to aortic pressure ratio, occurs in 55% of vessel dilations [43, 46]. Significant clinical improvement has been estimated at 35 to 50 % [46, 47]. Long term follow up is not available but midterm results out to 4 years suggest a 15% restenosis rate (10 month median follow up) [43]. Predictors of success have not been well established; however a balloon to lesion ratio of < 3 is a risk factor for failure [14, 43]. The effectiveness of dilation in sub-groups of patients, such as those with Williams or Alagille's syndrome, has not yet been defined.

Main Pulmonary Artery Stenosis

Main pulmonary artery stenosis or supra-valvar stenosis occurs both as a primary congenital lesion and as an acquired post operative lesion in patients following banding or arterial switch repair for transposition of the great arteries. The pathophysiologies of these two lesions are distinctly different, as one would suspect. Native congenital stenosis occurs just above the valve at the pulmonary sinotubular ridge and consists of both medial and intimal hypertrophy and tethering of the pulmonary valve leaflets in this area. Post operative lesions occur at the site of end to end anastomoses and are due to longitudinal stretching or circumferential proliferative scarring. Native lesions respond poorly to angioplasty, most likely because the ability to generate an adequate dilating force with a large enough balloon is limited by the proximity and size of the pulmonary annulus. Post-operative lesions due to stretching or kinking require stents. Post operative lesions due to circumferential scarring, on the other hand, can be responsive to angioplasty.

Procedure
After careful assessment of right heart hemodynamics, angiography in the MPA is performed to assess the significance of the stenosis. Generally straight lateral, and AP angiograms with cranial angulation, optimizes visualization of the lesion. Once measurements of the stenosis, distal MPA, and pulmonary valve annulus diameter are made, a balloon $\geq$ 2.5 times the lesion diameter but $\leq$ 1.4 times the pulmonary valve annulus is chosen. The wire can be placed in the distal lower lobe of either branch PA, preferably the one with the most direct course, which is most often the left. We typically use high pressure balloons. Because of a small incidence of aneurysm formation, repeat hemodynamics and angiograms should be performed over the existing guidewire with the use of a 'Y' adapter, and either a cut off pigtail or Gensini.

Results
There are no series reported of native supra-valvar stenosis dilation but our results have been largely unrewarding and we do not advocate dilation except in unusual circumstances. Successful dilation of post operative stenoses occurs in 50% if defined as either a $\geq$ 50% increase in angiographic diameter or $\geq$ 50% reduction in systolic pressure gradient [48]. Aneurysm or rupture occurs rarely, and may result in the development of an aorto-pulmonary window due to scarring of the aorta to the pulmonary artery after switch repair.

<u>**Homograft / Conduit Stenosis**</u>
Stenosis in RV to PA homografts or conduits occurs in all growing children, although the time from initial placement varies greatly depending on the age of the child, associated lesions, the state of the distal pulmonary bed, and other factors. The pathophysiology includes mechanical distortion such as kinking or sternal compression, bioprosthetic valve calcification, diffuse intimal hyperplasia and/or calcification, homograft "shrinkage", or scar formation at anastomotic sites. Most of these causes of obstruction will not respond to dilation alone, but will respond to stenting [49,50]. Stenosis within the homograft or conduit usually occurs at the RV or PA anastomotic sites if it is due to scar formation or mechanical

distortion, and at the valve or in areas of turbulent flow due to calcification or intimal hyperplasia. Many factors must be considered when deciding to palliate a homograft or conduit stenosis with balloon dilation. Often these stenotic lesions are associated with some degree of pulmonary insufficiency that may be exacerbated by dilation of the stenosis. Therefore, in addition to the site and presumed pathophysiology of the stenosis, assessment of right ventricular dilation and function are critical in deciding whether surgical replacement, balloon palliation, or stenting is the optimal treatment for a given patient. Moderate to severe stenotic lesions that are primarily valvar, or at anastomotic sites with minimal pulmonary insufficiency where right ventricular function is largely preserved, are appropriate for balloon dilation. If severe pulmonary insufficiency is present in the setting of significant right ventricular dysfunction, then we recommend surgical replacement.

Procedure
After a detailed right heart hemodynamic study, an AP angiogram with moderate cranial angulation and a straight lateral will often demonstrate the stenosis best. Because there is limited capacity for homografts or conduits to tear through intima into media we recommend balloon sizes limited to 110% of the implanted homograft/conduit diameter. Calcified lesions may require high pressure balloons.

Results
Although not curative, balloon dilation of stenotic conduit or homograft lesions can delay the need for surgical replacement in growing children. Dilation of stenotic valved homografts or conduits has been successful in up to 50% of cases with an average gradient reduction of 45% [51]. The increase in insufficiency that may occur with the use of stents in homograft or conduit stenosis, particularly if the valve must be crossed, must be weighed carefully against the potential benefit of stenosis relief. Aneurysm formation or conduit/homograft rupture has been reported and is of particular risk if oversized balloons are used to dilate calcified conduits or homografts.

Mustard / Senning Baffle Obstruction

Although uncommon, we still encounter patients with baffle obstruction following intra atrial repair of TGA. Baffle obstruction has been reported in up to 13% of patients following the Mustard repair [52] and 16% after Senning [53]. Stenosis is most often in the superior limb of the baffle, although it can occur in the inferior limb, and is presumed due to scar formation along the baffle suture line at the atrial septum. Pulmonary venous stenosis does occur, although quite infrequently. Careful assessment of the location of obstruction with echocardiography is essential prior to catheterization; in the older patient this may necessitate a transesophageal study. In general, stenting is the preferred therapy for these obstructions, although the principles derived from dilations apply directly to stent use.

Procedure

Femoral venous access is followed by hemodynamic measurements and angiograms, initially in the AP and lateral projection. Often repeat angled views are necessary. Additional access via subclavian or jugular veins can be helpful for simultaneous pressure measurements and to assure a stable wire position by externalization of the wire. Balloon positioning can be difficult because of the tortuous course of the baffle and the distortion that occurs when the guidewire is passed through the lesion. A repeat angiogram with the wire in place is often necessary prior to dilation to assure proper balloon positioning.

Because these lesions are quite compliant, the initial balloon diameter should be 5 times the lesion diameter but no greater than 2.5 times the normal SVC diameter. Simultaneous two balloon dilation is often required in older children[33] to achieve an adequate balloon diameter / lesion ratio. The balloon is inflated to low pressure and the waist inspected. If optimum, then the inflation pressure is increased until complete resolution of the waist or the maximal inflation pressure is reached. Although balloon angioplasty is often successful, stents have generally become the procedure of choice for those lesions.

Complications

Of the 25 cases in the literature there have been no reported complications. In our experience there have been no deaths. However, among 7 patients two developed significant tears in and around the heart. Although one resolved spontaneously, one required operative intervention which was successful. As with catheter-based relief of other compliant lesions, the use of stents has strongly replaced dilation alone.

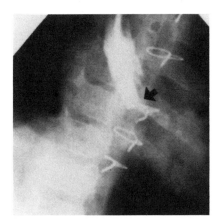 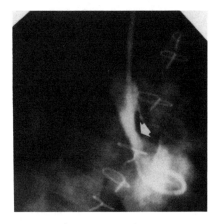

Figure 5-14: Successfully dilated systemic venous baffle obstruction (white arrow) following Mustard repair of transposition of the great arteries; near occlusion is seen in the predilation angiogram (left; black arrow)

144

Results

The two largest series reported [12,54], including our own experience, would suggest the procedure is successful in over 85% of cases (Fig. 5-14). Long term follow up is limited to a handful of patients but the restenosis rate is low out to 7 years [54]. With the judicious use of stents, we would expect the immediate success rate to increase and restenosis rate to decrease even further.

SVC / IVC Stenosis

Although extremely rare as a primary isolated lesion, SVC or IVC obstruction can occur in children with congenital heart disease after surgery such as caval pulmonary connection or prolonged cannulation such as with pacemaker or central line placement. The pathophysiology therefore varies from internal luminal thrombus with intimal proliferation to vessel distortion or stretch to, in rare cases, external compression. Indications for treatment of SVC obstruction include symptomatic SVC syndrome with plethora and venous congestion of the face and arms

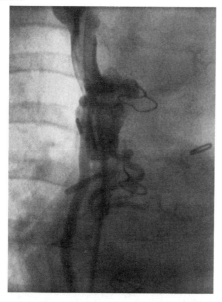

Figure 5-15: Large venous collaterals to the IVC due to SVC stenosis following total anomalous venous return repair.

In the setting of single ventricle physiology after either a Glenn or Fontan palliation even mild degrees of obstruction can be clinically significant. In patients with the need for chronic SVC cannulation, intervention may be needed to reestablish patency for repeat pacing or central line placement. Careful angiographic and hemodynamic evaluation is critical prior to intervention with particular attention to decompressing venous collaterals which may affect both the clinical significance of the stenosis and the severity of the measured pressure gradient. An example is the patient with a Glenn shunt stenosis who develops large SVC to IVC collaterals; these decrease the SVC gradient and reduce effective pulmonary blood flow causing worsening cyanosis (Fig. 5-15).

Procedure

Technical considerations are similar to those described for baffle obstructions. Vascular access from below and above the lesion, with simultaneous angiography, is mandatory if there is complete occlusion and a new communication must be reestablished. The complete obstruction can be crossed with either the stiff end of a .018" wire or a transseptal needle. Once the lesion is crossed, the small wire is snared from the opposite side and the lesion is sequentially dilated starting with a 4 mm balloon. Because of the compliant nature of the systemic veins, balloons with diameters 5 times greater than the stenosis (up to 2.5 times the normal surrounding vein) may be necessary, although angiograms after each dilation and before final stenting will reveal aneurysms that threaten to become transvascular tears.

Results

Post-operative venous stenosis dilation can be very effective, acutely reducing the mean gradient by >80% in up to 100% of patients [55]. However, restenosis is common, occurring in up to 65% of older patients by 1 year. Because of this high restenosis rate we now prefer to place stents in venous stenosis in most patients. In the very small child, too small to accept an adult size stent, we use angioplasty alone with repeat dilations as needed (Fig 5-16).

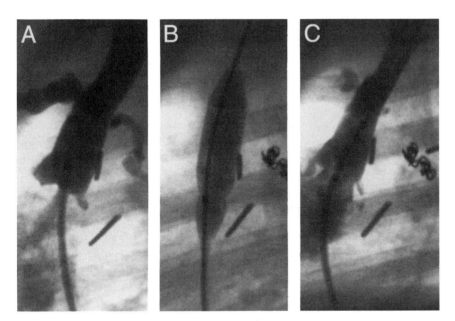

Figure 5-16: Successful dilation of severe SVC stenosis in an infant (A) = pre; (B) dilation; (C) post dilation.

Pulmonary Vein Stenosis

The pathophysiology of native pulmonary vein stenosis has generally been thought to be intimal proliferation, occasionally discrete medial hypertrophy, and often diffuse hypoplasia. Isolated vein stenosis can occur although more often multiple veins are affected. Post operative stenosis in patients with anomalous pulmonary venous return may be due to mechanical distortion, anastomotic site scar or diffuse intimal hyperplasia. The results of balloon dilation of unoperated pulmonary vein stenoses have been extremely disappointing [8] and have not been substantially improved with the use of stents. Although there are occasionally good immediate results, particularly with stent placement, restenosis rates approach 100%. We consider unoperated stenotic pulmonary veins to be undilatable lesions. Balloon dilation with stent placement may be a reasonable palliative bridge to lung transplant in select patients. Pulmonary venous stenoses following repair after infancy can be successfully dilated, and should be attempted when indicated.

REFERENCES

1. Dotter C.T. and Judkins MP. Transluminal treatment of arteriosclerotic obstruction. *Circulation* 1964, 30: 654-679.
2. Gruntzig A, and Hopff H. Perkutane Rekanalisation chronisher arterieller Verschlusse mit einem neuen Dilatationskatheter: Modification der Dotter-Technik. Deutsch Med. Wschr.1974, 99:2502-2505.
3. Gruntzig AR. Transluminal dilation of coronary artery stenosis. Lancet 1975, 1:263.
4. Casteneda-Zuniga WR, Formanek A, Tadavarthy M, et al. The mechanism of balloon angioplasty. Radiology 1980, 135:565-571.
5. Lock JE, Niemi T, Einzig S, et al. Transvenous angioplasty of experimental branch pulmonary artery stenosis in newborn lambs. Circulation 1981, 64: 886-893.
6. Lock JE, Niemi T, Burke BA, et al. Transcutaneous angioplasty of experimental aortic coarctation. Circulation 1982, 66:1280-1286.
7. Singer MI, Rowen M, Dorsey TJ. Transluminal aortic balloon angioplasty for coarctation of the aorta in the newborn. Am Heart J 1982, 103:131-132.
8. Driscoll DJ, Hesslein PS, Mullins CE. Congenital stenosis of individual pulmonary veins: clinical spectrum and unsuccessful treatment by transvenous balloon dilation. Am J Cardiol 1982, 49: 1767-1772.
9. Rocchini AP, Cho KJ, Byrum C, et al. Transluminal angioplasty of superior vena cava obtruction in a 15 month old child. Chest 1982, 82: 506.
10. Lock JE, Casteneda-Zuniga WR, Fuhrman BP. Balloon dilation angioplasty of hypoplastic and stenotic pulmonary arteries. Circulation 1983, 67:962-967.

11. Lock JE, Bass JL, Amplatz K, et al. Balloon dilation angioplasty of aortic coarctation in infants and children. Circulation 1983, 68: 109-116.
12. Lock JE, Bass JL, Casteneda-Zuniga WR, et al. Dilation angioplasty of congenital or operative narrowings of venous channels. Circulation 1983, 70: 457-464.
13. Hellenbrand WE, Allen HD, Golinko RJ, et al. Balloon angioplasty for aortic recoarctation: results of the valvuloplasty and and angioplasty of congenital anomalies registry. Am J Cardiol 1990, 65: 793-797.
14. Kan JS, Marvin WJ, Bass JL, et al. Balloon angioplasty-branch pulmonary artery stenosis: results of the Valvuloplasty and Angioplasty of Congenital Anomalies Registry. Am J Cardiol 1990, 65: 798-801.
15. Mullins CE, Balloon dilation of miscellaneous lesions: results of the Valvuloplasty and Angioplasty of Congenital Anomalies Registry. Am J Cardiol 1990, 65: 802-803.
16. Gentles TL, Lock JE, Perry SB. High pressure balloon angioplasty for branch pulmonary artery stenosis: early experience. J Am Coll Cardiol 1993, 22: 867-872.
17. O'Laughlin MP, Perry SB, Lock JE, et al. Use of endovascular stents in congenital heart disease. Circulation 1991, 83: 1923-1939.
18. Matsumoto AH, Barth KH, Selby JB Jr, et al. Peripheral angioplasty balloon technology. Cardiovascular and Interventional Radiology 1993, 16(3):135-43.
19. Abele, JE. Balloon catheters and transluminal dilation: Technical considerations. A.J.R. 1980, 135:901-906.
20. Sos T, Sniderman KW, Rettek-Sos B, et al. Percutaneous transluminal dilation of thoracic aorta postmortem. Lancet 1979, 2:970-71.
21. Lock JE, Casteneda-Zuniga WR, Bass JL, et al. Balloon dilation of excised aortic coarctation. Radiology 1982, 143:688-691.
22. Sohn S, Rothman A, Shiota T, et al. Acute and follow up intravascular ultrasound findings after balloon dilation of coarctation of the aorta. Circulation 1994, 90:340-347.
23. Tong A, Rothman A, Atkinson RL, et al. Intravascular ultrasound imaging of coarctation of the aorta: animal and human studies. American Journal of Cardiac Imaging 1995, 9:250-256.
24. Ino T, Okubo M, Akimoto K, et al. Mechanism of balloon angioplasty in children with arterial stenosis assessed by intravascular ultrasound and angiography. Am Heart J 1995, 129:132-138.
25. Stock JH, Reller MD, Sharma S, et al. Transballoon intravascular ultrasound imaging during balloon angioplasty in animal models with coarctation and branch pulmonary artery stenosis. Circulation 1997, 95:2354-2357.
26. Waller BF, Girod DA, Dillon JC. Transverse aortic wall tears in infants after balloon angioplasty for aortic stenosis: Relation of aortic wall damage to diameter of inflated angioplasty balloon and aortic lumen in 7 necropsy cases. JACC 1984, 4:1235-1241.

148

27. Edwards BS, Lucas RV, Lock JE, et al. Morphologic changes in the pulmonary arteries following percutaneous balloon angioplasty for pulmonary arterial stenosis. Circulation 1985, 71:195-201.
28. Marvin WJ, Mahoney LT, Rose EF. Pathologic sequelae of balloon dilation angioplasty for unoperated coarctation of the aorta in infants and children. JACC 1986, 7:117A.
29. Brandt III B, Marvin Jr. WJ, Rose EF, et al. Surgical treatment of coarctation of the aorta after balloon angioplasty. J Thorac Cardiovasc Surg 1987, 94:715-719.
30. Asahara T, Bauters C, Pastore C, et al. Local delivery of vascular endothelial growth factor accelerates reendothelialization and attenuates intimal hyperplasia in balloon injured rat carotid artery. Circulation 1995, 91:2793-2801.
31. Lee JS, Adrie C, Jacob HJ, et al. Chronic injury of nitric oxide inhibits neointimal formation after balloon induced arterial injury. Circ Res 1996, 78:337-342.
32. Reidy MA. Biology of disease: A reassessment of endothelial injury and arterial lesion formation. Lab Invest 1985, 53:513-520.
33. Mullins CE, Nihill MR, Vick III GW, et al. Double balloon technique for dilation of valvular or vessel stenosis in congenital and acquired heart disease. JACC 1987, 10: 107-114.
34. Fletcher SE, Nihill MR, Grifka RG, et al. Balloon angioplasty of native coarctation of the aorta: midterm follow up and prognostic factors. J Am Coll Cardiol 1995; 25:730-734.
35. Rao PS, Galal O, Smith PA, et al. Five to nine year follow up results of balloon angioplasty of native aortic coarctation in infants and children. J Am Coll Cardiol 1996; 27:462-470.
36. Shaddy RE, Boucek MM, Sturtevant JE, et al. Comparison of angioplasty and surgery for unoperated coarctation of the aorta. Circulation 1993, 87:793-799.
37. Shim D, Lloyd TR, Moorehead CP, et al. Comparison of hospital charges for balloon angioplasty and surgical repair in children with native coarctation of the aorta. Am J Cardiol 1997, 70:1143-1146.
38. McCrindle BW, Jones TK, Morrow WR, et al. Acute results of balloon angioplasty of native coarctation versus recurrent aortic obstruction are equivalent. J Am Coll Cardiol 1996, 28: 1810-1817.
39. Burrows PE, Benson LN, Babyn P, et al. Magnetic resonance imaging of the iliofemoral arteries after balloon dilation angioplasty of aortic arch obstructions in children. Circulation 1994, 90:915-920.
40. Rao PS, Galal O, Wilson AD. Feasibility and effectiveness of repeated balloon dilation of restenosed congenital obstructions after previous balloon valvuloplasty/angioplasty. Am Heart J 1996, 132:403-407.

41. Sweeney MS, Walker WE, Duncan JM, et al. Reoperation for aortic coarctation: techniques, results and indications for various approaches. Ann Thorac Surg 1985, 40:46-49.

42. Yetman AT, Nykanen D, McCrindle BW, et al. Balloon angioplasty of recurrent coarctation: A 12 year review. J Am Coll Cardiol 1997, 30:811-816.

43. Rothman A, Perry SB, Keane JF, et al. Early results and follow up of balloon angioplasty for branch pulmonary artery stenoses. J Am Coll Cardiol 1990, 15:1109-1117.

44. Baker CM, McGowan FX, Lock JE, et al. Management of pulmonary artery trauma due to balloon dilation. J Am Coll Cardiol 1998,31(Supp A):57A-58A.

45. Zeevi B, Berant M, Blieden LC. Late death from aneurysm rupture following balloon angioplasty for pulmonary artery stenosis. Catheterization and Cardiovascular Diagnosis 1996, 39:284-286.

46. Hosking MC, Thomaidis C, Hamilton R, et al. Clinical impact of balloon angioplasty for branch pulmonary arterial stenosis. Am J Cardiol 1992, 69:1467-470.

47. Zeevi B, Berant M, Blieden LC. Midterm clinical impact versus procedural success of balloon angioplasty for pulmonary artery stenosis. Pediatric Cardiology 1997, 18:101-106.

48. Nakanishi T, Matsumoto Y, Seguchi M. et al. Ballon angioplasty for postoperative pulmonary artery stenosis in transposition of the great arteries. JACC 1993, 22:859-866.

49. Hosking MC, Benson LN, Nakanishi T. et al. Intravascular stent prosthesis for right ventricular outflow obstruction. JACC 1992, 20:373-380.

50. Powell AJ, Lock JE, Keane JF, et al. Prolongation of RV-PA conduit lifespan by percutaneous stent implantation: Intermediate term results. Circulation 1995;92:3282-3288.

51. Lloyd TR, Marvin WJ, Mahoney LT, et al. Balloon dilation valvuloplasty of bioprosthetic valves in extracardiac conduits. Am Heart J 1987, 114:268-274.

52. Stark J, Silove ED, Taylor JFN, et al. Obstruction to systemic venous return following the Mustard for transposition of the great arteries. J Thorac Cardiovasc Surg 1974, 68:742-749.

53. DeLeon VH, Hougen TJ, Norwood WI, et al. Results of the Senning operation for transposition of the great arteries with intact ventricular septum in neonates. Circulation 1984, 70 (suppl):21.

54. Wax DF, Rocchini AP. Transcatheter management of venous stenosis. Pediatr Cardiol 1998, 19:59-65.

55. Wisselink W, Money SR, Becker MO, et al. Comparison of operative reconstruction and percutaneous balloon dilation for central venous obstruction. Am J Surgery 1993, 166:200-205.

6. CATHETER INTERVENTION: BALLOON VALVOTOMY

Scott B. Yeager, M.D.
Michael F. Flanagan, M.D.
John F. Keane, M.D.

Although use of transcatheter techniques [1,2] (Fig. 6-1), including a balloon catheter, [3] to perform valvotomies has been reported since the middle of this century, the first method to become widely accepted was the static balloon technique reported by Kan and associates [4]. Since the first edition of this text, balloon valvotomy has emerged as a mainstay of management in infants and children with stenosis of any heart valve. In the previous chapter, the technology of balloon catheters and their uses in vessel angioplasty were discussed. The same fundamental principles apply to the use of catheters for valvotomies within the heart.

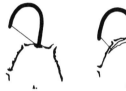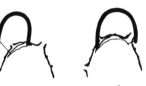

Figure 6-1: Original illustration of the first successful transcatheter valvotomy, reported from Mexico City in 1954, that lowered a pulmonary valve gradient from 90 mmHg to 30 mmHg. (Reprinted from Arch. Institut. Cardiol. Mexico 23: 183).

GENERAL GUIDELINES

Precatheterization evaluation for all patients should include history, physical examination, chest x-ray, electrocardiogram and echocardiogram (Chapter 1). In particular, all patients considered candidates for balloon valvotomy should have had a recent and complete echocardiographic evaluation to determine specific details of cardiac anatomy such as valve morphology, estimate of the annulus in two dimensions, and determination of pre-dilation gradient and regurgitation.

In children and adolescents, we use routine precatheterization sedation and analgesia, with additional sedation and local anesthesia administered prior to intervention to avoid movement during the procedure. For neonates and young infants, general anesthesia and controlled ventilation is usually preferable to provide more reliable sedation and to avoid complications of hypoventilation or apnea. We type and cross a unit of packed red blood cells for any patient in whom a valvotomy is contemplated. All patients are heparinized at 100 units/kg immediately after measuring baseline ACT and after line placement: for the experienced interventionalist, the risks of thromboembolism far outweigh the risks of bleeding. Additionally, all patients undergo a baseline diagnostic catheterization. This is not just a sterile exercise to check on our echocardiographic colleagues; measuring right heart saturations, filling pressures, gradients, and estimating valvar regurgitation and ventricular function will provide necessary clues as to the sense of urgency and the completeness with which a successful intervention is pursued.

For most dilation procedures, at least two experienced operators participate. In the case of double balloon procedures, particularly of the aortic valve, additional scrubbed hands are needed.

We do not routinely schedule surgical backup for any of these procedures, even in neonates, and our experience indicates that immediate surgical intervention is rarely required, even when complications occur. All patients other than those beyond infancy who have had a pulmonary valvotomy are admitted overnight post-dilation. Because of the large catheters and sheaths often required the puncture site dressing should be in view for at least eight hours and the patients continuously monitored during that period.

PULMONARY VALVOTOMY

As noted above, static balloon dilation of stenotic pulmonary valves was first reported in 1982 [4]. Subsequent reports documented the safety and efficacy of the procedure [5-8] and its application was extended to critical pulmonary stenosis in the neonate [9,10] and eventually to patients with pulmonary atresia and favorable anatomy [11-13].

Older Patients

Patient Selection
The child with an isolated peak to peak trans-valvar gradient over 30 mmHg should be considered a candidate for balloon valvotomy. A peak instantaneous gradient of greater than 50 mmHg as measured by continuous wave Doppler will usually identify patients with sufficiently severe obstruction to warrant dilation. Excellent results have been achieved using oversized balloons in the great majority with occasional success even in those with dysplastic valves. Thus patients should not be excluded based on the echocardiographic appearance of the leaflets or their apparent immobility.

The optimal patient size for elective dilation is dictated by the pulmonary annulus dimension, femoral vessel size, and the profile of appropriate balloons. The risk of injury or occlusion of femoral vessels is greatest in infants less than 5 kilograms. The use of low profile balloons, which can be passed through 7 F sheaths, reduces vascular trauma in the small patient. A pulmonary annulus dimension of 10 to 20mm and patient weight of greater than 10 kilograms will usually allow a technically straightforward procedure using a single balloon. Older and larger patients, including adults, often require a double balloon technique.

Technique

Pre-medication with sedatives and analgesics is usually adequate; general anesthesia should rarely be necessary. Following local anesthesia, the femoral vein is entered percutaneously and a 5 to 7F sheath with a diaphragm is introduced into the vein. A 3 to 5F arterial catheter may be omitted, especially if a patent foramen is present and right ventricular pressure is less than two thirds systemic level. After heparinization and hemodynamic measurements, the pulmonary valve can usually be crossed with a flow directed balloon tipped end-hole catheter, and a pullback done to document the gradient. An angiographic catheter is then placed in the right ventricular outflow tract and an antero-posterior and straight lateral angiogram is performed (1 cc/kg in 1 second) for measurement of the pulmonary annulus, right ventricle and valve anatomy. The lateral projection usually provides the optimal images of the valve hinge points with minimal foreshortening (Fig. 6-2).

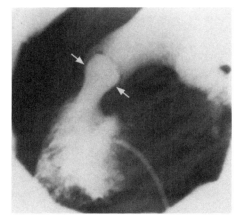

Figure 6-2: Lateral angiogram of a patient with moderate valvar pulmonary stenosis demonstrating the systolic doming of the valve. The annulus is measured at the hinge points of the valve (arrows), using the catheter diameter as an internal reference.

The catheter diameter can be used as an internal reference dimension for measurement of the annulus. The angiographic catheter is then replaced with a pulmonary wedge catheter; the balloon is inflated in the right atrium and advanced into the right ventricle to prevent passage of the catheter through the inter-chordal spaces of the tricuspid valve. The pulmonary valve is crossed and the catheter positioned in the left lower lobe branch of the left pulmonary artery. An appropriate exchange guidewire (0.018", 0.025" or 0.035" stiff wire depending on balloon selection) is placed in the peripheral pulmonary artery and the catheter replaced with a dilation balloon 120 to 140% of the measured annulus dimension. In young children, we generally use 2 cm long balloons to prevent damage to the right ventricular free wall. In older children and adults, 3 to 5 cm facilitate balloon positioning.

If the annulus size is too large for a single balloon dilation, a second balloon may be inserted through a sheath, usually placed in the opposite groin. The effective dilating diameter of the two balloons can be determined from Table 6-1.

EFFECTIVE DILATING DIAMETER (in mm)
DOUBLE BALLOON TECHNIQUE

	5	6	7	8	9	10	11	12	13	14	15	16	17	18	19	20	21	22	23	24	25	
5	8.2	9.0	9.9	10.7	11.6	12.5	13.5	14.4	15.3	16.2	17.2	18.1	19.1	20.0	21.0	21.9	22.9	23.9	24.8	25.8	26.8	5
6		9.8	10.7	11.5	12.4	13.3	14.1	15.1	16.0	16.9	17.8	18.7	19.7	20.6	21.6	22.5	23.5	24.4	25.4	26.3	27.3	6
7			11.5	12.3	13.1	14.0	14.9	15.8	16.7	17.6	18.5	19.4	20.3	21.2	22.2	23.1	24.1	25.0	25.9	26.9	27.8	7
8				13.1	13.9	14.8	15.6	16.5	17.4	18.3	19.2	20.1	21.0	21.9	22.8	23.7	24.7	25.6	26.5	27.5	28.4	8
9					14.7	15.6	16.4	17.3	18.1	19.0	19.9	20.8	21.7	22.6	23.5	24.4	25.3	26.2	27.2	28.1	29.0	9
10						16.4	17.2	18.0	18.9	19.7	20.6	21.5	22.4	23.3	24.2	25.1	26.0	26.9	27.8	28.8	29.7	10
11							18.0	18.8	19.7	20.5	21.4	22.2	23.1	24.0	24.9	25.8	26.7	27.6	28.5	29.4	30.3	11
12								19.6	20.5	21.3	22.1	23.0	23.9	24.7	25.6	26.5	27.4	28.3	29.2	30.1	31.0	12
13									21.3	22.1	22.9	23.8	24.6	25.5	26.4	27.2	28.1	29.0	29.9	30.8	31.7	13
14										22.9	23.7	24.6	25.4	26.3	27.1	28.0	28.9	29.7	30.6	31.5	32.4	14
15											24.5	25.4	26.2	27.0	27.9	28.8	29.6	30.5	31.4	32.2	33.1	15
16												26.2	27.0	27.8	28.7	29.5	30.4	31.2	32.1	33.0	33.9	16
17													27.8	28.6	29.5	30.3	31.2	32.0	32.9	33.7	34.6	17
18														29.5	30.3	31.1	32.0	32.8	33.6	34.5	35.4	18
19															31.1	31.9	32.7	33.6	34.4	35.3	36.1	19
20																32.7	33.6	34.4	35.2	36.1	36.9	20
21																	34.4	35.2	36.0	36.9	37.7	21
22																		36.0	36.8	37.7	38.5	22
23																			37.6	38.5	39.3	23
24																				39.3	40.1	24
25																					40.9	25

TABLE 6-1

Table 6-1: Effective dilating diameter using 2 balloons.

Pre-flushing of the balloon with carbon dioxide or dilute contrast is usually not necessary on the right side of the heart, and may make passage across a severely stenotic valve more difficult.

The balloon is centered across the valve annulus using lateral fluoroscopy and is rapidly inflated by hand with a mixture of approximately 25% contrast and 75% saline and the inflation is recorded on cine at a slow frame rate. If the balloon is appropriately positioned, a "waist" will be evident in the mid-portion of the balloon (Figs. 6-3 and 6-4).

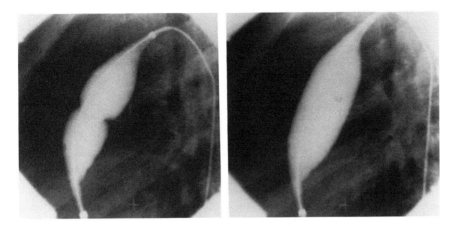

Fig. 6-3: An 18 mm balloon is inflated across a 14 mm annulus in a patient with valvar pulmonary stenosis. A moderate waist, seen at 1 atmosphere of pressure (left), is eliminated at 4 atmospheres of pressure (right).

Further inflation should result in obliteration of the "waist". Following full inflation, the balloon is immediately deflated and either advanced into the main pulmonary artery or withdrawn into the inferior vena cava. Transient systemic hypotension, sometimes associated with bradycardia, should be expected and is generally well tolerated and self-correcting. Following hemodynamic recovery, a second inflation verifies that no residual "waist" is encountered and that the balloon has been properly positioned. The dilation balloon is then removed with the guidewire remaining in the pulmonary artery. Passage through the sheath is facilitated by constant suction on the attached syringe and counter-clockwise rotation to re-wrap the deflated balloon on the shaft. The guidewire permits repositioning of an end-hole catheter into the distal pulmonary artery for repeat pressure measurements. Careful positioning of the catheter and multiple pullbacks may be necessary to identify a sub-valvar gradient if the right ventricular pressure is persistently elevated: a double lumen catheter is very helpful in this regard. A repeat estimation of cardiac output should be obtained. Post-dilation angiography is only necessary if significant sub-valvar obstruction is encountered, or if balloon-induced tricuspid regurgitation is suspected.

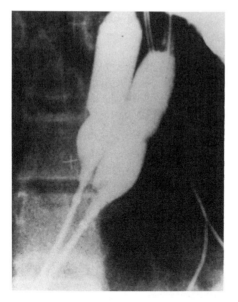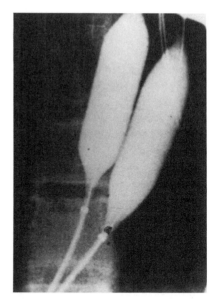

Fig. 6-4: Two 18 mm balloons (with an effective dilating diameter of 27 mm) are inflated across the pulmonary valve of an adolescent with a 23 mm annulus.

Complications

Extensive experience at many institutions has demonstrated pulmonary valvotomy in the older infant and child to be a very safe procedure. Transient complete heart block, right bundle branch block, or arrhythmias are rare. Post catheterization occlusion of the femoral vein may occur in smaller patients. Most patients are now discharged later the same day. Blood loss should be minimal and transfusion rarely required.

Results

A review of our initial experience using oversized balloons revealed an immediate reduction in gradient from 65.0 +/- 19.0 mmHg to 15.9 +/- 7.6mmHg and longer-term follow-up has shown persistent benefit [8]. Analysis of 533 patients in a multicenter registry demonstrated an association between suboptimal, long-term outcome and: (1) younger age at dilation, (2) dysplastic valve morphology, (3) smaller annulus size, (4) lower balloon-to-annulus ratio, and (5) higher immediate post dilation gradient [14]. The presence of more than mild residual pulmonary regurgitation was associated with: (1) dysplastic valves, (2) smaller annulus size, (3) the presence of associated cardiac lesions, (4) higher immediate residual gradients, and (5) higher balloon-to-annulus ratios. Using the technique described above, we have performed 313 dilations in infants, children and older patients at Children's Hospital between 1985 and 1998.

Critical Pulmonary Stenosis and in Neonates

While the original reports of balloon dilation of pulmonary valves involved infants and children, the technique has been successfully applied to the cyanotic neonate with severe obstruction as well as some patients with membranous pulmonary valve atresia.

Patient Selection
Neonates with severe valvar obstruction and cyanosis or those with evidence of suprasystemic right ventricular pressure are candidates for balloon dilation. Although several authors have suggested that patients with hypoplastic right heart structures are more likely to have an unsatisfactory outcome with persistent hypoxemia requiring surgical intervention [13,15], right sided hypoplasia is rarely a limiting factor in our experience in patients with valvar pulmonary stenosis. Similarly, the morphologic appearance of a dysplastic pulmonary valve, either by echocardiography or angiography, has not reliably predicted dilation outcome.

Our experience with true membranous pulmonary atresia is limited. We have crossed the valve with the soft end of a wire in patients without flow across the pulmonary valve. Therefore, we would attempt dilation with the usual technique in any patient with a normal or mildly hypoplastic right ventricle even if no trans-valvar flow can be demonstrated. We have limited yet successful experience with patients in whom an apparently atretic valve has been perforated using a stiff wire, laser tip, or a radio frequency catheter or wire. Although small RF ablation wires are very useful in these patients, they are not yet routinely available in the U.S. In patient selection, assessment of right sided hypoplasia and the details of coronary circulation, (including sinusoids and stenoses) is essential [16].

Technique
A detailed echocardiographic assessment of anatomy, including measurement of the pulmonary annulus, is performed prior to catheterization. Most neonates who are blue and especially those on prostaglandin E1 are intubated and ventilated prior to the procedure. Warming lights, heating blankets or other devices to avoid excessive thermal stress are important. Most patients will benefit from prostaglandin E1 infusion which increases systemic saturation and provides a stable wire position into the descending aorta. An umbilical artery catheter, or other arterial line, is introduced to monitor systemic blood pressure, saturation, and blood gases. The umbilical vein, if patent, can be used but is technically much more difficult. Thus, the right femoral vein is entered percutaneously and a 5F sheath with a diaphragm introduced. After routine heparinization and hemodynamic measurements, right ventricular angiogram using a 4 or 5F Berman catheter is performed in antero-posterior and lateral projections. A 0.025"

deflecting tip guidewire (Cook) or the hand modified stiff end of a guidewire may facilitate entry of the catheter into the right ventricle. The pulmonary annulus dimension is measured at the hinge points of the valve as seen in both projections. The angiographic catheter is replaced with an end-hole catheter which is manipulated into the right ventricle with the tip directed toward the right ventricular outflow tract.

We have used a variety of catheters, wires, and techniques to cross pulmonary valves in patients with critical pulmonary stenosis. As noted above, the safest approach is to inflate the balloon of a 5F end-hole catheter in the right atrium, advance it into the right ventricular outflow tract, and cross the valve with the soft end of a 0.018" torque wire. Although we start with this approach, the minimal flow across the tricuspid and pulmonary valves makes balloon floatation unhelpful. The most successful technique is to use a soft 4-5F relatively straight catheter with a short acutely-angled tip (e.g. 4F Bensor or Judkins right). With the stiff end of a guidewire bent to 60 degrees, and positioned 5-15 back from the catheter tip, the catheter can be advanced through the tricuspid valve toward the apex. After the curved stiff wire is replaced by the soft torque wire, gentle clockwise (or even counter-clockwise) rotation will position the angled catheter tip into the right ventricular outflow tract, pointing posteriorly toward the valve. This part of the procedure can be dangerous: if the tip is embedded in the free-wall myocardium, even the soft torque wire can perforate the heart. Further, unrecognized perforations or myocardial injury can weaken the wall, and undoubtedly contribute to the rare report of balloon dilation-induced myocardial rupture. Confirming the free intracavity position of the catheter tip, either with unconstrained wire movement of hand injections of small amounts of contrast, is essential in this most crucial part of the procedure. Under fluoroscopic guidance, the soft tip of 0.018" torque control wire is gently tapped against and through the pulmonary valve, and into a stable position in either the left lower lobe pulmonary artery or descending aorta across the ductus. An initial small 2 to 5mm, 2 cm long balloon is often used and advanced across the valve without pre-inflation (Fig. 6-5).

The guidewire must be held taut during balloon advancement to facilitate crossing the valve without buckling of the catheter in the right atrium or ventricle. The final dilating balloon should be approximately 120-130% of the measured annulus size, unless right ventricular outflow tract injury has occurred. Inflations are performed by hand, using 50-75% contrast in saline (these small balloons can be very hard to see), until the "waist" disappears and recorded on cine at slow frame rates. The balloon is immediately deflated. Two inflations are usually performed for each balloon size. Balloons up to and including 8mm diameter which fit through a 4F sheath are now available.

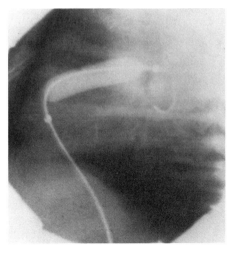

Fig. 6-5: A 2 cm long, 8 mm balloon is inflated across the pulmonary valve of a newborn with critical stenosis. Despite the short balloon length, the balloon fills the outflow track.

Following dilation, repeat measurements of pressures and saturations are obtained and the patient is maintained on prostaglandin E1 during transport back to the intensive care setting. We generally administer a dose of broad spectrum antibiotic (cefazolin 50 mgm/kg) during the procedure because of an apparent increased risk of post-procedure infectious complications in neonates.

Complications
Pulmonary valve dilation in the neonate is associated with a higher rate of complications than in older children and adults. Significant mortality and morbidity is reported in most reported series. In our initial experience with 36 neonates there was one death due to necrotizing enterocolitis and sepsis which developed 7 hours following a successful procedure [10]. Another infant developed Staphylococcal endocarditis requiring protracted intravenous antibiotic therapy. Other complications included right ventricular perforation, transient arrhythmias, right bundle branch block, loss of arterial pulse secondary to catheter placement, and occlusion of the femoral vein.

Results
The immediate result of 34 successful balloon dilations was a reduction in right ventricular/systemic pressure ratio from 150 +/- 32% to 83+/- 30% [10]. Nine babies demonstrated suprasystemic pressure immediately post dilation; 2 had surgery (26.5%) and the remaining 7 were managed medically with progressive reduction in gradient and good outcome, with only one requiring a repeat dilation at a later date. Most of the residual obstruction in this age group is at the infundibular level and both it and cyanosis resolve spontaneously in weeks to months. The longer-term outcome of the 31 managed medically alone was similarly good. All were acyanotic and well at a mean follow-up of 33 months (1-91 months) with 3 having required a repeat balloon dilation. The maximum instantaneous gradient as estimated by Doppler was less than 30mmHg in 28 patients and between 30 and 50mmHg in 3 patients. While right ventricular hypoplasia was uncommon (3 patients) in our series, others with a higher

percentage of underdeveloped ventricles have reported growth to normal dimensions during medium term follow-up, suggesting that these patients can also be anticipated to respond favorably to balloon dilation[17]. Through 1997, we have performed a total of 68 balloon dilation procedures on pulmonary valves in neonates, with only the one death already described.

Pulmonary Valvotomy In Pulmonary Atresia

We reserve this procedure for rare cases of membranous pulmonary atresia where the annulus and cavity are nearly normal in size, indicating that the infant will not require an RVOT patch for adequate gradient relief. In all other infants, balloon or surgical valvotomy alone will rarely relieve cyanosis, necessitating either prolonged PGE infusion or a surgical shunt. We believe the latter is a less morbid approach, and have used it with a surgical valvotomy or outflow patch in most of these neonates. The technique is virtually identical to that described for critical PS, with several additions: the optimum tool for crossing the pulmonary valve appears to be a 3F radiofrequency wire, and the location and anatomy of the main pulmonary artery must be well delineated prior to the application of any RF energy. Once the valve is crossed, the ablating wire is replaced with a standard 0.018" wire, and the valve dilated as described above.

AORTIC VALVOTOMY

Transluminal aortic valvotomy evolved from earlier techniques using technology adapted from vascular angioplasty and from pulmonary valvotomy. The clinical results of aortic valvotomy were initially reported in 1984 [18], with experimental data reported in 1987 (19).

Older Patients
Patient Selection (Beyond the neonatal period)
The risk for sudden death in children and young adults with congenital aortic valve stenosis is 1.2-1.3% per patient year when the peak systolic pressure gradient is greater than 50 mmHg, compared with one-third that risk for medically treated patients with a gradient less than 50 mmHg [20]. In general, a catheterization measured gradient greater than 50 mmHg with mild regurgitation at most are used as indicators for both surgical valvotomy and now dilation

At pre-catheterization echocardiographic evaluation, the mean gradient measured from the apical window tends to most accurately correlate with the pressure gradient determined in the catheterization laboratory, being approximately 2/3 the measured peak to peak systolic gradient. The echocardiographic maximum instantaneous gradient, particularly when measured from the right sternal border window, is frequently substantially greater than the peak to peak systolic gradient. We do not exclude patients because of "favorable" or "unfavorable" valve morphology, although careful echocardiographic assessment of the valve leaflet thickness, annular diameter, the number of commissures, the site of fusion, degrees of stenosis and regurgitation is obtained in every patient before valvotomy.

Technique
After routine pre-catheterization sedation and local anesthesia, a venous sheath and thermodilution catheter are inserted. In small children, the femoral artery is cannulated with a 5F sheath and those older with a 6F or 7F sheath, with a side arm for monitoring of femoral artery pressure. A pigtail catheter, one French size smaller than the sheath, is advanced through the sheath to the iliac bifurcation. Heparin is given. Simultaneous iliac arterial blood pressures are measured through the side arm of the sheath and the catheter to document that they are identical. The pigtail catheter is then advanced to the ascending aorta, and both arterial pressures re-measured to quantitate the standing wave effect (Chapter 3). The pigtail catheter is advanced over a guidewire into the left ventricle, followed by measurement of cardiac output and trans-valvar gradient. A left ventricular cineangiogram is recorded in a long axial oblique projection, and the aortic valve annulus diameter measured at the level of the hinge points of the leaflets (Fig. 6-6).

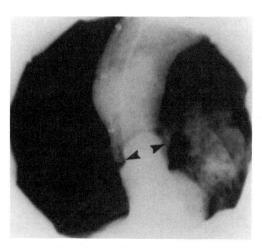

Fig. 6-6: Aortic valve annulus is measured from the hinge points (arrows) of the valve leaflets on a lateral aortogram or left ventriculogram.

The catheter is withdrawn to the ascending aorta to measure the gradient by direct pullback, and an aortogram performed to assess the degree of regurgitation.

If the patient is a candidate for balloon valvotomy, a second (4-5F) pigtail catheter is often placed in the other femoral artery and used to monitor arterial pressure, to measure transvalvar gradients after valvotomy and to assess aortic regurgitation.

The right femoral arterial catheter is re-advanced to the left ventricle and a 0.035" stiff or extra-stiff exchange guide wire, with a broad hand-curved tip (Fig. 6-7), advanced to the apex making sure on the lateral view that the wire course is anterior to the mitral valve apparatus. Since the orifice is commonly posterior

162

between the left and non coronary cusps, the wire as it crosses the stenotic valve may be directly posterior and pass through the mitral valve chordae.

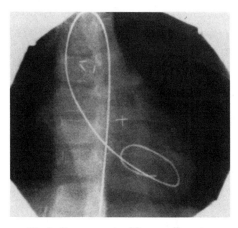

Fig. 6-7: The valvotomy guide wire is hand-curved so that a broad loop fills the left ventricle, allowing excess guidewire, and putting the stiff part of the wire across the aortic annulus.

A balloon inflated over this wire course will likely tear the anterior mitral valve leaflet. When using high profile balloons, sheaths as large as 10-11F may be needed. In children with a relatively small aortic annulus, or if a double balloon technique is used, low profile balloons up to 18 mm diameter may be advanced through a 7 or 8F sheath into the femoral artery. The valvotomy balloon should be 3 cm long for children 1-3 years old, 4 cm long for children 4-12 years old, and 5 cm long for adolescents and adults. It should be mounted near the end of a relatively stiff shafted catheter, and the initial balloon diameter should be at most 85 - 90% of the diameter of the aortic annulus. This initial balloon/aortic valve diameter ratio is chosen to reduce the risk of valve disruption which we have seen even at this low ratio. At this point, we administer extra sedation, local anesthesia, and enlarge the stab wound in the skin if necessary. The balloon catheter is then advanced over the wire into the descending aorta. During this maneuver, it is important to (1) hold the wire taut, (2) constantly aspirate the balloon to reduce its profile, (3) watch the left ventricular wire on fluoroscopy to insure a stable position, and (4) turn the balloon counter clockwise on the way through the sheath to further fold the balloon. With the balloon in the descending aorta, we flush it with CO_2 and then dilute contrast/saline to remove as much nitrogen as possible. The balloon is then advanced directly across the valve to the inflation position, with slightly more than half the balloon below the valve. It should not be advanced deep into the ventricle and then withdrawn to the dilating position, as this will tighten the catheter curve in the transverse arch and make it easier for the ventricle to eject the balloon during systole. The balloon is inflated a couple of times to a pressure of 4-6 atmospheres until the "waist" produced by the stenotic valve has been abolished (Fig. 6-8).

Each inflation-deflation cycle should last less than 10 seconds. The balloon is deflated and withdrawn over the guidewire to the descending aorta prior to the next inflation.

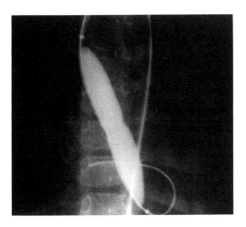

Fig. 6-8: A 5 cm long balloon dilation catheter is positioned across the aortic valve using the retrograde technique. A "waist" is demonstrated in the mid portion of the balloon prior to full inflation.

At this point, the pressure gradient (Fig. 6-9) and cardiac output are measured and an ascending aortogram done for regurgitation evaluation using the second arterial pigtail or by exchanging over the guidewire for a pigtail catheter.

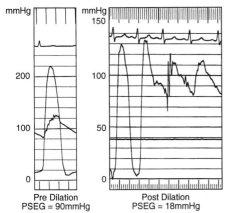

Pre Dilation
PSEG = 90mmHg

Post Dilation
PSEG = 18mmHg

Fig. 6-9: Pre (left) and post (right) valvotomy pressure tracings demonstrate a reduction in gradient across the aortic valve from 90 mmHg to 18 mmHg.

If the gradient has fallen 50% or less, and the degree of aortic regurgitation is largely unchanged, the next largest balloon is inserted. If the gradient reduction is satisfactory, or there is a clear cut increase in regurgitation, the valvuloplasty is terminated and hemodynamcs are re-measured.

This procedure can be difficult: balloon size position, and stability must be precisely controlled for optimum results. The degree of aortic damage and valvar regurgitation increase as balloon/annulus ratio increases, very significantly so at 1.25[10,21]. With currently available balloon sizes, the initial balloon may have little impact and the next available balloon size may result in considerable valve damage. This may be overcome using two appropriately sized smaller balloons inflated simultaneously, allowing an effective dilating diameter to within a millimeter or less of that desired [22], or by varying inflation pressures and hence actual balloon diameters [Table 6-1] and permitting better systemic and coronary flow during the dilation process [23,24].

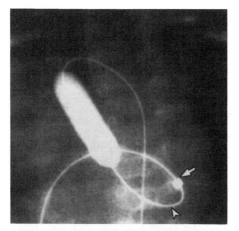

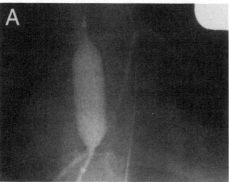

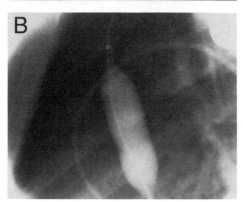

Fig. 6-10: Antegrade balloon dilation of valvar AS in infant showing tip of 5F sheath (arrow) in LV with preformed wire loop at LV apex (arrowhead).

Additionally, the hyperdynamic left ventricle forcibly ejects the inflating balloon into the ascending aorta, a process that is controlled by using stiff wires, longer balloons, and catheter advancement.

Although dilating the aortic valve antegrade (25) via the atrial septum can injure the mitral valve, using a pre-formed loop in a stiff wire makes this procedure safe and effective in younger children (Fig. 6-10). This loop is preformed prior to insertion in the patient. Without such a loop the hyperdynamic left ventricle will eject the inflated balloon and wire out the outflow tract and pulling back on the catheter will cause the draped stretched anterior leaflet to split (Fig. 6-11). Stiff guidewires passed antegrade across the mitral annulus without preshaping will also tent open the valve resulting in significant mitral regurgitation and hemodynamic instability throughout the duration of its presence there.

Fig. 6-11: (A) and LAT (B) views of balloon in valvar AS using antegrade approach showing loss of apical wire and catheter loop as balloon was ejected out aortic valve and catheter withdrawn to maintain position: anterior leaflet of mitral valve was torn, requiring surgical plication.

Complications
Among 150 patients 1 month to 20 years (mean 7 years) who underwent balloon aortic valvotomy at Children's Hospital between 1985 and 1991 serious complications occurred in fewer than 3% [26]. These included cardiac arrest requiring defibrillation or resuscitation, aortic intimal tear, aortic valve prolapse, mitral valve injury, rupture or pseudoaneurysm of the femoral artery, blood loss requiring transfusion and bacterial endocarditis. Mitral regurgitation occurred in 3% (4 patients; 2 dilated antegrade, 2 retrograde) and was successfully managed by surgical placation of the torn anterior leaflet. One infant with severe congestive heart failure died of ventricular fibrillation 1/2 hour after valvotomy, yielding a mortality rate of 0.7%. Other complications included transient arrhythmias, notably left bundle branch block in 13%, and asymptomatic femoral artery occlusion in 7%. The grade of aortic valve regurgitation increased immediately in 58% of the patients, and was at least 3+ in 13% immediately, increasing to 38% after a mean follow-up of 4 years, as noted also by others[27]. Patients 1-5 years of age, those with prior valvotomy, those with at least moderate (2+/4+) pre-valvotomy regurgitation, and perhaps those with unicommissural valves were more likely to have regurgitation of 3+/4+ or more after valvotomy [28]. These and other complications have been described at other institutions[21,27,29-31].

Results
Between 1983 and 1997, 228 children greater than 1 month of age underwent aortic dilation at Children's Hospital. In children over 1 month of age[26] gradient reduction of at least 40% was achieved in 85% of patients, the mean immediate residual gradient being 32 mmHg. Over a mean follow-up of 4 years, 17% had re-intervention for aortic stenosis (usually re-dilation), and another 8% for regurgitation. Overall, at 8 years 50% of patients were free of repeat intervention and patient survival was 95%. Excluding those under 2 years of age with other significant left heart obstructive lesions, there was only 1 late death (sudden) for a 99% survival rate. Similar results have been documented by others in children [21,27,29-31] and in young adults with non-calcific congenital aortic valve stenosis [32-33].

Critical Valvar Aortic Stenosis in Neonates

Patient Selection
These babies suffer from severe congestive heart failure and shock. Without intervention most will die within weeks. Mortality rates from balloon valvotomy and surgery are similar, both being higher than valvotomy in older children (34-37). Varying degrees of hypoplasia of the left ventricular chamber, mitral valve, left ventricular outflow, aortic annulus and arch are common, and profoundly influence survival following valvotomy [34,38]. The decision to proceed with valvotomy or other management options, such as a staged, single ventricle surgical

approach or cardiac transplantation, is often urgent and irreversible. Valvotomy is futile in those with prohibitively small left heart structures. Rhodes et al developed an incremental scoring system based on pre-catheterization echocardiographic threshold values for three risk factors: left ventricular long axis to heart long axis (0.8 or less), indexed aortic root diameter (3.5 cm/m2 or less), and indexed mitral valve area (4.75 cm2/m2 or less). The score correctly predicted outcome in more than 90% of patients. In patients with two or more risk factors the mortality with valvotomy, surgical or balloon, was 88-100%[39]. Using these criteria, the incidence of dilating aortic valves in neonates with hypoplastic left hearts has decreased from 30% of our initial 20 neonates to 5% in the most recent 20 babies.

When dilating these valves we use either an antegrade or a retrograde approach, both of which will be discussed in greater detail. Coming from the descending aorta, it is surprisingly easy to cross the stenotic aortic valve in these neonates, the femoral approach being technically easier than the umbilical arterial one. However pulse loss in the former approach is significant. We do not use a carotid artery cutdown approach because occlusion of this vessel can occur following cannulation, and central nervous system damage may result.

Technique – Retrograde Approach
Vigilant attention to technique, and optimization of the metabolic status, thermal environment, blood loss and respiratory status including intubation, ventilation, inotrope and PGE1 infusions as needed are essential to a favorable outcome. In babies less than 72 hours old, access from the umbilical artery is first attempted and a 3.2F pigtail placed in the ascending aorta and an 0.018" wire used to cross the valve: if the aortic valve cannot be crossed within 15-30 minutes, the femoral artery or transvenous approach is used. A 3.2F catheter is placed in the femoral artery and a 5F sheath and 5F Berman angiographic catheter in a femoral vein. After heparinization and routine hemodynamics, the pressure gradient across the valve is measured by simultaneous recording of left ventricular pressure (with the Berman catheter advanced antegrade through the foramen ovale) and ascending aortic pressure (with the pigtail catheter advanced retrograde). Biplane cineangiograms of the left ventricle and ascending aorta are recorded in long axial oblique and right anterior projections to measure the size of the aortic annulus, the degree of aortic regurgitation, the left ventricular size and systolic function, and to identify associated anomalies. The aortic valve is crossed retrograde with the soft tip of an 0.018" guidewire and the pigtail advanced to the apex of the ventricle. Prior removal of some of the pigtail tip may help direct the guidewire but is not usually necessary. The left non-coronary commissure is invariably patent. Therefore, the valve is crossed by dapping the wire leftward and posterior toward the angiographic jet of contrast. Care is taken to avoid damage to the coronary arteries or perforation of a valve leaflet. The initial guidewire is exchanged for a

0.018" wire with a terminal pre-shaped loop. If an 0.018" torque wire is used, it is important to initially shape the stiff mandril of this wire to the curve of the aortic arch prior to insertion to avoid arch wall damage. The wire is placed in the left ventricular apex along the septum anterior to the mitral valve chordae.

The pigtail catheter is exchanged for a balloon catheter with an inflated diameter at most 90% of the aortic annulus diameter as measured by angiography. Low profile balloon catheters up to 8 mm diameter fit through a 4F sheath (Meditech Sub-4, Boston Scientific Corporation: Tyshak, Braun Co.), reducing femoral artery trauma and facilitating hemostasis. The 2 cm long balloon is advanced retrograde over the guidewire to straddle the aortic valve and inflated for a few seconds by hand at 3-6 atmospheres inflation pressure, or until the "waist" in the balloon from the stenotic valve disappears. This is recorded on cine at a low speed for balloon diameter measurement and position. The balloon is immediately deflated and the catheter promptly withdrawn over the guidewire to the descending aorta under fluoroscopic guidance with care to maintain the position of the wire in the left ventricle. Since a "waist" may not be present in neonates and the balloon can move with cardiac ejection during the time to full inflation, 2 inflations are performed to ensure that an inflation in correct position is accomplished. The gradient, left ventricular end diastolic pressure and mixed venous O_2 saturation are remeasured to assess residual stenosis, and ascending aortography performed to evaluate aortic regurgitation. Since LV function is very compromised in most, initial gradients are often small and LVEDP high. Frequently improvement is manifest by decreases in a small gradient and LVEDP. Many will have a PDA which will later close, hence further reducing the gradient by elimination of this LV volume overload lesion. If adequate gradient relief has not been achieved (e.g., peak systolic gradient remains more than 50 mmHg or has been reduced less than 50%) and significant aortic valve regurgitation is not present, then valvotomy can be repeated with the next larger balloon size or by inflating the prior balloon to a higher pressure. Varying effective balloon diameter takes some practice, but can be very effective in improving neonatal valve dilations. With the inflating pressure kept relatively low (e.g. 3-4 atmospheres) the wire inside the balloon will be centrally located. As the inflation pressure increases, the balloon will a assume a banana-like shape, the wire will migrate to the inner curvature, and the actual diameter will increase as much as 0.5 mm. We re-measure hemodynamics and aortic regurgitation by angiography before each incremental increase in balloon size and at the end of the procedure. The babies are then transferred to the cardiovascular intensive care unit.

Technique – Antegrade Approach

Patient preparation and initial diagnostic catheterization are done as with the retrograde approach. A 3.2F pigtail catheter is placed in a femoral artery and a 5F sheath and 5F Berman angiographic catheter in a femoral vein. Using the left ventricular angiogram as a guide, a 5F Cook biopsy sheath is heated and shaped to course across the baby's foramen ovale and central mitral annulus to the left ventricular apex to avoid inducing mitral regurgitation. The shape and size can be double-checked prior to insertion by placing it over the chest in a sterile manner and using fluoroscopy. With the aid of a 5F balloon tipped end-hole catheter, the sheath is advanced from the femoral vein across the foramen ovale to the left ventricular apex. If the course or hemodynamic changes suggest that destabilizing mitral regurgitation is being induced, appropriate adjustments are made in the sheath shape. The end-hole catheter is advanced from the sheath and directed from the left ventricular apex to the ascending aorta and then descending aorta using a 0.028" tip-deflecting guide wire. This wire is then replaced with an 0.018" J-tipped guidewire with a pre-formed apical loop, advanced to the descending aorta and the catheter removed. Valvotomy is then performed with a trackable low profile catheter with a 2 cm length balloon. (Fig. 6-10) The initial balloon diameter is at most 90% of the aortic valve annulus. Simultaneous left ventricular and ascending aortic pressures are then measured using the sheath (with the wire in place using a Y-connector) and the pigtail catheter. Ascending aortography is repeated. If significant stenosis persists, and little or no aortic regurgitation is induced, the dilation process may be repeated using sequentially larger balloon diameters, or the same balloon inflated to a higher pressure.

Complications

Among 33 neonates who underwent balloon aortic valvotomy at Children's Hospital between 1985 and 1991 [36] there were 3 procedure related deaths (9%) due to: 1) endocarditis associated with a prolonged procedure through the umbilical artery, 2) perforation and subsequent dilation of a valve cusp, and 3) wire perforation of the left ventricle with tamponade. Possibly life threatening complications occurred in another 6 babies (18%), including cardiac arrest in 4 (all resuscitated), left anterior descending coronary artery occlusion in 1 and aortic arch flaps in 2. Additionally, all 20 babies with trans-femoral artery valvotomy initially had occlusion of the femoral artery, with patency reestablished in 35% with thrombolytic therapy, and none had clinical sequelae.

Results

In our series described above, babies with an echocardiographic score < 2^{38} had an early survival rate of 88% and probability of survival at 8.3 years of 88%. These results are at least as good as surgical intervention [34-36,39]. At 8.3 years the probability for re-intervention was 46%. At a mean follow-up of 4.3 years, 83% of survivors were asymptomatic, 65% had a Doppler maximum instantaneous gradient <50 mmHg and 14% had significant regurgitation (compared with 6% pre-valvotomy). Others [35,36,39,40] have achieved comparable results. Between 1983 and 1997, 70 neonates underwent aortic dilation at Children's Hospital.

Mitral Valvotomy

Our initial experience with mitral valvotomy was with rheumatic mitral stenosis [41]. Following promising results, this technique was extended to congenital mitral stenosis in infants and young children [42,43].

Patient Selection
Mitral valvotomy should be considered in the symptomatic patient with evidence of growth failure, exertional dyspnea, resting tachypnea or hemoptysis, or the asymptomatic patient with severe pulmonary hypertension. Patients with rheumatic mitral stenosis have a more favorable outcome and are technically easier. The anatomic appearance of the rheumatic mitral valve does not influence candidate selection for balloon valvotomy, although patients with more than a mild degree of mitral regurgitation are normally excluded. Patients with congenital mitral stenosis are a more complex and heterogeneous group. Outcome in these patients is strongly influenced by associated malformations. Of the various anatomic sub-groups of mitral stenosis, those with a supra-valvar mitral ring had the least satisfactory results [43]. Additionally, the few infants in whom we have attempted a second dilation because of re-stenosis have demonstrated high mortality and morbidity. The presence of more than mild mitral regurgitation is a relative contra-indication to valvotomy.

Technique
A thorough echocardiographic evaluation is performed prior to the procedure, with particular attention directed toward the identification of associated left-sided abnormalities (coarctation, aortic or sub-aortic stenosis, hypoplastic left ventricle, supra-mitral ring), left atrial thrombus, the anatomy of the mitral obstruction, and mitral annulus size.

Older patients may require only routine sedation and supplemental oxygen. In younger children and infants with congenital mitral stenosis, we routinely perform the catheterization under general anesthesia with positive pressure ventilation. After routine heparinization and hemodynamic measurements, left atrial entry using a Brockenbrough technique (Chapter 10) permits simultaneous measurement of left atrial and left ventricular end diastolic pressure.
A left ventricular cineangiogram is performed to evaluate mitral regurgitation and outline the annulus in the RAO view.
If initial hemodynamic and angiographic evaluation indicate that the patient is a suitable candidate, a 7F balloon end-hole catheter is positioned in the left atrium

and the mitral valve is crossed with the balloon inflated to ensure passage through the central orifice, and advanced to the apex. A pre-shaped 0.035" stiff exchange wire (Rosen wire) is advanced through the catheter to the apex and the catheter then removed. In patients requiring trans-septal puncture, predilation of the atrial septum with an angioplasty balloon (4 mm for infants, 6mm for older children and adults) is often necessary to facilitate passage of the dilation balloon.

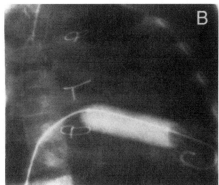

Fig. 6-12: Balloon inflation in stenotic mitral valve showing waist (A) and abolition of waist (B).

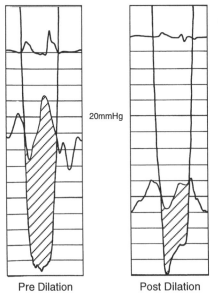

Pre Dilation   Post Dilation

20mmHg

Fig. 6-13: Showing simultaneous LA-LV pressures pre and post dilation of stenotic mitral valve.

Initial dilation is performed with a balloon 1 to 3 mm smaller than the echocardiographic estimate of the mitral valve annulus. The balloon is inflated by hand using dilute contrast and recorded on cine at a slow frame rate (Fig. 6-12). The balloon is then deflated immediately and removed. A repeat assessment of hemodynamics and mitral regurgitation is performed. If adequate relief is not achieved, progressively larger balloons are used until satisfactory reduction in gradient is accomplished or mitral regurgitation has increased, or 120% of the estimated annulus size is reached. A final hemodynamic evaluation (Fig. 6-13) is performed, including angiography with estimation of any left to right atrial shunt if the atrial septum has been dilated.

A post-procedure echocardiographic evaluation of the mitral valve is indicated to evaluate the status of the leaflets and provide a baseline for hemodynamic follow-up.

Complications

Older children and adults tolerate the procedure well. In our experience, complications in this age group have been confined to transient hypotension and arrhythmias, cardiac perforation without tamponade, increased mitral regurgitation, and small persistent atrial shunting. Infants, however, are a much more hemodynamically unstable group during the procedure particularly since they are symptomatic and ill to begin with. While we have not encountered mortality directly associated with a first procedure, instability can be anticipated. Profound bradycardia, heart block, and hypotension progressing to cardiac arrest requiring active resuscitation have occurred. Early repeat dilation for re-stenosis performed in three infants resulted in two dilation-related deaths. The use of relatively large sheaths increases the likelihood of venous thrombosis.

Results

Patients with rheumatic mitral stenosis generally respond favorably with excellent 3-5 year reduction of gradient, and resolution of symptoms. In our initial experience, balloon dilation reduced the gradient reduction from 21.2+/-4.0 mmHg to 10.1+/-5.5 mmHg and increased the mitral valve area index from 0.73+/-0.29 cm2/M2 to 1.34+/-0.32 cm2/M2 [41]. Several studies have shown persistent improvement in both symptoms and hemodynamics in patients followed for as long as 6 years post procedure [45-46]. The large majority of patients can expect significant and lasting clinical improvement; significant mitral regurgitation is uncommon.

Congenital mitral stenosis, on the other hand, has proven to be more intractable, particularly in infancy [42-44]. Of 18 ill patients less than 2 years of age who underwent balloon dilation, the mitral gradient was reduced from 20.3+/-8.2 mmHg to 10.9+/-4.9 mmHg [43]. 15 of 18 were felt to have a successful procedure (greater than 30% reduction in trans-mitral gradient). However, 7 (39%) developed significant mitral regurgitation related to the procedure and only 8 were alive and free of repeat procedures or surgery at one year follow-up. Among those with follow-up Doppler evaluations or catheterization, restenosis was common even in those with persistent clinical improvement. Patients with a supra-mitral ring had a particularly poor result: all required surgery for relief of gradient and most developed significant mitral regurgitation following dilation. Nevertheless, results were better than those of surgery [43]. At Children's Hospital, we performed 65 balloon dilation procedures in 55 patients between 1985 and 1998.

172

Tricuspid Valvotomy

There are a number of case reports and small series describing percutaneous balloon valvotomy for acquired tricuspid valve stenosis associated with rheumatic heart disease [47], carcinoid heart disease [48] and porcine bioprosthesis [49] in adults. In larger children and adults a double balloon technique may provide advantages over single balloon technique [24,50]. Congenital tricuspid valve stenosis is rare and usually occurs in association with critical pulmonary stenosis or pulmonary atresia with intact ventricular septum [51,52]. In these patients the range of tricuspid valve abnormalities can include severe dysplasia, annular hypoplasia and Ebstein's anomaly. The annulus diameter is proportionally underdeveloped. The leaflets are often thickened and the chordae and papillary muscles abnormal [53]. When severe tricuspid valve stenosis and an atrial septal defect coexist, flow through the right ventricle, and consequently growth of the right ventricle, are severely compromised [52]. In our experience intervention to relieve tricuspid valve stenosis can result in significant right ventricular growth [51]. To our knowledge, the technique for balloon valvotomy for congenital tricuspid valve stenosis in children has not been previously reported. In adults, only a possible single case report exists [54].

Patient Selection
At present, management of infants with pulmonary atresia without right ventricle-dependent coronary circulation appears best managed by surgical creation of an outflow from the right ventricle to the pulmonary artery in early infancy with a concomitant surgical shunt.
The severity of tricuspid valve stenosis will be underestimated by echocardiographic and catheter-derived hemodynamic measurements done when there is an atrial septal defect with right to left shunting. In this situation tricuspid stenosis is determined by hemodynamic measurements during temporary balloon occlusion of the atrial septal defect, as outlined below. Those with severe Ebstein's anomaly, particularly when associated with severe right ventricular hypoplasia, do not appear to be good candidates.

Technique
A catheter is placed in a femoral vein, a second in a femoral artery, and a complete diagnostic catheterization of the right and left heart is performed. When significant tricuspid valve stenosis is suspected and there is right to left shunting across an atrial septal defect, right heart hemodynamics are measured during temporary balloon occlusion of the atrial septal defect. Often, two venous sheaths are thereby required. Temporary occlusion of small atrial septal defects can be accomplished with a Berman angiographic catheter, and of larger atrial septal defects with an ASD sizing or septostomy balloon, inflated in the left atrium and gently pulled against the septum. During balloon occlusion, pressures are measured simultaneously in the right atrium and ventricle using the Berman

catheter for the right atrium and a second catheter via another venous sheath in the ventricle. Aortic pressure and heart rate should be closely monitored. If severe hypotension ensues, the aortopulmonary shunt may also need to be temporarily occluded. The adequacy of closure and the cardiac output during closure are determined using oxygen saturation measurements obtained in the right atrium and aorta during occlusion.

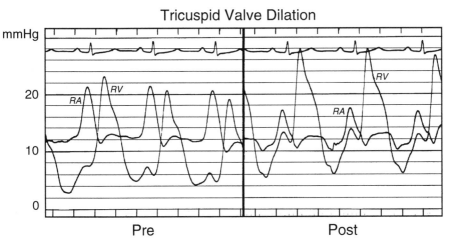

Fig. 6-14: Pre-(left) and post-(right) dilation gradient measured across the tricuspid valve of a patient with tricuspid stenosis. There is a marked reduction in the mean diastolic gradient between the right atrium (RA) and the right ventricle (RV).

Biplane angiography is performed with a Berman catheter in the right ventricle to assess the tricuspid annulus diameter and the competency of the tricuspid valve. Adequate angiographic measurement of the tricuspid annulus diameter is often difficult; we use echocardiographic measurements to aid in choosing the balloon size. A pulmonary wedge catheter is advanced through the sheath and, with the balloon inflated, through the right heart to the left lower pulmonary artery and exchanged for a guidewire, usually a 0.035" Rosen wire or a 0.018" Torque wire with a stiff shaft. We start with a balloon diameter of approximately 75 to 80% of the annulus diameter. Valvotomy is performed over the guidewire with an in-vivo pre-flushed balloon similar to pulmonary valvotomy. Hemodynamic measurements are repeated (Fig. 6-14).

Right ventriculography or echocardiography during the procedure can assess tricuspid valve regurgitation. If significant obstruction persists, and significant regurgitation has not been induced, the procedure is repeated with a larger balloon size. In our experience, successful cases have employed a maximum balloon diameter-tricuspid annulus diameter ratio of 85 to 125%. When a satisfactory result is achieved, hemodynamic measurements are repeated during temporary occlusion of the atrial septal defect, or after permanent occlusion of the ASD with an intracardiac umbrella.

Complications

Tricuspid regurgitation was increased in three of our 10 patients, ranging from trivial to moderate (2+/4+), two of whom had a successful valvotomy. Blood transfusion was given with ten of our 12 procedures. In one patient, balloon rupture was associated with a retained balloon fragment which remained in a left superior vena cava and produced no morbidity.

Results

Among ten patients who have undergone twelve valvotomies at our institution, pulmonary atresia or critical pulmonary stenosis was present in eight, one had Ebstein's anomaly and the other had tricuspid valve stenosis with a parachute-like abnormality and a single papillary muscle. They ranged in age from one month to 4.2 years (mean 1.7 ± 1.3 years) and body weight from 1.4 to 13.4 kg (mean 9.1 ± 4.0 kg). The eight with pulmonary valve disease had undergone prior surgery. Catheter access in four procedures was from jugular or subclavian veins because of femoral vein occlusion. Eight of the twelve valvotomies were associated with other procedures during the same catheterization, including pulmonary angioplasty (n=5), pulmonary valvotomy (n=2), coil occlusion of a right modified Blalock-Taussig shunt (n=2), closure of an atrial septal defect with a clamshell device (n=1) and mitral valvotomy (n=1). The tricuspid valvotomy was considered successful in five patients, decreasing the gradient from the right atrial A-wave to right ventricle end diastolic pressure from 12 ± 4 mmHg to 5 ± 2 mmHg with comparable cardiac output and tricuspid valve flow. The other seven procedures did not have a significant improvement. Important variations in the tricuspid stenosis anatomy may have affected the outcome in these cases. Among the 5 successful valvotomies four have remained free of re-intervention with a mean pressure gradient of 1.9 ± 0.7 mm Hg and $1.0 \pm 0.7 / 4+$ tricuspid regurgitation after 1.5-7.9 years (mean 5.1 ± 2.3).

REFERENCES

1. Rubio-Alvarez,V., Limon R.L. and Soni, J. Valvulotomias intracardiacas por medio de un cateter. *Arch. Inst. Cardiol. Mexico* 1953, 3:183-192.
2. Rubio-Alvarez V. and Limon, R.L. Comisurotomia tricuspidea por medio de un cateter modificado. *Arch. Inst. Cardiol. Mexico* 1955, 25:57-69.
3. Semb B.K.H., Tjonneland S., Stake G. et al. Balloon valvulotomy of congenital pulmonary valve stenosis with tricuspid valve insufficiency. *Cardiovasc. Radiol.* 1979, 2:239-41.
4. Kan J.S., White R.I. Jr., Mitchell S.E., et al. Percutaneous balloon valvuloplasty: A new method for treating congenital pulmonary valve stenosis. *New Engl. J. Med.* 1982, 307:540-42.

5. Kan J.S., White R.I. Jr., Mitchell S.E., et al. Percutaneous transluminal balloon valvuloplasty for pulmonary valve stenosis. *Circulation* 1984, 69:554-60.

6. Rocchini A.P., Kveselis D.A., Crowley D., et al. A. Percutaneous balloon valvuloplasty for treatment of congenital pulmonary valvular stenosis in children. *J. Am. Coll. Cardiol.* 1984, 3:1005-12.

7. Lababidi, Z. and Wu, J. Percutaneous balloon pulmonary valvuloplasty. *Am. J. Cardiol.* 1983, 52:560-62.

8. Radtke, W., Keane, J.F., Fellows, K.E., et al. Percutaneous balloon valvotomy of congenital pulmonary stenosis using oversized balloons. *J. Am. Coll. Cardiol.* 1986, 8:909-15.

9. Zeevi B., Keane J.F., Fellows K.E., et al. Balloon dilation of critical pulmonary stenosis in the first week of life. *J. Am. Coll. Cardiol.* 1988, 11:821-24.

10. Colli A. M., Perry S.B., Lock J.E., et al. Balloon dilation of critical valvar pulmonary stenosis in the first month of life. *Cath. Cardiovasc. Diagn.* 1995, 34:23-28.

11. Justo R.N., Nykanen D.G., Williams W.G., et al. Transcatheter perforation of the right ventricular outflow tract as initial therapy for pulmonary valve atresia and intact ventricular septum in the newborn. *Cath. Cardiovasc. Diagn.* 1997, 40:408-13.

12. Gournay V., Piechaud J.F., Delogu A., et al. Balloon valvotomy for critical stenosis or atresia of pulmonary valve in newborns. *J. Am. Coll. Cardiol.* 1995, 26:1725-31.

13. Fedderly R.T., Lloyd T.R., Mendelsohn A.M., et al. Determinants of successful balloon valvotomy in infants with critical pulmonary stenosis or membranous pulmonary atresia with intact ventricular septum. *J. Am. Coll. Cardiol.* 1995, 25:460-65.

14. McCrindle B.W., Independent predictors of long–term results after balloon pulmonary valvuloplasty. *Circulation*, 1994, 89:1751-59.

15. Talsma M., Witsenburg M., Rohmer J., et al. Determinants for outcome of balloon valvuloplasty for severe pulmonary stenosis in neonates and infants up to six months of age. *Am J Cardiol.* 1993, 71:1246-48.

16. Freedom R., How can something so small cause so much grief? Some thoughts about the underdeveloped right ventricle in pulmonary atresia and intact ventricular septum. *J. Am Coll. Cardiol.* 1992, 19:1038-40.

17. Tabatabaei H., Boutin C., Nykanen D.G., et al. Morphologic and hemodynamic consequences after percutaneous balloon valvotomy for neonatal pulmonary stenosis: medium term follow-up. *J. Am. Coll. Cardiol.* 1996, 27:473-78.

18. Lababidi Z., Wu J. and Walls J.T. Percutaneous balloon aortic valvuloplasty: Results in 23 patients. *Am.J. Cardiol.* 1984, 53:194-97.

19. Helgason H., Keane J.F., Fellows K.E., et al. Balloon dilation of the aortic valve; Studies in normal lambs and in children with aortic stenosis. *J. Am. Coll. Cardiol.* 1987, 9:816-22.

20. Keane J.F., Driscoll D.J., Gersony W.M., et al. Second natural history study of congenital heart defects. Results of treatment of patients with aortic valvar stenosis. *Circulation* . 1993, 87 [suppl I]:I-16--I-27.

21. Rocchini A.P., Beekman R.H., Ben-Shachar G., et al. Balloon aortic valvuloplasty: results of the Valvuloplasty and Angioplasty of Congenital Anomalies Registry. *Am. J.Cardiol.* 1990, 65: 784-89.

22. Yeager, S.B., Balloon selection for double balloon valvotomy. *J. Am. Coll. Cardiol.* 1987, 9:467.

23. Moore J.W., Slack M.C., Kirby W.C., et al. Hemodynamics and coronary blood flow during experimental aortic valvuloplasty: comparison of the dual versus the single catheter methods. *Am Heart J.* 1990, 119:136-42.

24. Mullins C.E., Nihill M.R., Vick G.W. III, et al. Double balloon technique for dilation of valvular or vessel stenosis in congenital and acquired heart disease. *J. Am. Coll. Cardiol.* 1987, 10:107-14.

25. Hausdorf G., Schneider M., Schirmer K.R., et al. Anterograde balloon valvuloplasty of aortic stenosis in children. *Am J Cardiol.* 1993, 71:460-62.

26. Moore P., Egito E., Mowrey B.S., et al. Midterm results of balloon dilation of congenital aortic stenosis: predictors of success. *J. Am. Coll. Cardiol.* 1996, 27:1257-63.

27. Shaddy R.E., Boucek M.M., Sturtevant J.E., et al. Gradient reduction, aortic valve regurgitation and prolapse after balloon aortic valvuloplasty in 32 consecutive patients with congenital aortic stenosis. *J. Am. Coll. Cardiol.* 1990, 16:451-56.

28. Sholler G.F., Keane J.F., Perry S.B., et al. Balloon dilation of congenital aortic valve stenosis: results and influence of technical and morphological features on outcome. *Circulation* 1988, 78:351-60.

29. Keane J.F., Perry S.B., Lock J.E. Balloon dilation of congenital valvular aortic stenosis. *J. Am Coll. Cardiol.* 1990, 16:457-58.

30. O'Connor BK., Beekman R.H., Rocchini A.P., et al, A. Intermediate-term effectiveness of balloon valvuloplasty for congenital aortic stenosis. *Circulation.* 1991, 84:732-38.

31. Kachaner J., Worms A.M., Bourlon F., et al. Percutaneous valvotomy of aortic valve stenoses in children *Arch. Mal. Coeur.* 1996, 89:525-31.

32. Arora, R., Jolly, N., Bhat, A., et al. Follow-up of balloon aortic valvuloplasty in young adults--a combined hemodynamic and Doppler echocardiographic study. *Ind. Heart J.* 1989, 41:314-17.

33. Rosenfeld H.M., Landzberg M.J., Perry S.B., et al. Balloon aortic valvuloplasty in the young adult with congenital aortic stenosis. *Am J. Cardiol.* 1994, 73:1112-17.

34. Zeevi B., Keane J.F., Castaneda A.R., et al. Neonatal critical valvar stenosis: a comparison of surgical and balloon dilation therapy. *Circulation* 1989, 80:831-39.

35. Mosca R.S., Iannettioni M.D., Schwartz S.M, et al. Critical aortic stenosis in the neonate: a comparison of balloon valvuloplasty and transventricular dilation. *J. Thorac. Cardiovasc. Surg.* 1995, 109:147-54.

36. Egito E.S., Moore P., O'Sullivan J., et al. Transvascular balloon dilation for neonatal critical aortic stenosis: early and midterm results. *J. Am. Coll. Cardiol.* 1997, 29:442-47.

37. Gildeur HP, Kleinert S, Weintraub RG, et al. Surgical commissurotomy of the aortic valve: Outcome of open valvotomy in neonates with critical aortic stenosis. Am Heart J 131: 1996, 754-59.

38. Rhodes L.A., Colan S.D., Perry S.B., et al. Predictors of survival in neonates with critical aortic stenosis. *Circulation* 1991, 84:2325-35.

39. Gatzoules M.A., Rigby M.L., Shinebourne E.A., et al. Contemporary results of balloon valvuloplasty and surgical valvotomy for congenital aortic stenosis, *Arch. Dis. Child.* 1995, 73:66-69.

40. Kasten-Sportes C.H., Piechaud J., Sidi D., et al. Percutaneous balloon valvuloplasty in neonates with critical aortic stenosis. *J. Am. Coll. Cardiol.* 1989, 13:1102-05.

41. Lock J.E., Khalilullah M., Shrivastava S., et al. Percutaneous catheter commissurotomy in rheumatic mitral stenosis. *New Engl. J. Med.* 1985, 313:1515-19.

42. Spevak P.J., Bass J.L., Ben-Sachar G., et al. Balloon angioplasty for severe congenital mitral stenosis. *Am. J. Cardiol.* 1990, 66:472-76.

43. Moore P., Adatia I., Spevak P.J., et al. Severe congenital mitral stenosis in infants. *Circulation,* 1994, 89:2099-2106.

44. Grifka R.G., O'Laughlin M.P., Nihill M.R., et al. Double-transseptal, double-balloon valvuloplasty for congenital mitral stenosis. *Circulation* 1992, 85:123-29.

45. Reyes V.P., Soma Raju B., Wynne J., et al. Percutaneous balloon valvuloplasty compared with open surgical commissurotomy for mitral stenosis. *New Eng. J. Med.* 1994, 331:961-67.

46. Dean L.S., Mickel M., Bonan R., et al. Four-year follow-up of patients undergoing percutaneous balloon mitral commissurotomy. *J. Am. Coll. Cardiol.* 1996, 28:1452-57.

47. Orbe L.C., Sobrino N., Arcas R., et al. Initial outcome of percutaneous balloon valvuloplasty in rheumatic tricuspid valve stenosis. *Am. J. Cardio.* 71:353-34. 1993.

48. Onate A., Alcibar J., Inguanzo R. et al. Balloon dilation of tricuspid and pulmonary valves in carcinoid heart disease. *Texas Heart Inst. J.* 1993, 20:115-19.

178

49. Feit F., Stecy P.J., Nachamie M.S. Percutaneous balloon valvuloplasty for stenosis of a porcine bioprosthesis in the tricuspid valve position. *Am. J. Cardiol.* 1986, 58:363-64.
50. Attubato M.J., Stroh J.A., Bach R.G., et al. Percutaneous double-balloon valvuloplasty of porcine bioprosthetic valves in the tricuspid postion. *Cath. Cardiovasc. Diagn.* 1990, 20:202-04.
51. Giglia T.M., Jenkins K.J., Matitiau A., et al. Influence of right heart size on outcome in pulmonary atresia with intact ventricular septum. *Circulation.* 1993, 88 [part 1]:2248-56.
52. Patel R.G., Freedom R.M., Moes C.A.F., et al. Right ventricular volume determinations in 18 patients with pulmonary atresia and intact ventricular septum. *Circulation* . 1980, 61:428-40.
53. Freedom R.M., Dische M.R., Rowe R.D. The tricuspid valve in pulmonary atresia and intact ventricular septum. A morphological study of 60 cases. *Arch. Pathol. Lab. Med.* 1978, 102:28.
54. Chen C.R., Lo Z.X, Haung Z.D., et al. Concurrent percutaneous balloon valvuloplasty for combined tricuspid and pulmonic stenosis. *Cath. Cardiovasc. Diagn.* 1988, 15:55-60.

7. DEFECT CLOSURE: UMBRELLA DEVICES

Albert Rocchini, M.D.
James E. Lock, M.D.

Although catheter-delivered devices to close intracardiac defects have been successfully deployed in humans for 25 years, their use has only become widespread during the past 2-3 years. While several devices are used routinely at this writing in Europe and elsewhere, no device has yet been approved by the U.S. Food and Drug Administration. Several factors have contributed to this delay; the combination of rare diseases, parents' and physicians' reluctance to submit children to randomized trials, a successful, albeit highly invasive therapeutic alternative (i.e. open heart surgery), safety and efficiency criteria for FDA approval based primarily on common adult diseases. Nonetheless, it seems clear that intracardiac occlusion devices are now necessary and vital tools in the management of simple and complex congenital heart disease.

This chapter will focus on the history of such devices, general comments on intracardiac umbrellas, a description of devices currently in use, and the techniques used to deploy them in ASDs, VSDs and other defects.

HISTORY

The first device used to close an ASD was a plastic button developed in 1959, by Hufnagel and Gillespie [1], which could be implanted in the atrial septum via a thoracotomy. The first successful transcatheter closure of an ASD was developed by King and Mills in 1974 [2-4]. This device was composed of two umbrella shaped discs of Teflon coated stainless steel and polyester fabric. Since all intracardiac closure devices have umbrella-like mechanisms in common, "umbrella" is not a bad generic term for such devices. Defects were closed by trapping the septum between the two halves of the umbrella device. Five patients underwent attempted closure of centrally positioned ASDs with 25-35 mm diameter devices. Follow-up (6-12 month) studies on all 5 patients revealed complete closure in 2, and a residual shunt in 3. The value of the device was in part limited by its 23F introducer that required a common iliac venous cutdown.

In 1983, Rashkind [5,6] developed a single disc device to close ASDs. Consisting of a single disc of polyurethane foam on a wire umbrella-like skeleton, the device closed the ASD by embedding in the atrial septum three small sharp "fish hooks" at ends of the wire skeleton. Results of device implantation were mixed. Rashkind reported successful device deployment in only 13/20 patients; however, 4 individuals required emergency surgery due to improper device deployment and 3 individuals had significant residuals shunts. Similarly, mixed results were reported by Beekman et al [7].
At the same time, Lock et al used the Rashkind PDA double umbrella device to successfully close a variety of intracardiac defects, including ASDs and PFOs [8], and VSDs [9]. This experience, confirmed by Reddington et al [10], led directly to the development of new intracardiac devices. While the devices of Hufnagle and Gillespie, King and Mills, and the two devices of Rashkind are no longer in clinical use to close intracardiac defects, they were crucial first steps.

THE IDEAL DEVICE
The recent proliferation of catheter-delivered devices used to close intracardiac defects emphasizes the complex nature of this therapeutic task.

Analyzing the results of intracardiac umbrella closure depends on the completeness and rigor of follow up, and the appropriateness of patient selection and comparison groups. Potential and real conflict of interest issues must be weighed in arriving at recommendations that best serve our primary customers, the patients.

Until more experience and more complete follow up narrows the therapeutic options, a theoretical discussion of the ideal intracardiac closure device will help focus attention on issues of considerable clinical importance. We have prepared a list of important device desiderata that should be considered as the multiple available devices are reviewed (Table 7-1).

TABLE 7-1

THE IDEAL INTRACARDIAC SEPTAL CLOSURE DEVICE

DURING CLOSURE

1. Small introducing catheter
2. Adjustable and retrievable prior to release
3. Flexible self-centering mechanism
4. Adjusts to variable septal topography
5. Inexpensive and easy to use

AFTER FAILED CLOSURE

1. Embolization produces minimal hemodynamic stress
2. Easily retrievable after release

AFTER SUCCESSFUL CLOSURE

1. Device lies flat against septum with a low profile
2. Covered with material that promotes full endothelialization
3. Reliable device integrity until full endothelialization
4. Minimal overlap to protect adjacent cardiac structures

RESULTS OF OPERATIVE MANAGEMENT

When evaluating the risks and benefits of a specific transcatheter device it is paramount to compare device closure with surgical closure in the following areas: the immediate peri-procedure morbidity and mortality, efficacy of defect closure, and long-term follow-up information, especially late complications.

Surgical closure of secundum atrial septal defects has been performed since 1951. During the past 47 years the average surgical mortality has declined from 12% in 1959 [11] to 0.4% in 1994 [12]. Relatively mild peri-operative complications, including gastrointestinal problems, urinary tract infections, fever, pleural and pericardial effusions, pulmonary atelectasis, and wound infections, occur in up to 70% of individuals following surgical closure (10). Moderate complications can occur in up to 10% of post-operative patients, including pneumonia, pleural and pericardial effusions requiring drainage, and arrhythmias such as junctional tachycardia and transient atrioventricular dissociation. Severe complications include sepsis, renal failure, pericardial tamponade, persistent bleeding requiring reoperation, neurological problems, cardiac arrest and heart block requiring pacing [12-14].

Surgery effectively closes the defect in more than 96% of cases [12,15]. As expected, contrast echocardiography can detect trivial or "absent" shunts in as many as 33% of post-operative patients [16].

Long-term cardiac status after surgical closure of atrial septal defects is also very good. Meijboom et al [15] reported that 92% of individuals were free from any medical or surgical intervention up to 20 years following atrial septal defect closure (mean follow up = 14.5 years). Long-term sequelae following atrial septal defect closure were primarily atrial and ventricular arrhythmias. Similarly, Murphy et al [17] reported that in patients 12-24 years of age at the time of surgery, late onset (24-32 years post-operative) atrial fibrillation and/or atrial flutter occurred in 17% of individuals.

In summary, surgical closure of secundum atrial septal defects is associated with a very low surgical mortality (< 1%), a high incidence of mild postoperative complications (70%), a 5-10% incidence of moderate to severe immediate postoperative complications, a >97% incidence of defect closure, and an 8-17% late incidence of problems, primarily arrhythmias.

GENERAL COMMENTS ON TECHNIQUES OF ASD CLOSURE

The most reliable method for delivering an ASD device into the atrial septum is with the use of both fluoroscope and transesophageal echocardiography [18]. Due to both the use of transesophageal echocardiography and the desire to minimize patient movement during device placement, intubation and general

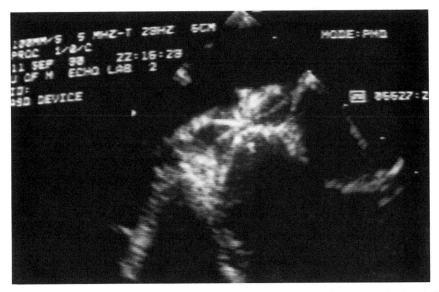

Figure 7-1: Transesophageal echocardiographic image of successfully placed clamshell device.

anesthesia are common. The femoral vein and artery are entered percutaneously. All patients receive heparin and prophylactic antibiotics. A right heart catheterization is performed. The ASD is crossed with an angiographic catheter and a left atrial angiogram is performed using 30-45 degrees left oblique with 10-15 degrees of cranial or caudal angulation.

For most devices, the defect is balloon-sized to obtain the stretched diameter. A 22mm balloon, Meditech (Mansfield, MA) follows a guidewire into the left atrium. The balloon is over-inflated in the left atrium, gently pulled back against the septum and then gradually deflated until it passes through the defect. The circumferential indentation of the balloon as it passes through the atrial septum is measured both angiographically and by transesophageal echocardiography. The stretched diameter of the atrial defect is usually 20-30% larger than the diameter measured by transesophageal echo [19].

An appropriate delivery catheter and sheath are placed on a guidewire and flushed outside the body to remove air. It is very important to remove all air from around both the wire and the dilator outside the body with vigorous flushing. The sheath and dilator are advanced over the guidewire into the left atrium. As the guidewire and dilator are removed slowly from the sheath, saline is infused through the sidearm to fill the sheath and prevent air from being sucked into the sheath. To eliminate the possibility of an air embolism, resulting from air trapped inside any device, the device is soaked in water before loading.
Before releasing the device, the position is checked primarily by transesophageal echo. Gentle pulling on the system will evert the distal arms or disc as they are pulled against the defect; by pushing, the proximal arms or disc will evert against the proximal side of the defect. Failure of the arms to move appropriately
suggests that either both discs are on the same side of the defect or that part of the umbrella is on the wrong side. The most reliable method of assuring that the device is properly positioned is transesophageal echo. (Fig. 7-1)

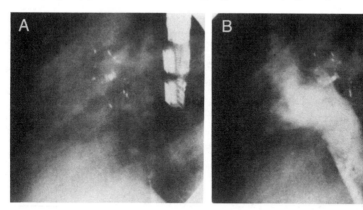

Figure 7-2:
A. A fluoroscopic image obtained in the left anterior oblique with cranial angulation that demonstrates the clamshell arms. The transesophageal echo probe is also visible.
B. A right atrial angiogram documenting the relation of the clamshell arms to the atrial septum.

With echo, each side can be visualized to insure it is correctly positioned. Echo also confirms that the device is not obstructing the pulmonary veins, inferior vena cava, superior vena cava or interfering with the atrioventricular valves. If

the device is satisfactorily positioned the umbrella is released using the release mechanism.
Following release, camera angles are adjusted so that one plane is parallel to the umbrella and the other is perpendicular. The plane which is parallel to the device helps to determine if the device is positioned correctly (Fig. 7-2A). The perpendicular plane helps to demonstrate the relationship of the device to systemic and pulmonary veins and atrioventricular valves. A right atrial angiogram is performed (Fig. 7-2B) and the contrast followed through to the levophase. Contrast and color Doppler echocardiography can also be used to test for residual shunts.
All patients are kept overnight after the catheterization, and a repeat transthoracic echocardiogram and chest x-ray are performed the day after the procedure. In the USA, the follow up for each device is performed as mandated by the FDA trial.

CURRENTLY AVAILABLE DEVICES

Although the device of King and Mills, the original Rashkind ASD device, and the original Lock Clamshell device are no longer in clinical use, there are five devices currently available either in clinical trials in the USA or in general use elsewhere. We will review these devices briefly; some of their characteristics are summarized in Table 7-2.

Table 7-2

Details On Introducer Size and Atrial Profile of the Currently Available Atrial Septal Defect Devices
10 mm Stretched ASD

Device	Size of Device (mm)	Sheath Size (French)	Size of LA Portion of Device (mm)	Size Of The RA Portion of Device (mm)
CardioSeal	23	11	23 – diagonal 17 – square	23 – diagonal 17 – square
Amplatzer	10	7	22- radius	18 – radius
Button	25	8	25	25
ASDOS	25	10	25 – radius	25 – radius
Angel-Wings	20	11	20 – square	20- square

20 mm Stretched ASD

Device	Size of Device (mm)	Sheath Size (French)	Size of LA Portion of Device (mm)	Size Of The RA Portion of Device (mm)
CardioSeal	40	11	40 – diagonal 29 – square	40 – diagonal 29 – square
Amplatzer	20	8	34 – radius	30 – radius
Button	40	8	40	40
ASDOS	40-45	10	40-45 – radius	40-45 – radius
Angel-Wings	40	11	40 – square	40 – square

Abbreviations: RA = right atrium; LA = left atrium

184

CardioSEAL Double Umbrella
Device and Delivery System: The CardioSEAL Septal Occluder (Nitinol Medical, Boston, MA) is a modification of the Bard Clamshell Device [20, 21]. The CardioSEAL septal occluder consists of a double umbrella. Each of the

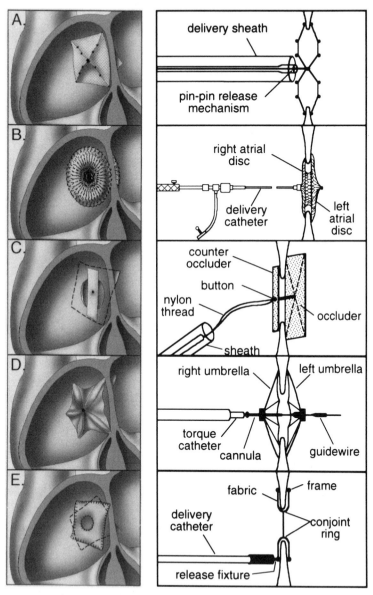

Figure 7-3: Schematic representation of the five currently available transcatheter atrial septal defect devices. (A=CardioSEAl; B= Amplatzer; C= Button; D = ASDOS; E = Angel Wings).

185

umbrellas has 4 spring-loaded arms. The arms are flexible, and flexibly attached to each other in the center, allowing arm separation when the septum is thick, and arm overlap when the septum is thin, creating a device with a low profile within the heart. The metal skeleton is covered with a woven Dacron fabric to promote early endothelialization. The CardioSEAL Septal Occluder has a square design and is available in 17, 23, 28, 33, and 40mm sizes.

The new device has several modifications: the metal used in construction has been changed to an alloy (MP35N) that is superior to the original stainless steel and mechanical stress to critical areas of the arms was reduced by adding an extra spring to each arm of the larger devices [22]. The extra hinges also improve septal positioning.

For delivery, the umbrella is connected to the release wire in the delivery catheter using a pin-pin mechanism (Fig. 7-3A).

Next, each umbrella is collapsed in the following manner: 1. the distal umbrella is collapsed by pulling the arms distally; 2. the umbrella is then pulled through a funnel shaped loading cylinder until the proximal umbrella collapses proximally; 3. finally, using the release wire the two collapsed umbrellas are pulled out of the loading cylinder and into the pod at the end of the delivery catheter.

The general procedure for ASD device implantation has been listed above. To deliver the CardioSEAL, a long 11 French sheath is used to advance the delivery catheter into the left atrium. The system can deliver the umbrella directly from the pod at the end of the delivery catheter. However, because of the pod is rigid and does not follow curves well, the pod is left at the IVC/right atrial junction and the umbrella is advanced out into the sheath using the release wire [23].

The umbrella is then advanced to the distal end of the sheath. The sheath is retracted until the arms supporting the distal umbrella spring open. The entire system, delivery catheter, umbrella and sheath, is then pulled back until only one of the distal arms begins to touch the left atrial side of the defect. Since the right atrial arms will begin to open well down into the right atrium, they will sweep the atrial septum towards the device, insuring ideal positioning. Without moving the umbrella, the sheath is retracted further until the arms supporting the proximal umbrella spring open on the right atrial side of the defect. The most common error in using this device is to retract the device too close to the septum, allowing one of the left atrial arms to prolapse through the ASD before release.

Once the device has been deployed so that the left atrial arms are on the left side and the right atrial arms are on the right side, the release wire is advanced to allow the pin-pin mechanism inside the cylinder to disengage, releasing the CardioSEAL.

186

Recent Modifications

The CardioSEAL design has recently been modified to allow for flexible self-centering.. This so called Starflex design (Fig. 7-4) has flexible nitinol springs attached to the proximal and distal umbrella tips, creating a cone-shaped device when positioning the left atrial arms, and a hammock-like self-centering system after release.

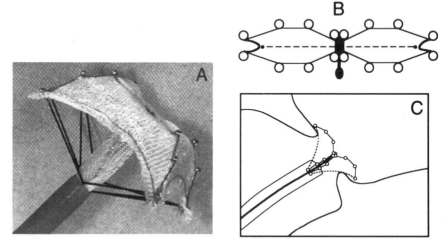

Figure 7-4: A: photograph of STARFlex™ with microsprings attached between distal opened and proximal unopened arms.
B: drawing of CardioSEAL® Occluder with STARFlex Centering System illustrating how the microsprings create a flexible "centering" hub.
C: drawing showing how STARFlex would center an ASD.

Amplatzer Septal Occluder

Device, Delivery System, and Delivery: The Amplatzer Septal Occluder (AGA Medical Corp., Golden Valley, MN) was developed by Amplatz in 1996 [24]. It's ingenious design is constructed from 0.004-0.005 inch Nitinol wires, tightly woven into two buttons with a 4 mm thick connecting waist (Fig. 7-3B). The device diameter is the diameter of the waist, and is available from 4-26 m sizes with 1 mm increments. For devices 4-10 mm (the diameter of the waist) the left atrial disc is 12 mm and the right atrial disc 8 mm larger than the waist; for devices sizes 11-26 mm, the left atrial disc is 14 mm and the right atrial disc 10 mm larger than the waist. Therefore, the diameter of the left atrial disc for the 20 mm device is 34 mm. The occluder is filled with fluffy polyester threads to enhance thrombogenicity. The surface is nitinol mesh; the Amplatzer is the only device that relies on endothelium covering a metal surface. The two buttons have a thickness of several millimeters, producing the highest profile of any currently available intracardiac devices. The device is connected to a delivery cable by a microscrew connection and withdrawn into a loader for introduction into the delivery catheter (7 French for devices less than 15 mm and 8 French for the larger devices).

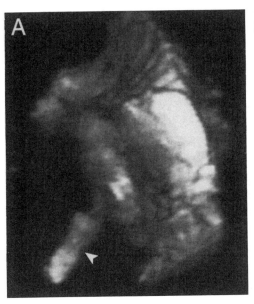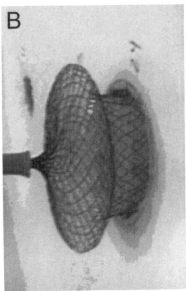

Figure 7-5: A: A three dimensional echo illustrating successful placement of a 15 mm Amplatzer septal occluder. The delivery cable is still attached to the device. The arrow is pointing to the delivery sheath.
B: A photographic illustration of the three dimensional image depicted in panel A. The 15 mm Amplatzer device on the delivery cable is positioned with the right atrial disc visible and the waist of the device positioned through a 14 mm hole.

The Amplatzer Septal Occluder device is designed to stent open the ASD, and thus the size is selected to be the same as the stretched diameter of the ASD (Table 1). A long 7 or 8 French sheath (AGA Medical Corp., Golden Valley, MN) is positioned in the left atrium. The delivery cable is passed through the loader, and the proper size device is screwed clockwise onto the tip of the delivery cable. The device and loader are immersed in saline solution as the Amplatzer Septal Occluder is pulled into the loader. The loader is then introduced into the delivery sheath and the device is advanced into the left atrium. The sheath is retracted until the left atrial disc and waist connection portion are opened in the middle of the left atrium, forming a cone which allows self-centering during deployment. The sheath with delivery cable are pulled back as one unit close to the left atrial side of the septum. With further retraction of the sheath, while maintaining constant tension on the delivery sheath and cable, the right atrial disc is deployed in the right atrium.

A unique advantage of the Amplatzer is that if both discs are incorrectly placed, both the proximal and distal parts of the device can be retracted back inside the delivery sheath, and the delivery steps repeated. Once proper device position is confirmed, the device is released by turning the cable counterclockwise using a pin vise (Figs. 7-5,6).

188

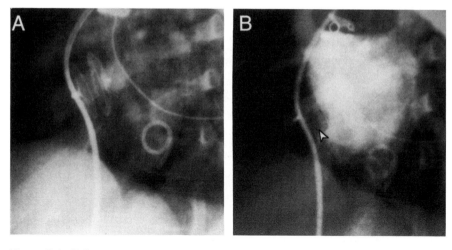

Figure 7-6: Pulmonary artery angiogram, obtained with left anterior oblique with cranial angulation, shows a successfully positioned 14 mm Amplatzer septal occluder.

Recent Modifications

The Amplatzer has been recently modified to have a thicker (7 mm) central spool and less bulky discs for closure of ventricular septal defects.

Button Device (Custom Medical Devices, Amarillo, TX)

Device, Delivery System and Delivery: In 1990, Sideris et al [25] developed the Button device, Custom Medical Devices, Amarillo, TX. The buttoned device system consists of 3 components: the occluder, counter-occluder and a delivery system. (Fig. 7-3C) The occluder is made of a Teflon-coated wire (0.018 inch) skeleton covered with 1/16 inch of polyurethane foam. The wire skeleton is x-shaped when open, and lies relatively flat against a smooth septal surface, with a low intracardiac profile. The wires can be rotated to a parallel position for introduction into an 8 French sheath. A 2 mm string loop is attached to the center of the occluder; the loop is closed by a 1 mm radiopaque knot (the button) [26]. The counter-occluder is composed of a single-strand, Teflon coated wire skeleton covered with a rhomboid-shaped piece of polyurethane foam. A latex rubber piece is sutured in the center of the counter-occluder and becomes the buttonhole. In individuals with a right-to-left shunt the counter-occluder has been modified to be near identical in shape and structure to the occluder [36]. The delivery system consists of: a Teflon-coated 0.035 inch guidewire (loading wire); a folded 0.008 inch nylon thread that passes through the guidewire whose rigid core has been removed (loop of thread passes through the loop in the center of the occluder); an 8 French long sheath with a side port; and an 8 French catheter (pusher) that is used to advance the occluder and counter-occluder within the sheath. The nominal size of each device is the length of the counter-occluder and the diagonal length of the occluder. Device sizes of 25, 30 35, 40, 45, 50 mm are available.

The Button device is selected to be at least twice the stretched diameter of the ASD and preferably >20 mm larger that the defect. This degree of oversizing is mandated by the lack of a self-centering mechanism and shrinkage of the polyurethane foam. (Table 7-2) A 8 French long sheath (9 French for 50 mm and some 45 mm devices) is positioned in the left atrium. The occluder is folded and advanced with the pushing catheter through the sheath into the left atrium. The occluder assumes a square shape when free in the left atrium, and is withdrawn to the left side of the atrial septum. With the sheath in the right atrium, the delivery wire is then passed through the latex "buttonhole" of the counter-occluder, and the counter-occluder is advanced out of the sheath into the right atrium, assuming a position roughly perpendicular to the sheath. The sheath is then advanced with traction on the delivery wire to position the counter-occluder along the right side of the atrial septum. Further traction on the delivery wire and advancement of the sheath causes the "button" to pass through the buttonhole, securing the counter-occluder to the occluder. Once in position, the device is released by opening the proximal end of the delivery wire nylon loop, pulling the guidewire shell off the nylon loop, and pulling gently on one link of the nylon loop until the other end passes out of the button loop and delivery sheath.

ASDOS Device

Device, Delivery System, and Delivery: Described by Babic in 1991, the ASDOS (Osypka Corp., Germany) consists of two major components: a delivery system that includes a 10 F introducer sheath, a 0.014 inch 450 cm ASDOS guidewire with a metal cone in the middle of the guidewire, a 7 French torque catheter, and a 20 gauge transseptal metal cannula; and two self-opening umbrellas made of Nitinol wire frame and a thin membrane of microporous polyurethane [28, 29]. The polyurethane on the outside of the device promotes closure and endothelialization (Fig. 7-3D). Each umbrella has 5 arms which assume a round shape in the open position. Umbrella sizes of 25, 30, 40, 45, 50, 55, and 60 mm are available.

After the 10 French transseptal sheath enters the left atrium, a 7 French balloon catheter is advanced from the left atrium to the ascending aorta and caught by a snare catheter. A 0.014 inch, 450cm Nitinol ASDOS J guidewire with a metal cone in the middle of the guidewire, is then advanced into the aorta, snared and exteriorized through the femoral artery. A 6 French catheter is then advanced over the wire from the femoral artery to the left atrium. A 20-gauge metal transseptal cannula is then introduced into a torque catheter and the right atrial umbrella is mounted over the tip of the metal cannula on to the torque catheter (creating the assembly unit). The left atrial umbrella and assemble unit are then introduced over the long guidewire into the long venous sheath. The left atrial umbrella is pushed with the metal cannula tip while the arms of the right umbrella are folded manually and pushed with the torque catheter. After the left atrial umbrella opens in the left atrium, the metal cone on the guidewire fixes the left atrial umbrella: by pulling back on the venous end of the wire, the left atrial umbrella is secured to the tip of the transseptal metal cannula. The long sheath is then retracted into the right atrium and the torque catheter is pushed over the metal cannula until the right atrial umbrella opens. The metal cannula is then rotated and the two umbrellas are approximated to each other by pushing the torque catheter. Using both right and left atrial angiography the umbrellas are manipulated until the appropriate place for anchoring is found. Keeping the left atrial umbrella against the metal cannula the torque catheter is then advanced over the cannula, engaging it into the slit of the right atrial umbrella. The two umbrellas are then screwed together using the torque catheter. The torque catheter and the metal cannula are then released from the umbrella and retracted into the lower right atrium leaving the interlocked umbrellas on the guidewire. If the umbrellas are not correctly positioned the metal cannula and torque catheter are then advanced up to the right atrial umbrella, the umbrellas are disconnected by counter-clockwise rotation of the torque catheter, and repositioned. Once the

190

umbrellas are secure in the appropriate location, the long guidewire is removed via the left atrial catheter out of the femoral artery.

Das-Angel Wings Device

Device, Delivery System, and Delivery: The Das-Angel Wings Device, (Microvena, Vadnais, MN) developed by Das in 1993, [30] consists of two square frames made of superelastic Nitinol wire (0.01 inch) with a radiopaque wire of platinum wound around it (Fig. 7-3E). Each square frame has four legs that are interconnected by flexible eyelets at the corners, with a flexible eyelet at the midpoint of each leg. The eight eyelets in each square frame function as torsion springs and permit the frame to be collapsed for loading the device. The wire frames contain Dacron fabric to promote closure and endothelialization. A circular hole, whose diameter is approximately half the size of the disk, is punched out of the right atrial disk. The margin of this orifice is sewn onto the fabric of the left atrial side to form a conjoint ring, causing self-centering. When properly positioned, the arms lay perfectly flat against the septum, with the lowest profile of any currently available device. The device is available in a range of sizes from 18 to 40 mm. Unlike the CardioSEAL device (where the measurements are diagonal), dimensions of the Das device are along the side of the square.

The delivery system consists of a control handle connected to a 10.5 French delivery catheter. A "Y" connector joins the delivery catheter to the control handle, permitting continuous flushing. A coaxial pusher connected to a thumbscrew is run inside the delivery catheter to its tip, permitting the tip to be drawn in or pushed out. At the tip of the coaxial pusher, a short length of stainless steel tubing is incorporated with a notch cut out. Within the lumen of this tube and the coaxial pusher, runs a 0.014 inch diameter Nitinol wire. The Nitinol wire runs from the tip of the stainless steel tubing, all the way back to the control handle where it is interconnected to a spring-loaded release trigger. One of the corner eyelets of the right atrial disc is positioned within the notch and the 0.014 inch diameter Nitinol wire is slid back through the eyelet, locking it in the release fixture.

The Angel Wings device is selected to be twice the stretched diameter of the ASD. The Angel Wings device, preloaded in its 10.5 French delivery catheter, is then advanced into an 11F sheath located in the left atrium. By rotating the thumbscrew, the left atrial disk is then extruded until the disk opens fully. The entire sheath assembly is then gently pulled back until the left atrial disc is snug against the atrial septum. While gentle traction is applied to the delivery catheter, the thumb-screw is rotated until the right atrial disc is extruded and deployed. The safety screw of the release trigger is then loosened, and the trigger is activated to release the device. Once the right atrial position of the device is extruded, it can no longer be retrieved.

RESULTS OF ASD CLOSURE WITH INTRACARDIAC DEVICES

A long and growing list of manuscripts report the results of catheter closure of ASDs [19,20,21,25-27,29,31-44]. As noted above, comparisons of these reports are difficult to interpret (Table 7-3).

TABLE 7-3

Comparison Of Various Transcatheter Devices That Are In Use To Close Atrial Septal Defects And Success Rate of Implantation, Incidence Of Severe Complications And The Rate Of Complete Closure

	Surgery	Amplatzer	Clamshell	Button	ASDOS	Angel-Wings
# Devices Implanted		>229	>400	>200	20	>50
Implantation Success Rate		100%	94%	87%	80%	92%
Incidence of Severe Comp*	5-8%	1.7%	6%	7%	20%	8%
% Complete Closure						
Immediate		52%	9%	20%	60%	70%
3 months		95%	35%	35%		
6 months			47%	48%		
>12 months			55%	52%		
>48 months	97%			74%		

* = Severe complications include: death, cerebral vascular accidents, need for emergent operation, tamponade, cardiac arrest and severe dysrhythmias. # = number.

The device with the largest and longest follow up is probably the original Clamshell device. Device embolization was common (11%) in the first report[40], rare (4.3%) in a later inclusive study, and not seen in the recent CardioSEAL experience [45]. Similarly, one stroke was reported in the initial experience [40]. Late inclusive follow up indicates an extremely low (< 1%) incidence of TIA's and arrhythmias in over 500 patients; endocarditis was not observed. Residual leaks were relatively common, with trivial leaks in 39% of patients [21], but significant leaks in 6%.

There are fewer reports of results of the Amplatzer [37,43]. In general, the closure rates are very good, and exceed 95% after 3 months of follow up [43]. Early complications were uncommon, but included both TIA and endocarditis.

Many studies report the results of the Button device [25-27,33,35,39]. Unsuccessful procedures were relatively common (5-10%), as was "urgent" surgery. Late unbuttoning resulting in late embolization has been described in several reports, although it is uncommon (1-6%). Residual shunts are common (26-48%) but almost always trivial. Late endocarditis is unreported.

Early trials of the Angel Wings device described embolization and surgical retrieval in 3 of 6 devices [31], although later studies achieved successful implantation in 92% [32]. Significant shunts were uncommon (9%) at 5 month follow up. The incidence of late complications is unknown. Finally, there are few reports of the ASDOS device [14,29,34], with occasional embolizations, rare late leaks and arrhythmias.

SUMMARY

Although FDA approval has yet to be obtained for any devices, continuing improvements in technique and device design have resulted in widespread and increasing international use. There is no question that these devices are important clinical tools for patients who are at increased surgical risk. Their utility in low risk patients will await longer-term follow up.

DEVICE CLOSURE OF VENTRICULAR SEPTAL DEFECTS

History

The first transcatheter device closure of a ventricular septal defect was accomplished in 1987-88 [9] when the Bard PDA Umbrella was used to close small ventricular septal defects. The closure of larger ventricular septal defects did not come until the development of the Clamshell Septal Occluder [46].

Indications For Device Closure Of Ventricular Septal Defects: A patient is considered a candidate for septal defect device closure with a device if they have one of the following: a muscular ventricular septal defect, a residual defect at the patch margins following surgery, a ventricular septal defect following a myocardial infarction. Due to their close proximity to semilunar and atrioventricular valves, the most common types of ventricular septal defects (perimembranous, inlet, and conal ventricular septal defects) cannot, except in rare cases, be closed using current transvenous techniques. Rigby and Reddington [47] did report a small series of patients who had a perimembranous ventricular septal defects closed using the Bard PDA Umbrella. However, these authors concluded that their results did not support the routine use of an Umbrella to close perimembranous defects. Another indication for transcatheter VSD closure of a ventricular septal defect is a patient with multiple ventricular septal defects in whom the muscular defects are closed at catheterization and the non-muscular defects or other complex heart disease is repaired in the operating room [46].

Techniques Used To Close Ventricular Septal Defects: As with the closure of atrial septal defects, a pre-catheterization echocardiogram is critical to determine the number, size and locations of the ventricular septal defects. In addition, the pre-catheterization echocardiogram is also crucial to determine the relationship of the defect to the atrioventricular and semilunar valves.

As with the closure of atrial septal defects, the procedure is usually done under general anesthesia with the assistance of transesophageal echocardiography. All patients are heparinized, undergo a complete diagnostic cardiac catheterization, one or more left ventricular angiograms and receive antibiotic prophylaxis. In almost all cases it is preferable to deliver the device using the venous side in order to avoid placing a large sheath in the femoral artery and across the aortic valve [23]. The ventricular septal defect is usually easier to cross from left to right ventricle, although the anterior muscular VSD is an exception. Depending on the location of the ventricular septal defect the left ventricle is either entered retrograde or transseptally (see Table 7-4).

TABLE 7-4

VSD Location	Catheter Approach	Catheter Used	Maneuvers
Anterior muscular	RA to RV to RVOT	5F, Judkins R, Cobra	Counter-clockwise rotation into RVOT sinus, torque wire through VSD
Apical Muscular	RA to LA to LV	7F balloon end hole	LPA twist to stiff end of 0.035" wire directs balloon toward VSD
Mid-Muscular	As for apical VSD	As for apical VSD	As for apical VSD, tighter wire curve
"Intramural" post-op VSD	Ao to LVOT	Judkins or Amplatz R	Catheter in LVOT, rotated anteriorly, withdrawn slowly

The ventricular septal defect can usually be crossed from the left ventricle using a balloon tipped, end-hole catheter either with the aid of a tip-defecting wire or a torque controlled guidewire. If the end-hole catheter fails, then a variety of preformed catheters and a torque controlled guidewire can be used. Once the catheter passes through the ventricular septal defect into the right ventricle and across the pulmonary or tricuspid valve an exchange guidewire is advanced out of the catheter and snared via the venous catheter. This guidewire now runs from either the femoral vein or artery through the heart across the ventricular septal defect and out the internal jugular or femoral vein. Undue traction on this wire can damage the heart or induce aortic or mitral regurgitation. For those reasons, extra stiff wires should not be snared and left pulled through the heart. This wire is used to take selective pictures in the ventricular septal defect, for balloon sizing and for positioning the long sheath used for device placement.

The only currently available devices that have been used to close a ventricular septal defect are the CardioSEAL and the Amplatzer device [48]. If the CardioSEAL device is used the device is chosen to be approximately two times the stretched diameter of the defect. If the Amplatzer device is used the device is chosen to be approximately the size (waist size) of the stretched diameter of the defect. Since the sides of the CardioSEAL are independently sprung, the thickness of the ventricular septum is not important in choosing this device. The center spool of an Amplatzer VSD device is 7 mm, corresponding to a 7 mm thick septum. How this device behaves in thinner or thicker septa is as yet unclear. Having determined device size based on defect size, one must determine if that device will fit in the heart without interfering with valves. A long sheath is then advanced across the defect, and the device is then loaded and delivered as discussed in the section on atrial septal defect closure. With the CardioSEAL device, failure of the left ventricular arms to open completely suggests entrapment in the free wall or other vital structures. To relieve this appearance, the still-attached device is withdrawn against the sheath after left ventricular arm deployment, insuring that the arms are fully deployed. In the right ventricle, arms commonly do not open completely due to the thickness of the septum and the presence of right ventricular trabeculae [23]. In the case of the Amplatzer device failure of the left ventricular disc to completely open suggests that the device may be entrapped in the free wall of the left ventricle or caught in the papillary muscles or other portion of the mitral valve apparatus. Prior to release, device position can be checked with angiograms, by manipulating the device, but the most reliable method is to use transesophageal echocardiography. Transcatheter closure of ventricular septal defects is technically a difficult procedure. In a study conducted by Laussen et al [49], at Boston Children's Hospital, 28 out of 70 ventricular septal defect closures were associated with significant hypotension requiring acute fluid administration in 12 and acute resuscitation in 16. Significant dysrhythmias occurred in 20/70. Blood transfusion was required in 38 individuals and the need for transfusion was directly related to the size of the patient. Despite that, there were no device or procedure related mortalities in 140 VSD closures using the Clamshell or CardioSEAL device. In certain cases, especially in individuals weighing less than 7 kg, intraoperative device closure of muscular ventricular septal defects has been performed [50].

Results of Transcatheter Closure Of Ventricular Septal Defects:
Boston Children's Hospital has the largest experience with closing ventricular septal defects with a transcatheter device. From February 1989 through July, 1998, 148 transcatheter ventricular septal defect closures were performed with no deaths or late morbidity due to catheterization related events. By echocardiography, 83% of the defects were either closed or had trivial residual leaks. They also reported that 20% of the defects were closed without actually straddling the defect. Rather, the Clamshell device was implanted in the right ventricular trabecula since this part of the "septum" was the most restrictive [23]. Complications associates with ventricular septal defect closure included: femoral vein thrombosis, asymptomatic hemothorax, and, in one case, umbrella impingement on the septal leaflet of the tricuspid valve [23].
There has been very limited experience with the use of the Amplatzer Septal occluder to close ventricular septal defects, none in Swiss cheese septa. Amin et al [48] reported on the use of this device to close experimentally created ventricular septal defects in animals, and the successful closure of an anterior muscular ventricular septal defect in a small child using the Amplatzer device.

General Comments On Device Closure Of Ventricular Septal Defects:
Only a small portion of individuals with a ventricular septal defect are candidates for device closure. Transcatheter closure of ventricular septal defects can be a technically difficult procedure: an experienced team of cardiologists, anesthesiologists and surgeons needs to be available to ensure that device closure of a ventricular septal defect can be performed with adequate safety. Even so, current results are very good, and support increasing use of this technique in appropriate patients.

TRANSCATHETER CLOSURE OF OTHER DEFECTS

Patent Foramen Ovale
The technique for closing these defects is very similar to that described for ASD. Since PFOs are largely tunnels rather than holes, self-centering devices will distort the septum and may not lie flat against the heart. For those reasons, the most commonly used devices have been the CardioSEAL and the Button device. The indications for and results of catheter closure of PFOs are discussed fully in Chapter 11.

Fenestrated Fontans

The increasing use of a baffle fenestration has created a large number of patients with small but significant defects in the lateral tunnel used to construct most Fontan pathways. The 17mm and 23mm CardioSEAL devices, with their low profiles and Dacron closure material, have been most commonly employed with success rates approaching 100%. Although the precise indications for closure are not yet established, we have recommended closure inpatients whose hemoglobin is elevated or whose O_2 saturation is below 90%.

Perivalvar Leaks

Although many perivalvar leaks are crescent shaped and therefore difficult to close using any of the currently available devices, we have successfully used either the Rashkind PDA occluder or the Clamshell to close over a dozen defects successfully [8]. These rather difficult procedures should only be performed by interventional cardiologists with considerable device experience, as the risk of causing mechanical valve dysfunction is real, and must be recognized prior to device release.

REFERENCES

1.   Hufnagel C ,Gillespie J   Closure of intra-auricular septal defects.   Bull Georgetown Univ Med Center 1959; 4:137-9.
2.   King T ,Mills N   Nonoperative closure of atrial septal defects.   Surgery 1974; 75:383-88.
3.   King T, Thompson S, Steiner C, Mills N   Secundum atrial septal defect: nonoperative closure during cardiac catheterization.   JAMA 1976; 235:2506-9.
4.   Mills N, King T   Nonoperative closure of left-to-right shunts.   J Thorac Cardoivasc Surg 1976; 72(3):371-8.
5.   Rashkind W   Transcatheter treatment of congenital heart disease.   Circulation 1983; 67:711-6.
6.   Rashkind W   Interventional cardiac catheterization in congenital heart disease.   Int J Cardiol 1985; 7:1-10.
7.   Beekman R, Rocchini A, Snider A, Rosenthal A   Transcatheter atrial septal defect closure: preliminary experience with the Rashkind occluder device.   J Intervent Cardiol 1989; 2:35-41.
8.   Lock J, Cockerham J, Keane J, Finley J, Wakely P, Fellows K   Transcatheter umbrella closure of congenital heart defects.   Circulation 1987; 75:593-599.
9.   Lock J, Block R, McKay R, Baim D, Keane J   Transcatheter closure of ventricular septal defects.   Circulation 1988; 78:361-368.
10.   Redington A, Rigby M   Transcatheter closure of inter-atrial communications with a modified umbrella device.   Br Heart J 1994; 72:372-7.
11.   McGoon D, Swan H, Brandenburg R, Connolly D, Kirklin J   Atrial septal defect: factors effecting the surgical mortality rate.   Circulation 1959; 19:195-200.
12.   Galal M, Wobst A, Halees Z, Hatle L, Schmaltz A, Khougeer F, De Vol E, Fawzy M, Abbag F, Fadley F   Peri-operative complications following surgical closure of atrial septal defect type II in 232 patients- a baseline study.   Eur Heart J 1994; 15:1381-1384.

13. Hovath K, Burke R, Collins J, Cohn L Surgical treatment of adult atrial septal defect: early and long-term results. J Am Coll Cardiol 1992; 20:1156-9.

14. Stansel H, Talner N, Deren M, Van Heckeren D, Glenn W Surgical treatment of atrial septal defect. Analysis of 150 corrective operations. Am J Surg 1971; 121:485-489.

15. Meijboom F, Hess j, Szatmari A, Utens E, McGhie J, Deckers J, Roelandt J, Bos E Long-term follow-up (9 to 20 years) after surgical closure of atrial septal defect at a young age. Am J Cardiol 1993; 72:1431-1434.

16. Santoso T, Meltzer R, Castellanos S, Serruys P, Roelandt J Contrast echocardiographic shunts may persist after atrial septal defect repair. Eur Heart J 1983; 4:129-31.

17. Murphy J, Gersh B, McGoon M, Mair D, Porter C, Ilstrup D Long-term outcome after surgical repair of isolated atrial septal defect. N Engl J med 1990; 323:1645-50.

18. Hellenbrand W, Fahey J, McGowan F, Weltin G, Kleinman C Transesophageal echocardiographic guidance of transcatheter closure of atrial septal defect. Am j Cardiol 1990; 66:207-13.

19. Boutin C, Musewe N, Smallhorn J, Dyck J, Kobayashi T, Benson L Echocardiographic follow-up of atrial septal defect after catheter closure by double-umbrella device. Circulation 1993; 88:621-627.

20. Latson L, Benson L, Hellenbrand W, Mullins C, Lock J Transcatheter closure of ASD-early results of multicenter trial of the Bard Clamshell Septal Occluder. Circulation 1991; 84 (Suppl II):II-544.

21. Prieto L, Foreman C, Cheatham J, Latson L Intermediate-term outcome of transcatheter secundum atrial septal defect closure using the Bard Clamshell Septal Umbrella. Am J Cardiol 1996; 78(11):1310-2.

22. Latson L Per-catheter ASD closure. Pediatr Cardiol 1998; 19:86-93.

23. Perry S, van der Velde M, Bridges N, Keane J, Lock J Transcatheter closure of atrial and ventricular septal defects. Herz 1993; 18:135-142.

24. Sharafuddin M, Gu X, Titus J, Urness M, Cervera-Ceballos J, Amplatz K Transvenous closure of secundum atrial septal defects: preliminary results with a new self-expanding nitinol prosthesis in a swine model. Circulation 1997; 95:2162-8.

25. Sideris E, Sideris S, Fowlkes J, Ehly R, Smith J, Guide R Transvenous atrial septal occlusion in piglets using a "buttoned" double disc device. Circulation 1990; 81:312-318.

26. Rao P, Wilson A, Levy J, Gupta V, Chorpra P Role of "buttoned" double disc device in the management of atrial septal defects. Am Heart J 1992; 123:191-200.

27. Rao R, Chandar J, Sideris E Role of inverted buttoned device in transcatheter occlusion of atrial septal defects or patent foramen ovale with right-to-left shunting associated with previously operated complex congenital cardiac anomalies. Am j Cardiol 1997; 80:914-921.

28. Babic U, Grujicic S, Popovic Z, Durisic Z, Vucinic M, Pejcic P Double-umbrella device for transvenous closure of patent ductus arteriosus atrial septal defect: First experience. J Interven Cardiol 1991; 4:283-294.

29. Sievert H, Babic U, Ensslen R, Scherer D, Spies H, Wiederspahn T, Zeplin H Transcatheter closure of large atrial septal defects with the Babic system. Cather Cardiov Diag 1995; 36:232-240.

30. Das G, Voss G, Jarvis G, Wyche K, Gunther R, Wilson R Experimental atrial septal defect closure with a new, transcatheter, self-centering device. Circulation 1993; 88:I-754-I 764.
31. Agarwal S, Ghosh P, Mittal P Failure of devices used for closure of atrial septal defects: Mechanisms and management. J Thorac Cardiovasc Surg 1996; 1112:21-6.
32. Das G, Hijazi Z, O'Laughlin M,Mendelsohn A Initial results of the VSD/PFO/ASD closure trial. J Am Coll Cardiol 1996; 27:119A.
33. Gutti R, Dronamraju D, Saha A Operative findings in failed button device closure of ASD (letter). Ann Thorac Surg 1995; 59:793-4.
34. Hansdorf G, Schneider M, Franzbach B, Kampmann C, Kargus K, Goeldner B. Transcatheter closure of secundum atrial septal defects with the atrial septal occlusion system (ASDOS): Initial experience in children. Heart 1996; 75:83-8.
35. Lloyd T, Rao R, RH Beekman, Mendelsohn A, Sideris E. Atrial septal defect occlusion with the buttoned device (a multi-instutional U.S. trial). Am J Cardiol. 73 1994; (286-93).
36. Magni G, Hijazi Z, Pandian N, Delabays A, Sugeng L, Laskari C, Marx G Two- and three-dimensional transesophageal echocardiography in patient selection and assessment of atrial septal defect closure by the new DAS-Angel Wings device. Circulation 1997; 96:1722-1728.
37. Masura J, Gavora P, Formanek A, Hijazi Z Transcatheter closure of secundum atrial septal defects using the new self-centering Amplatzer Septal Occluder: Initial human experience. Cathet Cardiovasc Diagn 1997; 42(388-393).
38. Prewitt K, Gaither N, Frab A, Wortham D Transient ischemic attacks after long-term clamshell occluder implantation for closure of atrial septal defect. Am Heart J 1992; 124:1394-1397.
39. Rao P, Sideris E, Hausdort G, Rey C, Lloyd T, Beekman R, Worms A, Bourlon F, Onorato E, Khalilullah M International experience with secundum atrial septal defect occlusion by the buttoned device. Am Heart J 1994; 128:1022-35.
40. Rome J, Keane J, Perry S, Spevak P, Lock J Double-umbrella closure of atrial defects. Initial clinical applications. Circulation 1990; 82:751-758.
41. Sievert H, Babic U, Ensslen R, Merle H, Osypka P, Rubel C, Scherer D, Spies H, Wiederspahn T, Zeplin H Occlusion of atrial septal defect with a new occlusive device. Zeitschrift fur Kardiologie 1996; 85:97-103.
42. Zamora R, Rao P, Lloyd T, Beekman R, Sideris E Intermediate-term results of phase I Food and Drug Administration Trials of Buttoned Device occlusion of secundum atrial septal defects. J Am Coll Cardiol 1998; 31:674-6.
43. Masura J, Lange PE, Wilkinson JL, Kramer HH, Alievi M, Goussous Y, Thanopulos B, Walsh KP, Hyazi Z. US/International Multicenter trial of atrial septal catheter closure using the Amplatzer Septal Occluder: Initial Results. J Am Coll Cardiol 1998; 31 (Suppl A): 57Å.
44. Lock J, Rome J, Davis R, van Praagh S, Perry S, van Praagh R, Keane J Transcatheter closure of atrial septal defects: Experimental studies. Circulation 1989; 79:1091-1099.
45. Moore p, Benson LN, Berman Jr W et al CardioSeal device closure of secundum ASDs: How effective is it? Circulation 1998:98:1-754 (Abstract).

198

46. Bridges N, Perry S, Keane J, Goldstein A, Mandell V, Mayer J, Jonas R, Castaneda A, Lock J Preoperative transcatheter closure of congenital muscular ventricular septal defects. NEJM 1991; 324:1312-1317.
47. Rigby M, Redington A Primary transcatheter umbrella closure of perimembranous ventricular defect. Br Heart J 1995; 73:368-71.
48. Amin Z, Gu I, Berry J, Bass J, Umess M, Amplatz K A new device for closure of muscular ventricular septal defects in a canine model. Circulation 1997; 96:I-373.
49. Laussen P, Hansen D, Perry S, Fox M, Javorski J, Burows F, Lock J, Hickey P Transcatheter closure of ventricular septal defects: hemodynamic instability and anesthetic management. Anesthesia and Analgesia 1995; 80:1076-82.
50. Fishberger S, Bridges N, Keane J, Hanley F, Jonas R, Mayer J, Castaneda A, Lock J Intraoperative device closure of ventricular septal defects. Circulation 1993; 88:II-205-9.

8. DEFECT CLOSURE - COIL EMBOLIZATION

Jonathan J. Rome, M.D.
Stanton B. Perry, M.D.

GENERAL PRINCIPLES

Vascular occlusions may be achieved using a wide variety of methods including device closure, coil embolization, and particulate embolization. For a particular lesion, the optimal closure technique is best determined by considering the anatomy in the context of the specific goals of the occlusion.

Goals of Embolization

Vascular embolization may be undertaken to occlude the entire arterial tree in part or all of an organ, to occlude only large arterial branches, or to occlude a vessel at a very localized point, similar to surgical ligation. Occlusion of the entire arterial tree, frequently for management of diseased organs prior to their surgical removal, requires the use of very small particles or solutions such as absolute alcohol. These microvascular embolization techniques are rarely required in cardiology practice and are generally used by interventional radiologists.[1,2] For occlusion of multiple arterial branches along their course (for example, vessels feeding an arteriovenous malformation, or arterial feeders to a source of hemoptysis) emboli must be large enough not to pass into the distal circulation and yet small enough to reach the end vessels. Gelfoam, Ivalon, microcoils, or combinations of these best meet these size criteria. Precisely localized interruption of vascular flow is far and away the most common goal of vascular embolization in the practice of the pediatric interventional cardiologist. This result is best accomplished by coil embolization or a closure device depending on vessel size and length. This chapter will focus on the use of coils and modifications of the coil; closure devices are described in chapter 7.

Materials

Table 1 outlines the types and sizes of coils commonly used by the interventional cardiologist. Coils of almost any diameter and length can be obtained (Cook, Inc.). Coils are available in wire diameters from 0.018 to 0.052", and extruded diameters from 2 to 20mm. Straight "coils" are also available. Versatile and inexpensive, the basic Gianturco coil (Cook, Inc.) remains the most used of the various coils now available. It is constructed of stainless steel with interwoven Dacron strands and comes preloaded in a stainless steel cylinder. The proximal 10 mm of the coil contains no Dacron strands so that they can not become entangled with the delivery wire. The coil is loaded from the cylinder into a delivery catheter using an appropriately sized guidewire. When extruded from the catheter the coil reforms to its stated size and shape. For simple helical coils the length of the coil and its diameter determine the number of loops. The extruded intravascular coil is thrombogenic and, if optimally positioned, will occlude even brisk arterial flow relatively rapidly.

Table 1. Coils and Coil-Based Occluders

Coil Type	Wire Size	Diameters (mm)	Lengths (cm)	Comments
Gianturco Coils[1]	0.025	2-5	1-5	The simplest and most versatile coils; simple helical shape.
	0.035	2-10	1-12	
	0.038	3-15	1-20	
	0.052	6-20	8-20	
Detachable Coils[1]	0.035	3-8	3-5	Same shape and as above also available in "tornado" shape; controlled release, less robust.
	0.038	3-8	4-10	
Amplatz Vascular Occluder[1]	0.052	9,13,15, 20		Useful for trapping coils in very large vessels.
Tracker Coils[2]	0.018	2-6	2-5	Deployed with a 3F catheter that will fit through most 5F catheters; useful for small tortuous vessels.
GGVOD		3-9mm		Nylon sack which is filled with coils and released; requires delivery sheath; for large high-flow vessels.

[1] Cook, Inc.
[2] Target Therapeutics, Inc.

Many modifications of this basic coil are now available. These modifications include coils of different shapes and materials, controlled delivery coils, and more complex coil-based occlusion devices. Controlled delivery or "detachable coils" are designed such that their proximal end locks into a delivery system. This delivery catheter is used in place of the usual guidewire to push the coil out an appropriately positioned end-hole catheter. When the extruded coil is deemed to be in a satisfactory position it may be unlocked and released from the delivery catheter. If the position is unsatisfactory, the coil can be simply removed by withdrawing the delivery catheter with the coil still attached. The detachable coil is particularly useful where there is high risk of inappropriate coil positioning during deployment either because of difficult vessel anatomy or because the site is particularly critical (for example coronary fistula where inappropriate coil positioning might occlude coronary branches). In this country, the currently available detachable coils (Cook,Inc.) are made with 0.018 inch wire; as a result they have decreased tensile strength and thrombogenicity.

Modified coil shapes include the "tornado" coil. These are coils that have a helical shape; however, the extruded diameter of the loops is larger at one end than the other. This shape is potentially more completely occlusive than standard coils.

The tracker coil, available in simple helical and complex cloverleaf shapes, are made of 0.18" wire and expensive. They are sold with a system of coil pushers and delivery catheters. The advantage of the tracker system is that the delivery catheter itself is small enough to fit through the lumen of any catheter that will accept an 0.038" guidewire. The larger catheter can thus be used as a guiding catheter and stable distal position achieved in even the most tortuous of vessels with the tracker catheter. Because of their complex design, the coils accommodate to vessels over a wide range of sizes. They are most useful for difficult to reach, relatively small vessels.

The Amplatz Vascular Occlusion Device, not a coil per se, is designed to be used in conjunction with coils. The device has several arms joined together at a central point looking something like the legs of a spider. When pushed out of a delivery catheter the arms open thereby fixing the device within the vessel. Coils put into the vessel upstream of the device are blocked by it from migrating distally. The Amplatz occlusion device can be helpful in embolizing particularly large vessels lacking stenoses.

The Gianturco-Grifka Vascular Occlusion Device (GGVOD) is a nylon bag, which, after positioning in the vessel to be occluded, is filled with a coil. The system must be advanced through a long 8F sheath to the vessel to be occluded. This device is useful in occluding relatively large vessels of limited length.[3] We have used it to occlude left superior venae cavae, patent ductus arteriosi, and complex Fontan baffle leaks involving right atrial trabeculations and enlarged Thebesian veins.

Basic Coil Embolization:

There are 2 basic approaches for positioning coils. The first involves packing 1 or more coils entirely within the lumen of the vessel. This is the technique used for most arterial and venous collaterals and shunts. The second involves straddling the defect with a coil and is most commonly used for the patent ductus arteriosus. The choice of coil size and the technique for delivery is different for the 2 approaches and will be described in the following sections.

Aortopulmonary Collaterals

Collaterals arising from the aorta or its main branches comprise one of the most common sites for coil embolization in patients with congenital heart disease.[4] There are 2 basic types of aortopulmonary collaterals. The first type, most commonly encountered in patients with tetralogy of Fallot and pulmonary atresia, are vessels not found in normals. The second type are actually "normal" vessels, though usually abnormally large and include bronchial arteries, intercostal arteries, internal mammary arteries and other branches off the subclavian artery. These are commonly referred to as "chest-wall" collaterals. The first type are commonly more difficult to coil embolize because they tend to be larger, shorter and may lack stenoses. The second type, though they may be difficult to enter, are easy to coil because they taper to capillary beds distally.

Precatheterization

There are few contraindications to the use of these devices. Patients who are bacteremic at the time of implantation are more likely to develop infection at the embolization site. One child in our experience underwent embolization during an active disseminated intravascular coagulopathy, and a clot did not form despite multiple coils and good positioning. Otherwise, precatheterization precautions are the standard ones.

Procedure

The preparations for coil occlusion are little different from those for standard catheterization. The access site, when possible, should provide the straightest and least complicated course to the vessel in question. The femoral artery is usually adequate and only rarely would it be preferable to use the femoral vein, the umbilical artery or the axillary artery. Studies in lambs have indicated that systemic heparinization at the time of coiling does not prevent clot formation; we therefore use heparinization at catheterization. Finally, since finding the ideal delivery catheter is important and may result in multiple catheter changes, we usually use a sheath for coil embolization procedures.

It is imperative to identify the vascular anatomy with considerable precision. In patients suspected of having collaterals we commonly start with an aortogram. The catheter is positioned in the distal transverse aortic arch and low-magnification is used to include the head and neck vessels and as much of the chest and upper abdomen as possible. In newborns and infants the initial angiogram is often a balloon occlusion angiogram in the descending aorta using a Berman catheter from the vein. Subsequent angiograms are selective hand injections in or near the origin of the individual collaterals. These catheterizations require a lot of contrast and the initial aortogram can often be avoided. Thus, if a patient had an aortogram at a previous catheterization, simply repeating what has already been done is a waste of contrast. Even if there is no previous aortogram, one could proceed with finding and coiling collaterals and then perform an aortogram at the end to see what is left. Several details of the collaterals must be defined. The entire *length* of the vessel should be demonstrated. In some cases, this may require more than 1 selective angiogram. *The diameter* of the vessel to be embolized should be seen throughout its course. If the vessel/coil "fit" is borderline and the potential for dislodgment to a normal vessel is considerable, it can be useful to determine the diameter in both its native and distended (occluded) condition (see below). *The shape* of the segment to be occluded should be outlined.

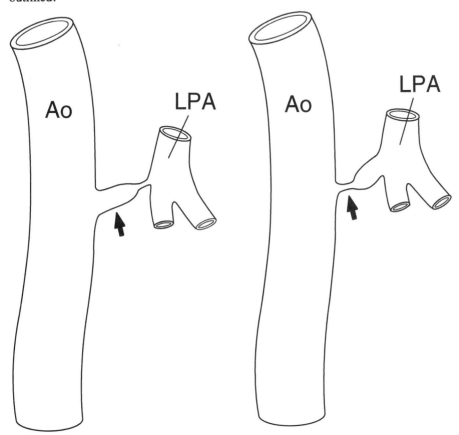

Figure 8-1 (left): Diagram of a collateral with length and a downstream stenosis (arrow) prior to its anastomosis with the pulmonary circulation.

Figure 8-2 (right): Diagram of a very short "Potts-like" collateral where the communication (arrow) between the aorta and the left pulmonary artery is less than 5 mm in length.

The easiest vessels to close with coils are those that funnel to a narrow segment (Fig. 8-1) or end in a nonvital capillary bed. Vessels that have a relatively long segment of even diameter before opening up into a larger vessel can also be closed safely, although considerable care must be taken to identify vascular diameter. Most collaterals are closed by positioning the coil or coils entirely within the vessel, but this is not possible if the collateral is very short (Fig. 8-2). It may be possible to close these short collaterals using the straddling technique if the vessel proximal and distal to the collateral is large enough to accept the coil loops.

The distribution of the vessels distal to the site being embolized, and the likelihood of unwanted tissue ischemia, must be assessed. In other words, is the segment of lung supplied by the collateral also supplied by the native pulmonary artery? Due to competitive flow, sequential contrast injections in the collateral and the native pulmonary artery may not be adequate to answer this question. It is commonly necessary to balloon occlude 1 vessel and inject the other to definitively demonstrate the presence or absence of dual supply. Though collaterals supplying small segments of lung without dual supply can be safely embolized, those supplying large segments without dual supply are better unifocalized.

The hemodynamic effect of coil occlusion may need to be measured. If a child with cyanotic heart disease is undergoing occlusion of systemic-pulmonary collaterals prior to definitive repair, closing the vessels may produce an increase in cyanosis. If it appears possible that the increase in cyanosis might be considerable and life-threatening, test occlusion of the collateral with a balloon-tipped catheter and assessment of the degree of cyanosis are mandatory before permanent occlusion. In general, test occlusions producing no more than a 10% fall in saturation or resulting in a saturation of more than 75% are reasonably well tolerated. If anticipated, systemic saturations below 75% can often be managed with intubation and ventilation and by sending the patients directly the operating room for definitive repair. If not all collaterals can be closed, we generally attempt to close the collaterals that would be most difficult for the surgeon to reach.

Once the anatomy has been defined, one must choose the proper coil and delivery catheter. For aortopulmonary collaterals which are almost always closed by positioning the coil entirely within the lumen of the vessel, the coil diameter should be 10-20% larger than the diameter of the vessel. If the coils are the same size as the vessel, they will reform completely upon extrusion and, if short, form a circle when the vessel is imaged from the side, and if long, form a circle when the vessel is viewed on end. Neither configuration is likely to occlude flow (Fig. 8-3), just as migration of a single coil into a normal vessel is unlikely to cause vascular occlusion and both, in fact, are likely to migrate. If the coil is too large it will remain relatively straight and attempts to deliver it will either force it distally or, more likely, force the catheter out of the vessel. The appropriately sized coil assumes a tortuous, noncylindrical, yet compact shape. The coils themselves tend to be slightly larger than their stated diameter.

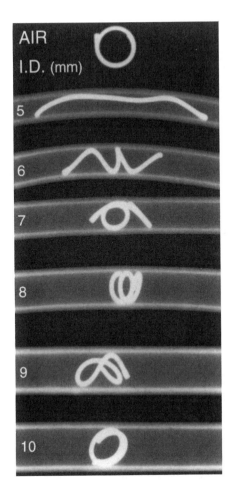

Figure 8-3: Ten coils were extruded into tubing of known diameter (5-10 mm), and X-rays were taken. When larger than the tubing (top) the coil lengthens; when the same or smaller than the tubing, it reforms into a perfect circle (bottom).

The 0.018 and 0.025" coils can be delivered through catheters as small as 3F and the 0.035 and 0.038" coils through catheters as small as 4F. The smaller coils are less robust and more easily forced to coil in undersized vessels but they are also more susceptible to distal embolization in high flow sites. Coil length (the length of the coil when it is straightened or packed in its cylinder) is perhaps the least important variable. Longer coils, when properly positioned, are more likely to occlude the vessel and less likely to migrate. In general, it is easier and safer to use short coils in these vessels realizing that several may be needed to occlude flow. The ideal inner diameter of the catheter is equal to or, at most, slightly larger than the coil caliber. If the delivery catheter has a lumen too large for the coil, the coil will spring open slightly making it difficult to advance the coil through the catheter. The guidewire may also wedge itself inside the coil if the catheter is too large. One must be sure that the delivery wire passes easily through the tip of the delivery catheter without altering catheter position before coil insertion. Ideally, one should fix the tip of the catheter with a preformed curve to provide better control and increase the chances that the slightly oversized coil will form a compact mass at the time of extrusion.

The loaded coil cylinder is held firmly inside the catheter hub and the stiff end of the appropriate sized guidewire is used to advance the coil into the catheter shaft (e.g., 10-20 cm). With the coil inside the catheter, the guidewire and cylinder are removed and the cylinder is bent to identify it as empty. The floppy end of the guidewire is used to deliver the coil. The stiff end will straighten the delivery catheter, causing the tip to move. The catheter is then straightened as much as possible (without moving the tip) to reduce friction and the coil is advanced until it begins to extrude from the catheter tip. The "natural" catheter course must be kept constant as the coil comes out. If the tip is pushed back by the extruding coil, the catheter can buckle in the aorta and flip out of position with the coil partially extruded; this should always be avoided by withdrawing the catheter shaft over the guidewire during delivery if the tip begins to move proximally. Occasionally, the coil gets stuck in the catheter when partially extruded and cannot be delivered. This happens frequently with balloon-tipped end-hole catheters, which have an uneven lumen at the balloon. Even though it is tempting to use these catheters because the tip can be fixed with balloon inflation, we no longer use them for coil delivery. Many catheters have a slightly tapered tip, which allows passage of the guidewire but not the coil embedded with Dacron strands. Finally, the guidewire may get jammed inside the coil when the catheter lumen is too large or has been stretched slightly by delivery of multiple coils. If this happens, forcing the wire will only make matters worse. Rather, one should repeatedly and gently tap the coil with the wire. If this fails, a vigorous injection of saline using a 1 cc syringe may deliver the coil. One may also pull the catheter hoping that the coil remains in the vessels, which is unlikely, or that the coil comes with the catheter. The latter is more likely if the wire can be jammed inside the coil. The risk, of course, is that the coil will flip out of the vessel and the catheter and embolize elsewhere. Another option is to position a balloon-tipped catheter along side the partially extruded coil and inflate the balloon to trap the coil while the delivery catheter is pulled. Finally, after removing the catheter hub, we have advanced a small snare over the guidewire and catheter shaft and into the body. The snare tracks along the delivery catheter until it reaches the distal tip and the partially extruded coil can then be snared and removed.

More than one coil may be needed to completely occlude flow. To allow time for thrombosis, we wait 5-10 minutes after coil delivery before performing an angiogram. In general, the first coil should be the largest, preventing distal embolization, with subsequent smaller coils delivered to "pack in" the occlusion site. It is usually possible to readvance the catheter so that the tip is inside the first coil for delivery of subsequent coils. In our experience, vessels with trivial residual flow will be completely closed at follow-up. If there is more than trivial residual flow and no room for more coils, temporary balloon occlusion of the vessel will interrupt flow and frequently produce complete occlusion.

Chest wall (type 2) collaterals are frequently encountered in patients who have undergone thoracotomies, who have reduced pulmonary blood flow, or who have pulmonary vein stenosis or atresia. The flow through these enlarged internal mammary and intercostal arteries is difficult to quantify, but we have closed them when segments or lobes fill entirely from these vessels rather than antegrade from the native pulmonary arteries. Because they are long and taper to "normal" capillary beds, there is no risk of distal coil migration. Because these chest wall collaterals interconnect, they should be occluded as extensively as possible. When closing an internal mammary, for instance, we commonly inject gelfoam or Ivalon particles to occlude the small distal branches. The entire length of the artery is then filled with coils. If coils are only placed at the take-off of the internal mammary, the artery will fill retrograde from the intercostals. In concert with closing these vessels, attempts should be made to correct any underlying problems. For example, a patient with a Glenn shunt with pulmonary artery stenosis distally should have the stenosis dilated and stented if necessary to enable a later Fontan operation. The largest collaterals are seen in patients with pulmonary vein atresia. Coiling collaterals in these patients is generally futile (they will recur), but may reduce the surgical risk of lung transplantation.

Postcatheterization
It is our practice to administer 3 doses of intravenous antibiotics and obtain a radiograph for documentation of coil position prior to hospital discharge. Otherwise patients receive routine post catheterization care. Low-grade fevers and occasionally chest pain are seen in the first 24-48 hours after coil embolization, and are more common in those who have undergone extensive closure of chest wall collaterals.

Complications
The most commonly encountered complication is inadvertent migration of the coil, which occurred in 1.4% of coils in our initial experience in 58 patients with collaterals[4]. When this occurs, the coil will assume its circular or helical shape and move distally in the arterial tree. The coil is relatively low profile in this configuration and rarely occludes the vessel. In most instances the embolus has been to the distal pulmonary artery tree. Errant coils are relatively easily removed with standard vascular retrieval techniques (see below). Substantially rarer, but more serious, complications include hemolysis and endarteritis. Both have occurred, but only in vessels with significant residual flow; we have not encountered either in embolization of collaterals. Hemolysis has occurred only in high flow lesions with significant residual flow after coil placement. It is best treated by completely occluding the lesion or removal of the coil.

Results
Embolization of aortopulmonary collaterals has resulted in complete occlusion or only trivial residual flow in 96% of vessels[4]. Follow-up angiography has demonstrated recanalization in only 5% of vessels that were completely occluded immediately following coil embolization[4]. On the other hand, almost all collaterals with trivial residual flow go on to complete thrombosis.

Patent Ductus Arteriosus (PDA)
Precatheterization
The majority of restrictive PDAs outside the newborn period can be closed by coil embolization. The great majority of PDAs <2.5-3 mm in diameter can be closed with a single coil, whereas those larger than 3 mm generally require 2 or more coils. The precatheterization echocardiogram can be used to screen patients based

on the size of the PDA. Sizing based on the color-flow jet is generally easier than measurements from the 2-dimensional images. With experience, the anatomy of the PDA can usually be defined, but we have not found this particularly useful in screening patients.

The larger the diameter and shorter the length of the ductus, the more likely there is to be a residual shunt after coiling. In addition, larger PDAs require placement of multiple coils in order to achieve complete closure. For optimal results, an adequate-sized ductal ampulla should be present in patients with larger PDAs (>3mm). Though coil embolization can be accomplished in shorter PDAs of this diameter, a significant amount of coil material will almost invariably protrude into the aorta, pulmonary artery, or both. Coiling the small PDA appears to be the procedure of choice. It is likely that PDAs, which require several coils, will be better managed with other devices.

Procedure

There are many approaches for coil occlusion of a PDA. The coil can be delivered using the venous or arterial catheter and multiple coils can be delivered simultaneously or sequentially. The simplest approach involves a single arterial catheter without a sheath and no venous access. This catheter (we usually use a 4 F Cobra that can deliver a 0.038" coil) is used for angiography and coil delivery. With the tip positioned in the aorta just distal to the PDA, a hand injection of contrast will show the anatomy of the ductus. The catheter is then advanced into the pulmonary artery with or without a guidewire and the pulmonary artery pressure measured. The coil is delivered and contrast injections by hand demonstrate closure. Because the procedure commonly takes 15 minutes or less, no heparin is given. This approach is ideal for the patient with a small (<3 mm) PDA by echo.

Another approach is to place both arterial and venous catheters. Complete hemodynamics are performed followed by an aortogram. The coil can be delivered using the venous or arterial catheter and an aortogram is performed following coil placement. Compared with the former approach, this approach requires access to two vessels, increased fluoro time, increased catheter manipulation and increased charges to the patient.

We choose the coil to be twice the diameter of the narrowest portion of the PDA, which is almost always the pulmonary end of the PDA. We prefer a coil with approximately 4 loops (#loops=coil length/(coil diameter x π)). The goal is to end up with 1 to 1.5 loops on the pulmonary artery side of the PDA and the rest in the ampulla or aorta. The retrograde arterial approach is simplest and ideal for small PDAs. A 4F catheter with a preformed curve that will accept an 0.038" wire is advanced retrograde to the ductal ampulla. A variety of preformed catheters can be used including cobras, headhunters, and right or left coronary catheters. A floppy-tipped guidewire is advanced through the PDA into the main pulmonary artery and followed with the catheter. The coil is advanced out the catheter until approximately 1 loop is deployed in the pulmonary artery. The catheter, coil and guidewire are withdrawn as a unit until the loop of coil deforms at the pulmonary end of the PDA. The lateral projection is almost always better than the AP view and the best landmark is the anterior border of the trachea, which usually identifies the pulmonary end of the PDA. There are 2 approaches for delivering the rest of the coil. One is to simply withdraw the catheter and guidewire leaving the coil, i.e. pull the catheter off the coil. This generally works because the resistance to pulling the pulmonary loop through the PDA is greater than the resistance to pulling the 0.038" coil out of the catheter. The other option is to pull the catheter over the guidewire without moving the coil. The most common error with this technique is to inadvertently advance the coil so that too much ends up in the pulmonary artery. With either method the coil can be released from the catheter in the descending aorta following which it will spring back into the ampulla. Alternatively, when the proximal end of the coil is at the distal end of the catheter, the catheter can be readvanced into the ampulla and the coil released by pushing the guidewire. The latter approach is more controlled. Once released, the loops of the coil in the aorta or ampulla can be gently moved or compacted using the catheter.

The coil can also be delivered using the venous catheter although very small PDAs are more easily crossed from the arterial side. From the pulmonary artery it is easiest to cross the PDA using a straight, soft-tipped guidewire and a relatively straight catheter such as a balloon-tipped wedge or multipurpose catheter positioned in the main pulmonary artery. If the PDA cannot be crossed directly from the pulmonary artery, it can be crossed retrograde with an exchange wire, which is then snared and brought out the vein. The venous catheter is positioned so its tip is just at the mouth of the ductal ampulla in the descending aorta. All but 1.5 loops of the coil are delivered out the catheter and the catheter is then pulled through the PDA to the pulmonary side. The coil is thereby pulled into the aortic end of the PDA. Further withdrawal of the catheter allows one loop to be delivered on the pulmonary artery side of the ductus pinning the coil in place.

An angiogram is performed approximately 10 minutes after coil placement. If there is more than trivial residual flow, the PDA is carefully recrossed and a second coil delivered.

Recrossing a coiled PDA is surprisingly easy and we have not dislodged the first coil with this maneuver. We have found the TAD wire particularly useful for this purpose. With the first coil as a landmark, the second coil is easy to position. The second coil is commonly chosen to have a smaller diameter than the first. PDAs larger than 3 mm virtually always require 2 or more coils for complete occlusion. When a larger duct is present, particularly in a smaller patient, we have found simultaneous delivery of two coils the best approach. This method permits one to use smaller diameter coils than would otherwise be possible.

210

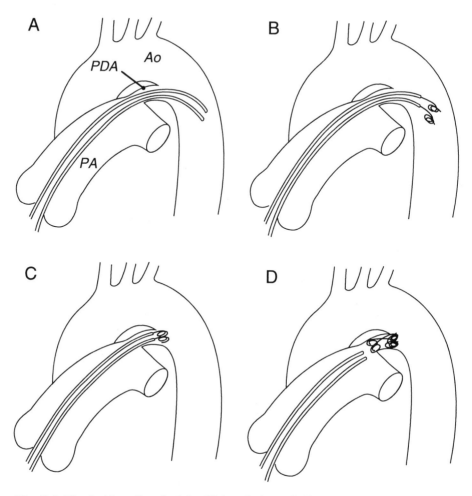

Fig. 8-4: The double coil method for PDA occlusion. (A) Two transvenous catheters are advanced across PDA to the descending aorta. (B) With the tips of each catheter free in the aorta, all but 1.5 loops of the coils are delivered. (C) Both catheters are pulled into the aortic ampulla of the PDA allowing the coils to intertwine. (D) Each catheter is pulled through the PDA into the pulmonary artery delivering the remainder of the coils across the ductus.

We usually deliver both coils transvenously. Two transvenous catheters are positioned across the PDA into the descending aorta. All but 1.5 loops of each coil are delivered out the catheters and then they are each pulled into the aortic end of the PDA. With the two coils intertwined inside the PDA, the pulmonary ends are sequentially delivered (Fig. 8-4). Another option is to balloon occlude the PDA from the venous side and deliver sequential coils from the arterial side. A guidewire is advanced through a balloon-tipped end-hole catheter in the main pulmonary artery through the PDA into the descending aorta. The arterial catheter is advanced through the PDA, a single loop of coil is extruded and the arterial catheter is then pulled back until the coil contacts the pulmonary end of the PDA. The venous catheter with the balloon inflated is advanced over the guidewire to occlude the pulmonary end of the PDA. The aortic end of the coil is then delivered. If necessary, the balloon can be pulled back slightly when recrossing the PDA for subsequent coils. When the PDA is closed the guidewire is pulled prior to deflating the balloon. The 0.052" coils are ideal for PDAs larger than 3.5 to 4 mm[5]. They are delivered using a 6F guiding catheter or a 4F long sheath.

Postcatheterization
We routinely give 3 doses of antibiotics. Patients are discharged after a 4-6 hour observation period in the recovery room. A chest x-ray or brief fluoroscopy is performed prior to discharge. SBE prophylaxis is continued until color-flow Doppler, 3-6 months following the procedure, demonstrates complete occlusion.

Complications
Potential complications after coil embolization of patent ductus arteriosus are identical to those described above for general embolization procedures. Hemolysis, which has been reported after incomplete occlusion, has resolved following subsequent repeat coil complete occlusion of the PDA[6]. There have also been reports of mild left pulmonary artery stenosis in cases where multiple coils were used (generally with large PDAs). The only complication we have encountered in this population has been embolization of coils to the distal pulmonary artery tree. The embolized coils were successfully retrieved, usually with a snare.

Results
In our experience with PDA coil embolization, 75% of patients leave the cath lab with complete occlusion of the ductus; the remainder had trivial residual flow by angiogram. All of the PDAs with trivial flow had closed on follow-up echocardiography by color Doppler resulting in a complete closure rate of 94%. In published reports occlusion after coil embolization of PDA is greater than or equal to 90% at follow-up[7,8]. Recently there have been reports of recanalization after documented complete occlusion in short PDAs[9] which also occurred in one of our patients. Comparable results have been reported by others, including simultaneously placed coils [10, 11].

Shunts
Coil embolization of surgical shunts may be performed when these shunts are no longer needed for pulmonary blood flow. The most common indication is the patient with pulmonary atresia and an intact ventricular septum who underwent right ventricular outflow reconstruction and a Blalock-Taussig (BT) shunt as a newborn. When the right ventricular size and compliance improves, the shunt can

be closed (Chapter 13). In addition, our surgeons prefer that we close left BT shunts whenever possible. If, for example, a patient has at least 2 sources of pulmonary blood flow, one of which is a left BT shunt, and is going to the operating room for definitive repair, we would coil the left BT, if tolerated, just prior to surgery.

Precatheterization
Several special considerations apply to shunt embolizations. It is important to coordinate the procedure with other planned interventions. This is particularly true in palliated patients with shunts and other sources of pulmonary blood flow scheduled for surgical correction. Needless to say, these patients will be more cyanotic after embolization. Where possible we plan the interventions so that surgery follows immediately after the embolization. Patients who become significantly more cyanotic can usually be managed with intubation and ventilation on supplemental oxygen between the two procedures.

Procedure
We obtain venous as well as arterial access for virtually all shunt embolizations. Angiograms of the shunt should show the entire length of the shunt as well as the size and presence of any stenoses within the shunt. More than one angiogram is commonly needed to get this information and selective angiograms are almost always preferable to aortograms. The first picture is usually a hand injection with the tip of the catheter at the mouth of the shunt. The shunt is crossed with the arterial catheter (a cut-off pigtail or Berenstein is commonly used) and an exchange wire positioned distally in the pulmonary artery. The shunt is test-occluded using a balloon wedge catheter over the wire to be sure the patient does not become excessively cyanosed following closure. An angiogram performed after removing the wire and with the balloon inflated will demonstrate the distal anatomy of the shunt very nicely. If balloon-occlusion is tolerated, the shunt is embolized. Ideally coils are positioned proximal to narrowings within, or at the distal anastomosis of, the shunt. Modified (Gore-Tex) shunts are more difficult to embolize because they rarely have stenoses along their length and, unlike vessels, are non-compliant. Therefore, coils are more likely to embolize from a modified shunt. Because of this, it is very helpful to occlude the distal end of the shunt while delivering the coils. This can be accomplished by advancing an appropriately sized angioplasty or occlusion balloon catheter anterograde from the vein to the shunt insertion site in the pulmonary artery (Fig. 8-5). With the occlusion catheter in place, the coil delivery catheter is advanced over the previously placed arterial exchange wire into the shunt. The occlusion balloon is inflated and one or more coils delivered into the shunt. Because the shunt will not distend, a short coil only slightly larger than the shunt should be chosen.

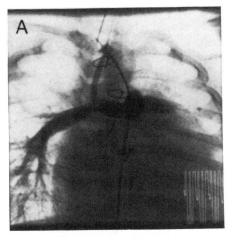

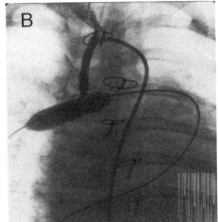

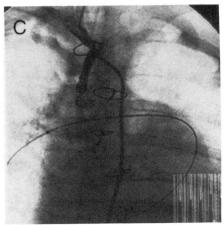

Fig. 8-5: Technique for coil embolization of modified Blalock-Taussig shunt. (A) The shunt is relatively long but lacks discrete stenoses. (B) An inflated angioplasty balloon, advanced over an anterograde wire into the right pulmonary artery, occludes shunt flow. (C) After embolization, the occlusion balloon is deflated and angiography demonstrates the shunt has been successfully occluded.

The occlusion balloon is kept inflated for several minutes after coil delivery to allow thrombus formation. The balloon is then partially deflated while the coils are observed for stability. If there is any movement of the coils, the balloon is reinflated and additional coils delivered.

Complications
The complications are identical to those described above for embolization procedures; however, because of the problems discussed, distal coil embolization is more common. The one instance of intravascular hemolysis we have seen after coil embolization occurred in a patient who had undergone (intentional) partial shunt occlusion with coils.

Results
All shunts we have coil embolized were classical or modified Blalock-Taussig shunts. In one patient with a large left modified Blalock-Taussig shunt to a

discontinuous left pulmonary artery, the procedure was unsuccessful. Because of the anatomy, the shunt could not be occluded during coil delivery, resulting in distal embolization of coils of multiple different sizes. The coils were retrieved by catheter and the shunt ligated at surgery. Overall, coil placement has resulted in successful occlusion of 90% of shunts in our experience.

Other Lesions
Venous Collaterals

The most commonly coiled vein is the small left superior vena cava (LSVC) in a patient with single ventricle. The LSVC to coronary sinus will result in cyanosis following a Glenn anastomosis and in Fontan patients in whom the coronary sinus drains to the left atrial side of the Fontan baffle. We routinely look for a LSVC in all patients prior to a Glenn anastomosis by performing a balloon occlusion angiogram in the innominate vein with an end-hole catheter. We usually coil the LSVC from the innominate vein because catheter access is a little easier but they can be coiled from the coronary sinus. The latter approach may be marginally safer because the catheter partially occludes the LSVC and coronary sinus and the coil is not likely to embolize past the catheter into the systemic circulation. Because the LSVC is unusually small (if large, a bilateral bi-directional Glenn is performed), it is easily coil occluded. There are, however, 2 important points to remember. First, although rare, one should remember to look for atresia of the os of the coronary sinus because coiling the LSVC will result in occlusion of the coronary sinus. Second, the left azygos enters the LSVC. If the LSVC is coiled between the azygos and innominate vein, the azygos will continue to drain to the coronary sinus and result in cyanosis after a Fontan. Thus the coil should be positioned between the coronary sinus and the azygos or positioned in the LSVC to straddle the azygos. A final option is to coil the azygos and then position a second coil in the LSVC between the azygos and the innominate vein.

Rarely, a LSVC will drain to an unroofed coronary sinus resulting in cyanosis in an otherwise normal person. The degree to which occlusion of the LSVC raises venous pressure depends on the number and size of venous connections in the head and neck to the RSVC or IVC. This can be tested with balloon occlusion of the LSVC. In our experience the increase in venous pressure is rarely more than a few mm Hg and it tends to decrease following occlusion as venous collaterals enlarge. As opposed to pre-Glenn patients, these LSVC tend to be large and require either multiple coils with or without an Amplatz "spider" occluder device, a Grifka bag (Fig. 8-6), or other devices. Because veins are more distensible than arteries, it is a good idea to measure these large LSVC while occluded with a balloon. Veno-venous collaterals are one of the more common causes of cyanosis in patients with cavopulmonary anastomoses. In patients with a bi-directional Glenn, the abnormal venous channels connect the right or left innominate veins or its tributaries to either the pulmonary veins or the IVC. The veins draining to the pulmonary veins should be coiled (Fig. 8-7), but those draining to the IVC need not be coiled if a Fontan is to be undertaken in the near future.

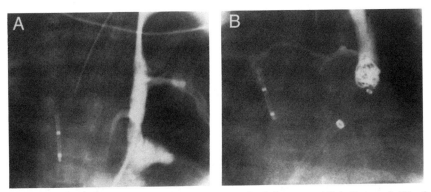

Fig. 8-6: A left superior vena cava connecting to the left atrium (A) before and (B) after occlusion with a Grifka bag.

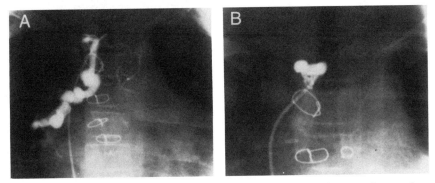

Fig. 8-7: Selective injection in a venous collateral arising from the innominate vein and connecting to the right pulmonary vein (A) before and (B) after coil occlusion.

In a Fontan patient, cyanosis will result from any connection between the systemic and pulmonary veins, some of which arise from the hepatic veins. These veno-venous collaterals tend to be small and tortuous and the most difficult part of the coiling procedure is gaining access to the vessel. This can usually be done with the appropriate pre-shaped catheter, based on angiograms of the vessel, and a torque-controlled wire. The venous access site can also be critical. For example, some collaterals from the SVC are easily entered from the internal jugular vein but nearly impossible to enter from the femoral vein or vice versa. We have also encountered collaterals off the hepatic veins that were very difficult to enter from the internal jugular and femoral veins, but easily entered using a transhepatic approach.

216

Coronary Fistulae

Prior to embolization, the anatomy of the fistula and its relationship to coronary side-branches must be carefully delineated. The arteries often become very tortuous in this condition and multiple angiograms may be required to clarify these anatomic relationships.

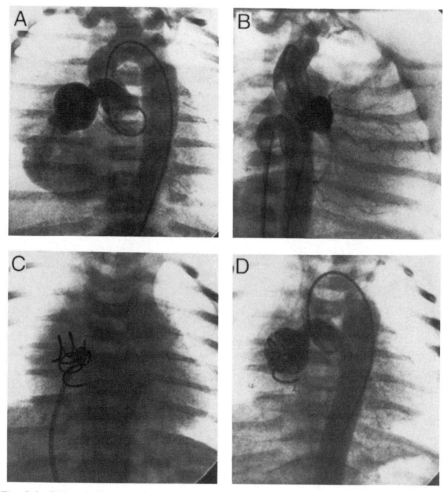

Fig. 8-8: Coil embolization of a coronary cameral fistula in a neonate. (A) A retrograde aortic root injection demonstrates a fistula from the right coronary artery to the right atrium, but the anatomy of the right coronary anatomy is not well demonstrated due to runoff through the fistula. (B) Repeat angiography, following balloon-occlusion with an end-hole balloon catheter over a wire into the fistula from the right atrium, demonstrates the right coronary artery anatomy. (C) The transvenous route was used to deliver coils into the fistula. (D) After several coils, the fistula was completely occluded.

It is very important to identify all of the normal coronary branches and when the fistulous connection and resultant run-off is substantial this may not be possible without balloon occluding the fistula distally during angiography (Fig. 8-8).

Stable positioning of the coil delivery catheter is particularly important in coronary fistulae but often difficult because of the tortuosity of the arteries. We have found coronary guiding catheters helpful in such cases. An appropriately-curved coronary guide catheter is advanced into the origin or proximal portion of the enlarged coronary. This coaxial system usually allows one to manipulate the coil delivery catheter into position with the aid of a high-torque, floppy wire. In smaller patients, the same system can be created by advancing a tracker catheter through a standard 4 or 5F coronary catheter. In some cases (particularly where the fistula connects to right atrium) the most stable course for coil delivery is anterograde into the fistula from the vein (Fig. 8- 8).[12] When it is difficult to enter the fistula directly from the vein, it is usually possible to advance an exchange guidewire retrograde through the fistula and snare it transvenously.
Coils can be positioned within the vessel itself or delivered to straddle the fistulous opening (similar to the technique used for coiling a PDA). When the vessel involved in the fistula is quite large, it may not be possible to position the multiple coils needed for occlusion without closing distal side-branches. The latter technique avoids this problem and even when the vessel is large the opening is usually relatively small.

Pseudoaneurysms and Vascular Rupture
Vascular rupture or dissection with pseudoaneurysm formation is a rare but serious complication of angioplasty or endovascular stenting; coil embolization is often the best means of treatment. Therapy must be decided on a case by case basis considering the feasibility of embolization and the surgical alternatives to it. Vessel rupture during pulmonary artery dilations most commonly involves small distal vessels and can be due to over-distention with the balloon or to perforation with the guidewire. Although many of these are self-limiting, they can be life threatening. Balloon occlusion of the vessel involved can be used to stop the hemorrhage, but if the bleeding recurs when the balloon is deflated coil embolization should be considered. Coil embolization will result in sacrifice of some distal vessels. However, since the alternative may well be lung resection or worse, the catheter approach is usually preferable.
The technique of aneurysm embolization is relatively straightforward. Generally we place several larger coils first and then fill in this scaffolding with as many small coils as possible. The goal is thrombosis of the entire aneurysm (Fig. 8-9). These patients should be followed closely and re-evaluated after the coil procedure. The coils cast artifact on MRI images and therefore we have always brought these patients back for subsequent angiography to follow the aneurysms after coil placement. Other lesions which have been coil occluded include Fontan fenestrations, Fontan baffle leaks, pulmonary arteriovenous malformations, leaks

around artificial aortic and mitral valves, muscular ventricular septal defects, and left ventricular to descending aortic conduits.

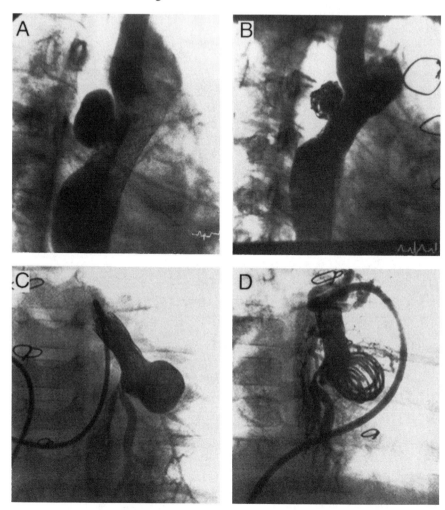

Fig. 8-9: Angiograms demonstrating coil embolization of pseudoaneurysms. (A) Descending aortogram demonstrating a pseudoaneurysm after stenting of a coarctation. (B) The aneurysm was packed with multiple coils. Several weeks later on repeat angiography the aneurysm is thrombosed without further extension. (C) Left pulmonary arteriogram demonstrating a large aneurysm just distal to a previously implanted stent. (D) After multiple coils were deployed, the majority of the aneurysm had thrombosed. Lateral branches to the left lower lobe were lost, however there is still flow to the medial portion.

Coil Retrieval

One of the advantages of coils is that they are relatively easy to retrieve. The most common indication for coil retrieval is inadvertent migration. Occasionally, it is necessary to retrieve a coil that has not migrated but is malpositioned as, for example, a PDA coil which hangs too far into the aorta or pulmonary artery. Snares, baskets, biopsy forceps, grasping forceps, and tip-defector wires have all been used to retrieve coils. A snare is the preferred retrieval device in most situations. The Microvena snares are available in multiple snare diameters and fit through catheters as small as 4F. Biopsy and grasping forceps can be effective but are more difficult to position and are more likely to damage the vessel. It is easy to grab coils with baskets, but, due to their relatively large size, they can be difficult to position for coil retrieval.

Coils that are malpositioned, but have not embolized are usually very easy to snare because at least one end is hanging into another vessel and exposed. Coils that have migrated to another vessel are somewhat more difficult. In order to snare these coils it is usually necessary to get a wire and then a catheter past the coil. With the catheter past the coil the snare is opened by withdrawing the catheter. The snare is usually chosen to be at least slightly larger than the coil. One attempts to intertwine the snare in the coil by rotating it with gentle pushing and pulling. The catheter is intermittently readvanced to check if the coil has been snared. Ideally one would like to snare a single strand of the coil rather than snaring the coil as a bundle. When snared as a bundle, it will be difficult, if not impossible to pull the snare through the sheath or skin. It is common to snare the Dacron strands, but this rarely allows removal of the coil from the body. The most common mistake in attempting to retrieve a coil is to jam the coil more distally into the vessel. If this happens one can attempt to position a tip-deflector wire beyond the coil and hook the coil. Although this will rarely allow one to remove the coil from the body, it can be used to pull the coil free and then further attempts can be made with a snare. There is some risk of vessel damage with the tip-defector wire. Another trick for a jammed coil is to use an 0.018" torque-controlled wire. This wire is usually relatively easy to maneuver past the coil and, because the tip is very soft, is safe. With the wire tip past the coil, the torque wire is twisted several times to entwine the Dacron strands on the coil. Again, this will rarely allow retrieval of the coil, but can be used to free the jammed coil.

Coil retrieval usually involves removing the coil from the body but this is not always necessary. On several occasions we have snared a coil and repositioned it in the vessel to be embolized. An attempt to coil a left BT shunt in a patient whose only sources of pulmonary blood flow were right and left BT shunts, resulted in coil migration to the LPA. The left BT shunt was directed anteriorly making it very difficult to enter the distal LPA. The coil was, therefore, snared from the right BT shunt and pulled back to the insertion of the left BT shunt. While holding it there, it was snared with a catheter through the left BT shunt and pulled into the shunt where it was successfully released.

Being able to manage complications is an integral part of any procedure. Most coils migrate to the pulmonary arteries and it can be argued in many cases that retrieval is not absolutely necessary. First, most do not occlude flow. Second,

220

occlusion of a small segment of an otherwise normal pulmonary bed will not be hemodynamically significant. Nevertheless, we have taken the approach that all coils should be retrieved and only rarely, early in our experience, have we left coils. The experience gained has been invaluable when retrieving coils that could have caused major problems. For example, we have retrieved a coil from the middle cerebral artery within 4 minutes of embolization and the patient suffered no neurologic problems.

REFERENCES

1. Athanasoulis CA, Pfister RC, Green RE, Robertson GH. Interventional Radiology. Philadelphia: W.B. Saunders, 1982.
2. Katzen BT. Interventional Diagnostic and Therapeutic Procedures. New York: Springer-Verlag, 1980.
3. Grifka RG, Miller MW, Frischmeyer KJ, Mullins CE. Transcatheter occlusion of a patent ductus arteriosus in a Newfoundland puppy using the Gianturco-Grifka vascular occlusion device. J Vet.Intern.Med. 1996; 10:42-44.
4. Perry SB, Radhke W, Fellows KE, Keane JF, Lock JE. Coil embolization to occlude aortopulmonary collateral vessels and shunts in patients with congenital heart disease. J.Am.Coll.Cardiol. 1989; 13:100-108.
5. Owada CY, Teitel DF, Moore P. Evaluation of Gianturco coils for closure of large ($\geq$ 3.5 mm) patent ductus arteriosus. J Am Coll Cardiol 1997;30:1856-62.
6. Shim D, Wechsler DS, Lloyd TR, Beekman RH. Hemolysis following coil embolization of a patent ductus arteriosus [see comments]. Cathet Cardiovasc Diagn 1996; 39:287-290.
7. Shim D, Fedderly RT, Beekman RH, Ludomirsky A, Young ML, Schork A, et al. Follow-up of coil occlusion of patent ductus arteriosus. J.Am.Coll.Cardiol. 1996; 28:207-211.
8. Rothman A, Lucas VW, Sklansky MS, Cocalis MW, Kashani IA. Percutaneous coil occlusion of patent ductus arteriosus. J.Pediatr. 1997; 130:447-454.
9. Daniels CJ, Cassidy SC, Teske DW, Wheller JJ, Allen HD. Reopening after successful coil occlusion for patent ductus arteriosus. J.Am.Coll.Cardiol. 1998; 31:444-450.
10. Hijazi ZM, Geggel RL: Results of antegrade transcatheter closure of patent ductus arteriosus using single or multiple Gianturco coils. Am J Cardiol 1994:74:925-929.
11. Alwi M, Kang LM, Samion H, Latiff HA, Kandavel G, Zambahari R: Transcatheter occlusion of native persistent ductus arteriosus using conventional Gianturco coils. Am J Cardiol 1997:79:1430-1432.
12. Perry SB, Rome JJ, Keane JF, Baim DS, Lock JE. Transcatheter closure of coronary artery fistulas. J.Am.Coll.Cardiol. 1992; 20:205.

9. STENTS.

Jacqueline Kreutzer, M.D.
Stanton B. Perry, M.D.

INTRODUCTION

Following animal studies demonstrating the feasibility of stent implantation in pulmonary arteries and systemic veins[1], the first stents in a pediatric patient were implanted in a patient with branch pulmonary artery stenosis in 1989. Over the last 10 years stents have proven to be among the most significant advances in transcatheter therapy of congenital heart disease. Stents are now the treatment of choice for many branch pulmonary artery and systemic venous stenoses and an accepted form of palliation for conduit or homograft stenoses. Stents are also being used with increasing frequency in native and post-operative coarctation of the aorta. In addition, they have been used in left and right ventricular outflow tract obstruction, aortopulmonary collaterals, shunts, and in pulmonary vein stenosis. Stents have also been used to maintain patency of atrial and ventricular septal defects and of the patent ductus arteriosus[2-6].

Intravascular stents are an ideal adjunct for treating those lesions not responsive to conventional balloon dilation. Such lesions include compliant obstructions, stenoses due to kinking, external compression, and intimal flaps, stenoses presenting in the early post-operative period, relatively mild stenoses and restenoses following successful dilation. The results of stenting are almost always better in terms of increase in diameter and reduction in gradient than for balloon dilation alone. However, not all lesions are ideally suited to stenting. Peripheral pulmonary artery stenoses are often difficult to stent without covering and possibly obstructing side-branches. Even though sequential redilation of stents is often possible, implanting stents in small, growing pediatric patients remains a problem.

Despite the availability of self-expanding stents,[7] balloon expandable Palmaz stents, manufactured by Johnson and Johnson, have been used almost exclusively in children. Although self-expanding stents offer advantages during implantation and in dealing with malposition, the Palmaz stents are more versatile with respect to achievable diameters and redilation and are associated with less intimal hyperplasia. The Palmaz stent is a stainless-steel tube with staggered rows of slots, which become diamond shaped with expansion. The most commonly used sizes in pediatrics are the hepatobiliary stents, 2.5 mm in unexpanded diameter and 10, 15 or 20 mm in length, and the iliac stents, 3.4 mm in unexpanded diameter and 12, 18 or 30 mm in length. The length decreases as the stent expands (Fig. 9-1). Although the manufacturer recommends maximum expanded diameters of 8 mm for the hepatobiliary and 12 mm for the iliac stent, in our experience, the hepatobiliary stent can be expanded to 12 mm and the iliac stent to over 18 mm in diameter. We have rarely used a coronary stent in a small branch of the pulmonary artery. Larger Palmaz stents designed primarily for the aorta have been used on a compassionate use basis in the main pulmonary artery.

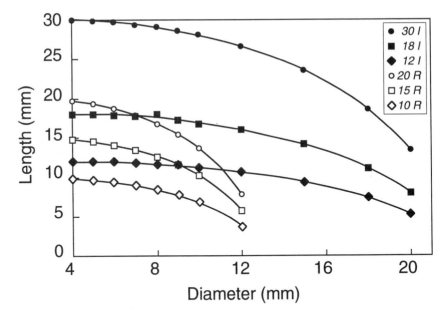

Figure 9-1. The graph plots stent length as a function of stent diameter. Open dots =: hepatobiliary (A) stent; solid dots = iliac stent(I)

GENERAL CATHETERIZATION CONSIDERATIONS

Prior to the catheterization, the medical and surgical history, chest x-ray, electrocardiogram, echocardiogram are reviewed. Patients with branch pulmonary artery stenoses undergo lung perfusion scans. We cannot stress enough the importance of carefully reviewing previous angiograms. Many of these procedures push the limits for contrast, and dye should not be wasted replicating available data. Most patients do not require hospitalization prior to catheterization, but all are hospitalized overnight following stent implantation. Most stents are implanted using routine sedation but general anesthesia is used in difficult to sedate patients or in those likely to have hemodynamic compromise during stent implantation. After obtaining arterial and venous access, 100 units/kg (maximum 5000 units) of heparin is given and repeated as needed to maintain the activated clotting times above 200 seconds. The patient is given 3 doses of a broad-spectrum antibiotic, cefazolin, 1 dose prior to and 2 following stent implantation.

With rare exceptions, a complete hemodynamic study is performed first. Stenoses are identified and localized using pressure pullbacks and angiography. Pressure pullbacks can be performed with an end-hole catheter, a double lumen catheter, or a cut-off pigtail with Y-adaptor over a wire. The latter is usually preferred because it can also be used for angiography and avoids the need for crossing the lesion repeatedly. Angiograms, optimally angulated to avoid foreshortening and overlapping with other structures, are needed to define the anatomic characteristics of the lesion.

The decision to implant a stent is based on thorough evaluation of the patient's condition and the risks and benefits of stents versus other therapeutic options. Many of the indications are lesion specific and will be considered below. Stents should not be implanted in lesions which are not balloon expandable although, fortunately, this is very rare. There is some controversy regarding stent implantation in infants and children in whom adult-sized vessels cannot be achieved. Although we consider this a relative contraindication, in our experience, many infants have benefited from stent implantation. If the stents are placed in locations accessible to the surgeon, they can be removed at a subsequent surgery when, in many cases due to the stent, the surgical risk is less and more likely to be successful.

Stent Type and Size

Based on the patient's size and the anatomic characteristics of the lesion, a hepatobiliary or an iliac stent will be selected for implantation. In general, hepatobiliary stents are used if the final diameter is expected to be less than 10 mm, and iliac stents for larger diameters. The length of the stent is determined by the length of the lesion and the presence of adjacent structures such as vessel branches or valves, etc. The final length also depends on the diameter to which the stent will be expanded (Fig 9-1).

Balloons

Ideally, the balloon should have a profile large enough to prevent slipping of the crimped stent. Although many balloons can be used, balloons with a slippery surface, e.g. "Terumo" coated balloons, are less than ideal. Scratch resistant balloons minimize the risk of balloon rupture during inflation. Initially, VACAS balloons (Mansfield, Boston Scientific Coorporation, Watertown, MA) were used. The Ultrathin balloons from Meditech (Boston Scientific Corporation), which we used to implant stents with diameters of ≤10 mm, are being replaced with Marshall balloons (Meditech, Boston Scientific Corporation) for stent implantation. The Marshall balloons were designed for stent implantation and have increased scratch resistance and a non-slippery surface. We use Z-Med balloons (B. Braun Medical Inc., Bethelehem, PA) and XXL balloons (Meditech, Boston Scientific Corporation) when implanting stents with diameters > 10 mm.

The balloon diameter should be large enough to insure stent fixation, which is usually 10-20% larger than the caliber of the "normal" vessel on either side of the stenosis. Once implanted, a larger balloon can be used to enlarge the stent or flare the ends if they are not in contact with the vessel wall. Markedly over-expanding the stent is usually counter-productive because intimal proliferation tends to "fill-in" the over-expanded segment so the diameter of the lumen on follow-up is no greater than the lumen of the flanking vessel. Choosing the appropriate balloon length is more difficult. The advantage of a longer balloon, excluding the taper, is that the stent is less likely to slip off the balloon during positioning and expansion. When longer than the stent the two ends of the balloon expand followed by the center and thus, the stent. The stent can puncture the balloon as the ends inflate, especially if the course involves a curve. Short balloons avoid this problem but are more likely to be associated with stent slippage. Generally, we choose a balloon somewhat longer than the stent.

Long Sheaths

There are 2 basic techniques for stent implantation. The conventional technique is to advance the long sheath and dilator beyond the obstruction, remove the dilator and advance the balloon and stent over the wire through the long sheath.

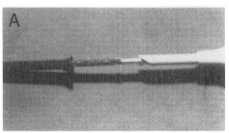

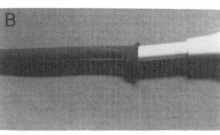

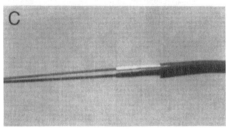

Figure 9-2: Conventional delivery technique showing A: stent or balloon via "side-arm adaptor" being introduced into long sheath and B: side arm adaptor bevelled end advanced into distal sheath for hemostasis, C: frontloading technique with stent end of sheath on delivery balloon (lowe images due to shadows each frame)

However, if a relatively small sheath is being used, if the course involves curves, or if the sheath kinks, the stent may slip off the balloon as it is advanced through the sheath. The alternative technique is "front-loading". This involves pushing the balloon through the sheath outside the body. The stent is then mounted on the balloon and pulled into the sheath leaving the distal tip of the balloon to serve as the dilator. The balloon, stent and long sheath are then advanced as a unit over a wire to the lesion. To ease passage through the skin and subcutaneous tissues a standard length sheath, 1 or 2 Fr sizes larger than the long sheath, should be used.

With the "front-loading" technique, smaller diameter sheaths can be used, the problem of stent slippage is avoided and there is less blood loss. The French size of the long sheath depends on the profile of the balloon and stent and the technique being used. Hepatobiliary stents can be implanted with sheaths as small as 6 F and iliac stents with sheaths as small as 8 F.

A side arm adaptor at the proximal end of the long sheath prevents blood loss and allows contrast injections during implantation of the stent. However, advancing a mounted stent through the valve in the side-arm adaptor risks altering the position of the stent on the balloon. Therefore, the side-arm adaptor is placed on the balloon shaft prior to mounting the stent and inserted in the sheath after the balloon. Side-arm adaptors can be purchased or created using a trimmed standard length sheath with backstop either the same or 1 Fr size smaller than the long sheath (Fig. 9-2 A).

Wires

Stiff exchange wires are usually required for positioning the long sheaths. In infants we use a moderately stiff 0.035 inch Rosen wire (Cook , Blomington, IN), and in larger patients, a very stiff 0.035 inch Superstiff wire with a 1 cm floppy tip (Meditech, Boston Scientific Corporation, Watertown, MA). It is helpful to pre-shape the guidewire to conform to the curves in the catheter course. This should be done using smooth curves rather than discrete bends as passage of a balloon-mounted stent can force the tips of the stent against the balloon, promoting balloon puncture.

Pre-Dilation

Even when committed to stenting, inflating a balloon in the lesion prior to stent implantation can be useful. It will demonstrate lesion expandability and the location of the waist or waists. Further, it will determine if the balloon moves during inflation and whether balloon rupture is likely to occur in calcified lesions or by adjacent stents. This information can be important in properly positioning the stent. Thus, although not absolutely necessary, we continue this practice in most patients.

Assembly And Methods Of Implantation

Negative pressure is applied to the balloon lumen using a syringe with 1/3 strength contrast. The side-arm adaptor is placed on the balloon shaft (Fig. 9-2 A). The stent is mounted and crimped on the balloon being careful not to damage the balloon. A few drops of contrast on the balloon prior to mounting the stent makes the balloon "sticky" and may prevent stent slippage during positioning and

226

inflation. We crimp the stent by rolling it between the fingers rather than using a crimping tool. The stent is usually centered on the balloon, but in certain situations an off-center stent is preferable. First, if the stent slips as the balloon is advanced through the sheath it will slip proximally and, therefore, it may be better to crimp the stent towards the distal end of the balloon. Second, if there is a stenosis distal to the targeted lesion, which will cause the balloon to move proximally during inflation, it is better to mount the stent more distally on the balloon.

The balloon and stent are positioned across the lesion by advancing through a previously placed long sheath or using the front-loading technique (Fig. 9-2). Withdrawing the sheath exposes the balloon and stent. Hand-injections of contrast through the side-arm adaptor in the end of the long sheath are used to insure proper positioning of the stent. Two operators should always be involved, one to inflate the balloon and one to control the stent position. The initial phase of balloon inflation should be slow. During this phase one watches for both ends of the balloon to inflate. If only one end inflates, the stent may be pushed in the opposite direction off the balloon. After both ends of the balloon are inflated there is still an opportunity to adjust the position of the stent. This is accomplished by advancing the guidewire to move the stent proximally or pulling the wire to move the stent distally. If the stent is correctly positioned, the inflation is completed and the balloon deflated and removed. If part of the stent is not in contact with the vessel we use a larger balloon to enlarge the entire stent or to flare one or both ends. We believe it is important to leave stents in contact with the vessel wall to promote endothelialization and avoid late complications.

Post-Catheterization Care And Anti-Coagulation

Patients are heparinized overnight with an intravenous infusion of 20 units/ kg/hour (maximum dose 1,000 units/hour). A chest X-ray in anteroposterior and lateral projections is obtained the following morning to determine stent position and for comparison during follow-up. In general, patients with pulsatile flow through their stent are placed on aspirin (40 mg to 80 mg per day) for 6 months. Patients with non-pulsatile flow are placed on coumadin. Patients with Fontan lateral intra-atrial tunnels and no history of atrial arrhythmias are switched to aspirin at 6 months. Although no stent has clotted in our experience, no study has been performed to determine the optimal anticoagulation regimen.

Problems and complications:

Even with meticulous attention to detail, problems with stent implantation can, and do, occur. The stent can slip off the balloon during positioning or during expansion and the balloon can rupture during inflation. These problems as well as balloon movement during inflation can lead to stent malposition. Rarely, a stent, which seems to be in good position, will embolize either within a few minutes or after leaving the cath lab. Side-branches in vessels which are covered by the stent can be occluded. It is rarely possible to retrieve a stent and attempting to move an expanded stent in contact with the vessel wall will almost certainly damage the vessel. Although Palmaz stents are not nearly as forgiving as most implantable devices, many of these problems can be overcome without abandoning the procedure or resorting to surgery.

One of the more frequently encountered problems with stent deployment is movement of the stent on the balloon as the balloon/stent are advanced through the long sheath to the lesion. In all these cases, the stent slips proximally on the balloon. The most common offending site is at kinks in the long sheath. Even in the absence of an actual kink, the sheath lumen can assume an oval configuration at significant curves thereby reducing the lumen. There are several techniques for overcoming this problem. First, the sheath and dilator can be preformed using heat or by gently stripping between the fingers to assume the configuration of the guidewire prior to introduction. Larger diameter sheaths, "front-loading" and stainless steel reinforced sheaths (Super-Arrow-Flex, Arrow, Reading, PA), which are more kink resistant than conventional sheaths (Cook, Bloomington, IN) can also be used. Using a longer balloon, one with a larger profile or one with non-slippery surface and crimping the stent more distally and with a slight curve will also help. Slightly inflating both ends of the balloon prior to putting the balloon/stent in the long sheath will help prevent slipping both during delivery and during inflation of the stent. This is accomplished by gently applying pressure to the syringe until one end of the balloon begins to inflate. This end is then squeezed between the fingers until the other end begins to inflate. The slight inflation of both ends is maintained using a 3-way stopcock positioned between the syringe and inflation port.

If, however, the stent does slip on the balloon while it is still inside the sheath, there are 2 options. First, one may remove the balloon and stent and start over. Second, one may position the balloon across the lesion and withdraw the sheath to uncover the stent and balloon. Then the sheath is readvanced until it catches the proximal end of the stent and the sheath is used to push the stent onto the balloon. The latter approach is obviously riskier.

The stent can also slip off the balloon during balloon inflation. This happens when only one end of the balloon inflates and the stent is pushed in the opposite direction. Most balloons have a single opening between the inflation lumen and the balloon and to our knowledge this is always at the proximal end. Therefore, the proximal end of the balloon is more likely to inflate, especially in the presence of a tightly crimped stent. This problem can be avoided by slightly inflating both ends of the balloon before advancing it through the sheath. Some manufacturers recommend inflating and deflating very tight fitting balloons prior to mounting the stents. Another trick we have used is to position the sheath mid-stent, inflate the balloon slightly to expand the distal end and then fully withdraw the sheath to finish balloon inflation. Worries that the stent could get stuck in the sheath have been unfounded but we have not used sheaths with distal markers for this maneuver. It is relatively easy to deal with a stent that has slipped proximally, but much more difficult to deal with one that slips distally. As soon as the stent starts to slip, inflation should be stopped. If it has slipped proximally, the sheath is readvanced to catch the proximal end of the stent and hold it while the balloon is repositioned. The balloon should be deflated enough to allow repositioning of the stent but not enough to allow the stent to embolize. If the stent slips distally but has been expanded enough to remain in position one can deflate the balloon and try to readvance it through the stent. This may work if the balloon deflates to a low profile but exchanging for a smaller balloon is usually preferable. If the stent slips distally and is not stable, attempting to reinsert the balloon will simply push it distally. Care must be taken to keep the stent on the guidewire and avoid jamming the stent into the vessel distally. Once the original balloon or, preferably, a new balloon is through the stent it is inflated enough to catch the stent but not enough to expand it. One then attempts to pull the balloon and stent back into position. A more complicated, but sometimes useful technique is to use a second catheter to prevent the stent from moving distally. One can place a snare around the guidewire or inflate a balloon distal to the stent to maintain its position during balloon reinsertion.

There are several options for dealing with a stent that has embolized and is free in a vessel or chamber of the heart: a) Reposition the stent to the proper site. b) Expand the stent in a harmless position. c) Remove the stent in the catheterization laboratory. d) Entrap and fix the stent with a second stent. e) Remove the stent in the operating room. If the stent is free one should maneuver a guidewire and then a balloon catheter through the stent. With the balloon inflated just enough to catch the stent without expanding it, the stent can be moved. If it cannot be repositioned in the lesion it can often be left in a harmless position. We have expanded and left stents in the iliac veins and arteries, the branch pulmonary arteries and the descending aorta where they have remained for years without problems. For patients who do not otherwise need to go to the operating room, this option seems preferable. Retrieving partially or fully expanded Palmaz stents is rarely possible, but we have successfully done this on 2 occasions. In one adult patient, a 30 mm iliac stent had been expanded to 15 mm in a right atrium to right ventricle conduit and embolized to the right atrium. Using a series of snares and baskets the stent was crushed and removed through a 24 Fr sheath. In another adult, a 30 mm iliac stent was expanded to 15 mm in the proximal left pulmonary artery before it embolized to a very large main pulmonary artery. The stent was subsequently expanded to 25 mm, and became extremely short with a ring-like appearance. A guidewire was passed through the stent and snared, catching the stent. It could then be pulled out through a 14 Fr sheath. Over the years, there have been a few stents that slipped out of the proximal left pulmonary artery into the main pulmonary artery shortly after implantation. Because the stents were fully expanded, the stents could not be readvanced into the left pulmonary artery. In these cases we passed a long sheath and longer stent through the original stent. The sheath was retracted and used to hold the original stent against the orifice of the left pulmonary artery as the second stent is expanded. The second stent was long enough to overlap the first and fix its position. If a stent has embolized, and cannot be dealt with or if the patient needs surgery anyway, removing the stent in the operating room may be the best solution.

A major consideration when implanting stents in the pulmonary arteries and the aortic arch is the presence of side-branches. Covering a large side-branch coming off at right angles will rarely result in occlusion; however, covering a small vessel coming off at an acute angle will usually result in occlusion.

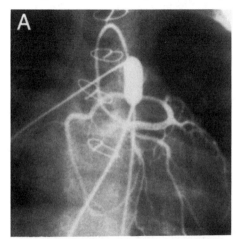
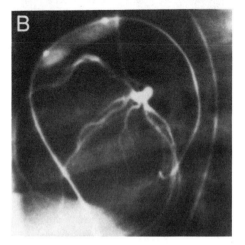

Figure 9-3: Patient with tetralogy of Fallot and single left sided coronary artery: right coronary artery arises from left and closes anterior to right ventricular outflow (RVO): balloon inflated in RVO does not obstruct flow in right coronary: A=A-P, B= LAT projection.

Whenever possible one should avoid covering side-branches, but there are rare cases in which occluding a small side-branch while relieving a stenosis to a large segment of lung will prove beneficial. Covering a side-branch usually occurs because the stent is malpositioned by a few millimeters rather than from intentionally attempting to cover the branch. If the stent is barely covering the branch, further dilation will shorten the stent and may uncover the branch. If a wire can be passed into the branch without traversing the stent, a small balloon can be used to flare the stent at the origin of the branch. If a wire can be passed through the stent and into the branch, a small balloon may open the branch even if it remains covered or may push one edge of the branch off the end of the stent. The balloon

230

can also be used to pull that part of the stent away from the branch. These maneuvers, however, risk getting the wire or catheter caught in the stent, especially if the balloon ruptures.

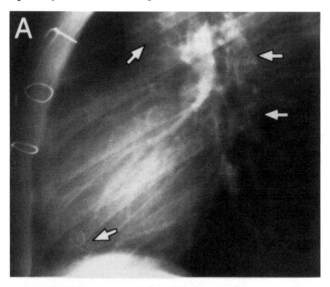

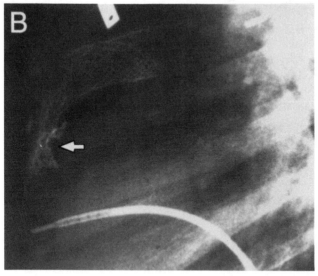

Figure 9-4: (A), A chest X-ray in another patient shows pieces of a fractured stent that have embolized to the pulmonary arteries and right ventricle (arrows).
(B), Spot cine demonstrates a compressed and fractured stent in a right ventricle to pulmonary artery homograft immediately underneath the sternum (arrow).

Occasionally, a stent will compromise an adjacent structure. The most common example is covering the valve in a right ventricle to pulmonary artery homograft. The relative trade-off between gradient reduction and increased pulmonary insufficiency remains to be determined. In most cases, structures that could be compromised by stents are less obvious than the valve in homografts and the consequences of failing to anticipate these could be disastrous. Examples include the criss-crossing systemic and pulmonary venous pathways in Mustards and Sennings, or coronary arteries, especially when aberrant, when stenting right ventricle to pulmonary artery homografts, right ventricular outflow tracts in Tetralogy of Fallot or unusual Fontan baffles. The effects of the stenting can be tested prior to implantation by performing an angiogram in the adjacent structure with a balloon inflated in the lesion to be stented (Fig. 9-3). In some cases, dilating or stenting the compressed structure may be an option, but most will require surgery.

Balloon rupture during stent deployment is the most common cause of stent malposition. The balloon may rupture on a calcified homograft, on adjacent stents or on the stent being deployed. If the balloon has a small hole, rapid inflation may result in enough stent expansion to fix it in position. If not, attempts should be made to replace the balloon as discussed above. If the balloon cannot be pulled out of the stent, the patient needs to go to surgery.

In addition to stent malposition, the ruptured balloon itself is often a problem, because most have circumferential tears. As the balloon is removed the distal half parachutes and makes it very difficult to pull the balloon through the skin. Pieces of the balloon can also be torn off the shaft and embolize. It is usually necessary to use large sheaths or cutdowns to remove the balloon. If a piece is missing, it is often, due to its configuration, trapped on the guidewire. In these cases, the fragment can be removed by snaring the end of the guidewire.

Stent Fracture

Spontaneous fracture of the stent at follow-up has not been seen in pulmonary or systemic arteries or veins. However, approximately 15% of stents in contact with beating myocardium (right or left ventricular outflow tracts) and stents in right ventricle to pulmonary artery homografts or conduits, fracture, resulting in restenosis (Fig. 9-4A). In a few cases stent fracture can be recognized on chest X-ray due to stent compression or embolization of pieces (Fig. 9-4B) but in most cases fluoroscopy is needed. All articulated renal stents, used early in our experience, fractured at the articulation. One pulmonary artery stent fractured during attempts to redilate it. Stent fracture usually results in restenosis, but, with the exception of one patient who developed hemolysis, has otherwise been asymptomatic.

Restenosis And Redilation

Stents in contact with a vessel wall become endothelialized within weeks. Although not true for all stent design, for Palmaz stents this intimal layer rarely reduces the lumen by more than 1 or 2 mm. With the exception of pulmonary veins, intimal hyperplasia rarely progresses during follow-up. Consequently, significant restenosis due to intimal hyperplasia is rare ($\leq$ 3%) [4,6,8,9], but more likely to occur in stents with a small diameter or when the stent is hyperexpanded to a diameter larger than that of the proximal and distal vessel (Fig. 9-5).

With the exception of homografts and ventricular outflow tracts, restenosis due to stent collapse or fracture is rare. In patients with congenital heart disease, the most common cause of restenosis is patient growth relative to the fixed diameter of the stent.

Animal studies of stents in pulmonary arteries and the aorta have shown that stents can be successfully redilated up to a year following implantation. In one study,[12] balloon to stent ratios of 2 resulted in aortic rupture whereas a ratio of 1.4 did not, suggesting gradual sequential dilations are safer. Clinical experience is accumulating to show many stents can be redilated to keep pace with patient growth [6,8,10,11]. In a study involving 33 redilations up to 2½ years following implantation, the average increase in diameter was 28% [8]. Another study of pulmonary artery stents redilated between 1 and 4 years following implantation found an average increase in stent diameter of 25%.[13]

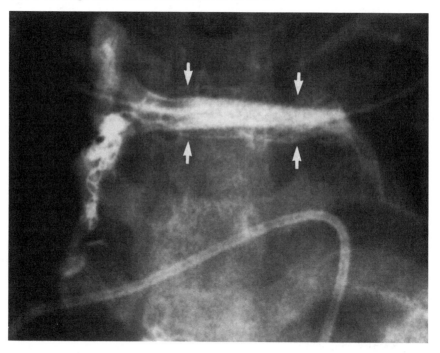

Figure 9-5- Neointimal proliferation is demonstrated in an innominate vein stent (arrows) at a follow-up catheterization. At the time of implantation the stent had been expanded to a diameter larger than that of the vessel on either side of the stenosis.

Experience has shown stents can often be redilated using pressures no higher than used at implantation, suggesting remodeling of the vessel wall. On the other hand, further dilation is most consistently accomplished using high-pressure balloons. The Blue Max balloons (Meditech, Boston Scientific Corporation, Watertown, MA) have the highest inflation pressures currently available and a 12 mm maximal diameter. If very high pressures are needed, 2 or more of these smaller balloons can be used to redilate larger stents. The stent, which will be oval-shaped following 2 balloons, can be rounded again using a single large balloon. In terms of anticoagulation and endocarditis, we treat redilated stents as if they were new stents. If stent restenosis occurs secondary to stent fracture, redilation alone is unlikely to be effective and restenting or surgery is usually required.

SPECIFIC LESIONS: TECHNICAL ASPECTS AND RESULTS

Between 9/89 and 1/98, 477 patients underwent stent implantation at Children's Hospital, Boston. There was no procedural related mortality. The most common locations were pulmonary arteries in 246 patients, obstructed right ventricular to pulmonary artery conduits or homografts in 108, and coarctation of aorta in 32. Other sites included obstructed Fontan baffles or conduits in 21 patients, pulmonary veins in 18, systemic ventricular outflow tract obstructions in 14, stenotic aortopulmonary collaterals in 12, and systemic venous obstructions in 16. Uncommon, though often successful, uses of stents in our patients have included treatment of peripheral arterial obstructions, the creation and maintenance of ventricular and atrial septal defects and Fontan fenestrations, stenotic or thrombosed Blalock-Taussig shunts and in the patent ductus arteriosus to maintain patency in duct-dependent lesions.

Pulmonary Artery Stenosis

Following experimental studies in animals [1,14,15] stents have been used in branch pulmonary artery stenoses since 1989 [2-6]. A report by O'Laughlin et al[3] in 1993 described 80 stents implanted in 58 patients with pulmonary artery stenoses, resulting in an increase in diameter from 4.6 ± 2.3 to 11.3 ± 3.2 mm and a reduction in gradient from 55.2 ± 33 to 14.2 ± 13.5 mm Hg. In those patients with unilateral stent implantation the lung perfusion to the ipsilateral lung increased from 26.4% to 51.1%. Other reports have confirmed these results[4,6,16]. The immediate increase in diameter following stenting is higher than for conventional balloon dilation of pulmonary arteries[17]. Complications including fractures, thrombosis, aneurysm formation and stent migration are extremely rare. Significant restenosis due to endothelialization occurred in less than 4% [8].

There are several indications for stents in branch pulmonary artery stenoses. The most common indication is stenosis of the proximal left and/or right pulmonary artery resulting in a right ventricular pressure greater than half-systemic. A unilateral stenosis associated with hypertension in the contralateral lung or resulting in less than 20% of pulmonary blood flow to the affected lung is also an indication for stenting. The patient's age, size, response to conventional balloon dilation, and need for further surgery must also be considered. An infant with isolated left pulmonary artery stenosis, excellent hemodynamics and adequate response to conventional dilation should not be stented even though the short term result may be better. Rather, the patient can be followed and, if necessary, stented when larger. On the other hand, consider an infant with tetralogy of Fallot with pulmonary atresia who has undergone a right ventricle to pulmonary artery homograft and is left with severe bilateral branch pulmonary artery stenoses that have responded poorly to dilation alone. Stents in the proximal pulmonary arteries in this patient will provide palliation and allow for somatic growth prior to subsequent surgeries. Stents implanted in infants should be in a location accessible to the surgeon. When proximal to the take-off of the right upper lobe pulmonary artery and in the left pulmonary artery at or proximal to the left main stem bronchus our surgeons have not found it difficult to cut through the stents and patch over the vessel or remove the stent entirely. Stenting in the early post-operative period is less likely to rupture the pulmonary artery than conventional balloon dilation due to the smaller balloon to lesions ratios required. Although some centers implant stents in the operating room[16], we do not. It is largely a blind procedure and, therefore, difficult to avoid trauma from the distal end of the balloon and to optimally position the stent relative to the stenosis and to side-branches.

Advancing the long sheath and positioning the stent can be difficult when using femoral venous access due to the tortuous catheter course. Although these difficulties can usually be overcome using stiff guidewires and pre-shaping the long sheath, there are advantages to using subclavian or internal jugular venous access. The catheter course from these vessels has a single curve through the right atrium and ventricle as compared with the s-shaped curve from the femoral vein and it is easier to get the sheath to follow the single curve. The internal jugular vein is larger than the femoral vein in young patients. If the femoral approach proves difficult, the internal jugular vein can be easily accessed by positioning a catheter from the femoral vein in the internal jugular vein and using it as a target for the needle. A transhepatic approach can also be used when other vessels are not available.

The major limitation to stenting pulmonary arteries is the presence of branches. For this reason, the majority of stents in our 246 patients are in the proximal right or left pulmonary artery. The few distal stents have been implanted in either the right intermediate pulmonary artery (just distal to the take-off of the right upper lobe), the right upper or middle lobe, or one of the lower lobes. Stents can also occasionally be placed in branches that have been unifocalized. Implanting these stents without covering side-branches requires selective angiograms in multiple views, careful selection of the stent length in relation to diameter and precise positioning. In some cases, the problem of branches can be overcome by implanting 2 stents simultaneously, 1 in each branch. Due to the relatively small size of currently available stents, they are not routinely used in the main pulmonary artery. Over the last 10 years we have placed 11 main pulmonary artery stents including 6 following arterial switch, 3 following repair of tetralogy of Fallot and 1 following a pulmonary artery band take-down. Of these, 9 were successful. Of the 2 failures, 1 was due to stent embolization in a patient with unoperated tetralogy of Fallot. In the other patient, stenting of supravalvar pulmonary stenosis after an arterial switch resulted in supravalvar aortic stenosis. The patient went to surgery where the stent was removed and the pulmonary artery patched.

Obstructed Conduits

Conduit or homograft obstruction can develop as a result of external compression, intimal proliferation, calcification, kinking, shrinking or due to patient growth. As opposed to conventional balloon dilation, stents are effective in palliating conduit obstructions[2,9,18,19]. As of January 1998, 108 patients have had stents implanted in right ventricular to pulmonary artery conduits or homografts at Children's Hospital, Boston, resulting in a 50% reduction in gradient. The actuarial freedom from reoperation was 65% at 30 months[9] (Fig. 9-6). Stent fractures were observed in 16% of patients during follow-up (Fig. 9-4). All stent fractures resulted in restenosis, but, with the exception of 1 patient who developed hemolysis, patients were otherwise asymptomatic. In 3 patients pieces of the stent embolized to the pulmonary arteries, but did not obstruct flow in the 2 patients who were catheterized.

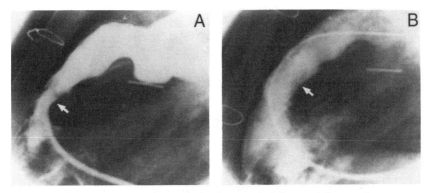

Figure 9-6: Cineangiograms of a severely obstructed right ventricle to pulmonary artery homograft before (A) and following stent implantation (B).

Due to the high incidence of homograft rupture, we do not dilatehomografts with balloons more than 1 or 2 mm larger than the nominal size of the homograft. Dilating calcified homografts not infrequently results in cracking of the calcification with extravasation of contrast outside the wall. This rarely results in problems, presumably due to post-operative scarring around the homograft and often, proximal stenosis. However we have had one fatality in a child a few hours after catheterization in the intensive care unit when rupture occurred acutely at such a fractured site at systemic pressure without any proximal stenosis.

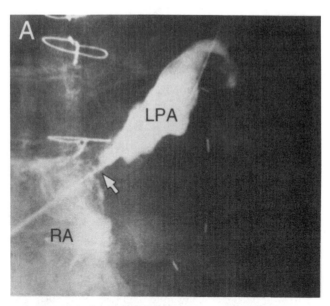

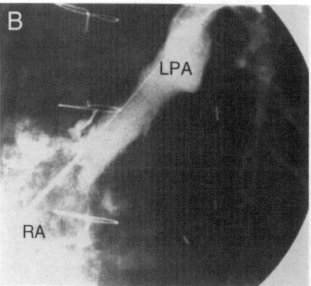

Figure 9-7: A = patient with complete occlusion of a right atrium (RA) to main and left pulmonary artery conduit and a right classic Glenn, a tract is created (arrow) between the right atrium and the left pulmonary artery (LPA) using a Brockenbrough needle. Following balloon B = dilation and stent implantation there is significant angiographic improvement.

Calcification also increases the risk of balloon rupture. It is seldom possible to relieve homograft stenoses without covering the homograft valve with the stent, but usually by the time the homograft needs gradient relief, the valve is already incompetent.

Conduits in other positions have also been managed with stent implantation [6,7,20] (Fig. 9-7).

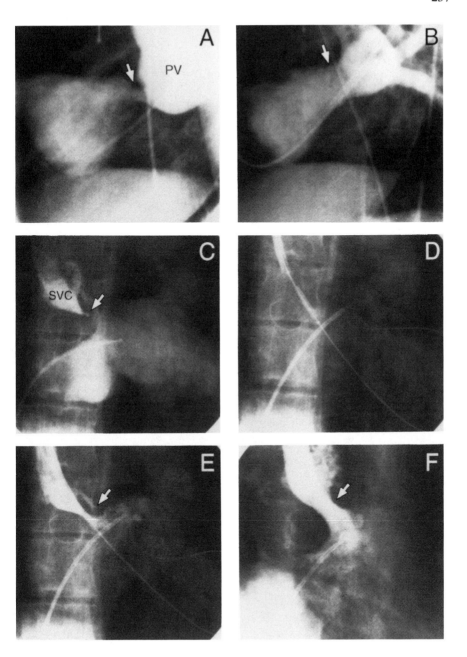

Figure 9-8 Following Mustard operation, complete occlusion of the SVC anastomosis (C, arrow) and severe stenosis of the pulmonary venous pathway (PV) are demonstrated (A, arrow). An angiogram just prior to SVC stent expansion demonstrates position of the stent relative to the narrowing (E, arrow). After stent implantation in PV there is significant angiographic improvement (B, arrow). Utilizing a Brockenbrough needle, a tract is created

between the SVC and the right atrium (D), followed by balloon dilation and stenting of this pathway (F, arrow). (SVC: superior vena cava).

We have implanted stents in 21 patients with obstructed Fontan conduits. Immediate results demonstrated signfiicant reduction in gradients, from 11.4 +/- 5.1 mmHg to 2.8+/- 2.1 mmHg (peak gradients), and 7.0+/- 4.4 mmHg to 1.4 +/- 1.3 mmHg (mean gradients). Many had the old-style right atrial to right ventricular conduits. The actuarial freedom from reoperation for these patients was 50% at 3 years following stent implantation. Complications included two stent embolizations; one was retrieved and another expanded in the proximal left pulmonary artery. Restenosis from a fractured stent occurred in a patient with a substernal atrio-pulmonary anastomosis and required restenting

Stenotic Systemic Veins

Since 1989, 16 patients have undergone stent placement for systemic venous obstructions at our institution including 7 with stenotic systemic venous pathways after a Mustard operation. The procedure was successful in 15 of the 16 patients. The immediate results demonstrated significant improvement in diameter (3.9±4.6 mm to 11.8±5.7 mm) and gradient (14.6±9.4 mm Hg to 1.6±1.5 mm Hg). Others have reported comparable success rates[6]. In general, venous obstructions are compliant, allowing high balloon to vessel ratios and excellent luminal diameters post stent implantation. In 4 patients, 2 with an occluded SVC and 1 with an occluded IVC following a Mustard and 1 following a classic Glenn anastomosis, right atrial to vena caval continuity was reestablished using a transseptal needle and subsequent dilation followed by stenting (Fig. 9-8). In 1 patient a superior vena caval stent embolized to the right atrium 6 hours after stent implantation and was subsequently surgically removed.

Coarctation Of Aorta

Stents are being used with increasing frequency in patients with native or post-operative coarctation and have also been used for diffuse systemic arteriopathies (i.e., Takayasu's, Williams' or Rubella syndrome) [21,22]. Indications for stents in the aorta continue to evolve as experience is gained. Initially, stents were used in patients who had failed conventional dilation and were considered to be at increased risk for surgery. More recently, patients with relatively mild gradients and left ventricular dysfunction, primarily diastolic dysfunction, have undergone stenting.[21] There is little surgical experience with this group and conventional balloon dilation rarely succeeds because the mild stenosis limits the size of the balloon that can be used for dilation. Primary stenting, often with staged dilation, is being used in older patients with native coarctations in whom conventional dilations have been associated with an increased incidence of aortic tears and dissections. In 32 patients with native or recurrent coarctation, stenting decreased the gradient from an average of 25 to 5 mm Hg and increased the diameter from 8 to 13 mm. In 16 patients with follow-up catheterizations, the end-diastolic pressure decreased significantly from 19 to 12 mm Hg.

Although most native and postoperative coarctations are at or just distal to the left subclavian artery, associated transverse arch hypoplasia is common and it is, therefore, important to localize the arch gradients using angiography and an end-hole or multi-purpose catheter. It is usually relatively easy to avoid the left subclavian artery when stenting the coarctation, but more difficult to avoid the innominate and left carotid arteries when stenting the transverse arch. In an occasional patient the left vertebral artery will also arise directly from the aorta. Multiple stents may be needed to avoid the head and neck vessels. Though usually not needed, a second wire or catheter can be left in a branch to mark it and allow access to the vessel if the stent impinges upon it. This can be done transvenously using a Brockenbrough transseptal approach if the branch is proximal to the stent. Positioning of the stent is also aided by the use of very stiff wires, pre-inflation with a balloon to look for movement and multiple angiograms through the long sheath during positioning. Covering intercostal arteries has not yet presented a problem. With a stenosis just distal to the left subclavian artery the stent can be positioned to partially overlap the origin of that vessel. Following implantation, inflating a balloon in the subclavian artery will flare the stent and enlarge the orifice.

The guidewire can and should be left in the right or left subclavian artery rather than the ascending aorta or left ventricle if these vessels are large enough or far enough from the lesion to allow balloon inflation. There are several advantages to the straighter catheter course this provides. A curved balloon will be punctured by the sharp ends of the expanding stent. Expansion of a stent around a curve can result in crushing and shortening of the part of the stent on the inside of a curve. A curved catheter course has more play than a straight catheter course, making positioning more difficult.

One study of experimental coarctation of the aorta demonstrated aortic rupture in 2 of 7 animals at stent redilation [12]. In both animals, a balloon/coarctation diameter ratio of 2 was used, compared with a ratio of 1.4 in the remaining 5 animals. Other animal studies[10,23] have demonstrated the feasibility and safety of stent redilation, which correlates with our clinical experience to date. Gradual enlargement of the aorta using a staged approach to stent implantation and redilation would seem prudent.

Miscellaneous Sites

Both conventional balloon dilation and stenting have been found to relieve pulmonary vein stenosis in the short-term. In our experience, however, pulmonary veins have uniformly restenosed within 6 to 8 weeks following conventional balloon dilation. Restenosis commonly occurs within 3 months following stenting. Only 3 of 18 patients (none less than a year of age) received long-term benefit from a stent. Most stents restenosed due to tissue ingrowth and covered stents were used in 2 patients in an attempt to overcome this problem. Although neither developed restenosis at the stent, both developed progressive stenosis beyond the stent. Currently we do not advise the use of stents in infants with pulmonary vein stenosis except as a way of prolonging life in those pursuing lung transplantation.

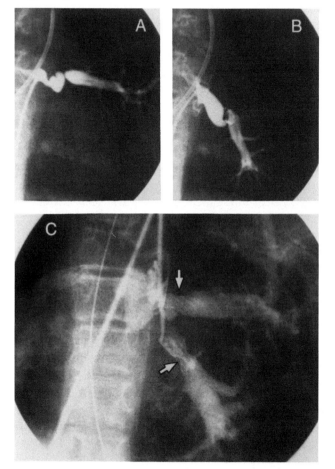

Figure 9-9 Severely stenotic aortopulmonary collaterals (A, B) are stented (C; arrows) prior to a unifocalization procedure.

Aortopulmonary collaterals are very rigid and balloon dilation, even with high-pressure balloons, is rarely successful. Even the modest increases in diameter attainable with stents can be beneficial in inoperable patients whose only source of pulmonary blood flow are these collaterals[24]. Stents have also been used to increase blood flow prior to unifocalization (Fig. 9-9) in the hope this will promote growth of the segment and increase the patency rate following surgery. We have implanted stents in 14 patients with systemic ventricular outflow tract obstruction. These have included patients with a restrictive bulbo-ventricular foramen in single ventricle, a subaortic stenosis in Shone's complex (Fig. 9-10), a repaired transitional atrioventricular canal, a left ventricular to descending aortic conduit and double outlet right ventricles. In the group with double outlet right ventricle, stents were implanted in restrictive ventricular septal defects, one created at the catheterization, in a subaortic conus or in the baffle from the VSD to the aorta.

All but one had immediate improvement in the diameter and the gradient. Several had dramatic improvement in left ventricular function in the months following stents. At present, this procedure should be reserved for selected patients at high risk for surgery or as a bridge to surgery for those with poor ventricular function. More routine use of stents in this location will await stents more resistant to fracture, which has occurred in 27% of cases.

The available techniques for creating atrial defects, blade and balloon septostomy and balloon dilation, do not allow one to precisely control the size of the defect. Stenting the atrial septum or atrial baffles creates a round hole and allows precise control of the size. Because the septum is relatively thin and mobile positioning the stent can be difficult. The easiest method is to stain the septum with contrast when performing the transseptal puncture and then to immediately implant the stent before the contrast disappears. We have stented an atrial septum in an adult with pulmonary hypertension and a newborn with hypoplastic left heart syndrome and an intact atrial septum. In the newborn the stent was removed 3 days after implantation during Stage 1 surgery. Stents have also been implanted in the atrial baffle in 3 Fontan patients with newly created fenestrations.

Covered Stents

We have implanted 5 covered stents made with expanded polytetrafluoroethylene (EPTFE) surgical membrane (W. L. Gore & Associates, Flagstaff, AZ) covering Palmaz stents. The EPTFE is sewn into a tube, the diameter and length of which conforms to the eventual diameter and length of the stent following implantation. The Gore-Tex tube is fastened to the middle of the stent using a single suture and then folded and rolled around the stent for insertion. In addition to pulmonary veins, these covered stents have been used to simultaneously dilate an LPA and close a Potts' shunt and to close an iatrogenic aortopulmonary window in a patient with transposition who had undergone an arterial switch[25].

Conclusions

It has now been nearly 10 years since the first stent was used in a patient with congenital heart disease. The results have demonstrated that stents provide effective relief or palliation for many lesions and the indications continue to expand. During this same period many of the shortcomings of stents have been

242

identified. These include the technical difficulties of implantation, a nontrivial incidence of fracture in certain lesions and limited ability to expand stents as the patient grows. It is likely many of these shortcomings will be solved in the next few years as new stent designs emerge.

REFERENCES

1. Mullins CE, O'Laughlin MP, Vick CWIII, et al. Implantation of balloon expandable intravascular grafts by catheterization in pulmonary arteries and systemic veins. Circulation 1988;77(1):188-199.
2. O'Laughlin MP, Perry SB, Lock JE, Mullins CE. Use of endovascular stents in congenital heart disease. Circulation 1991;83:1923-1939.
3. O' Laughlin MP, Slack MC, Grifka RG, Perry SB, Lock JE, Mullins CE. Implantation and intermediate-term follow-up of stents in congenital heart disease. Circulation 1993;88:605-614.
4. Fogelman R, Nykanen D, Smallhorn JF, McCrindle BW, Freedom RM, Benson LN. Endovascular stents in the pulmonary circulation. Clinical impact on management and medium term follow-up. Circulation 1995; 92:881-885.
5. O'Laughlin MP. Balloon-expandable stenting in pediatric cardiology. J Interv Cardiol 1995;8:463-475.
6. Shaffer KM, Mullins CE, Grifka RG, O'Laughlin MP, McMahon W, Ing FF, Nihill MR. Intravascular stents in congenital heart disease: short and long term results from a large single-center. J Am Coll Cardiol 1998; 311:661-7.
7. Redington AN, Well J, Somerville J. Self expanding stents in congenital heart disease. Br Heart J 1994; 72:378-383.
8. Ing FF, Grifka RG, Nihill MR, Mullins CE. Repeat dilation of intravascular stents in congenital heart disease. Circulation 1995;92:893-897.
9. Powell AJ, Lock JE, Keane JF, Perry SB. Prolongation of RV-PA conduit life-span by percutaneous stent implantation: intermediate term results. Circulation 1995;92:3282-8.
10. Morrow WR, Palmaz JC, Tio FO, et al. Re-expansion of balloon-expandable stents after growth. J Am Coll Cardiol 1993;22:2007-2013.
11. Grifka RG, Vick GWIII, O'Laughlin MP, et al. Balloon expandable intravascular stents: Aortic implantation and later further dilation in growing minipigs. Am Heart J 1993;126:979-984.
12. Mendelsohn AM, Dorostkar PC, Moorehead CP, Lupinetti FM, Reynolds PI, Ludomirsky A, Lloyd TR, Heidelberger K, Beekman RH. Stent redilation in canine models of congenital heart disease: Pulmonary artery stenosis and coarctation of the aorta. Cath Cardiovasc Diagnosis 1996; 38:430-440.
13. Be'eri le, Preminger TJ, Keane JF, Lock JE., Perry SB. Feasibility of stent redilation more than one year post-implantation in children with congenital heart disease. Circulation 1994;90:I-641 (abstract).

14. Benson LN, Hamilton F, Dasmahapatra H, et al. Percutaneous implantation of balloon-expandable endoprosthesis for pulmonary artery stenosis: an experimental study. J Am Coll Cardiol 1991;18:1303-1308.

15. Rocchini AP, Meliones JN, Beekman RH, et.al. Use of balloon-expandable stents to treat experimental peripheral pulmonary artery and superior vena caval stenosis: Preliminary experience. Pediatr Cardiol 1992;13:92-96.

16. Mendelson AM, Bove EL, Lupinetti FM, Crowley DC, Lloyd TR, Fedderly RT, Beekman RH. Intraoperative and percutaneous stenting of congenital pulmonary artery and vein stenosis. Circulation 1993;88(Part 2):210-217.

17. Rothman A, Perry SB, Keane JF, Lock JE. Early results and follow-up of balloon angioplasty for branch pulmonary artery stents. J Am Coll Cardiol 1990;15:1109-1117.

18. Hosking MCK, Benson LN, Nakanishi T, Burrows PE, Williams WG, Freedom RM. Intravascular stent prosthesis for right ventricular outflow tract obstruction. J Am Coll Cardiol, 1992;20:373-380.

19. Almagor Y, Pregosti LG, Bartorelli AL, et al. Balloon expandable stent implantation in stenotic right heart valved conduits. J Am Coll Cardiol 1990;16:1310-1314.

20. Kreutzer J, Perry SB, Keane JF, Mayer JE, Jonas RA, Lock JE. Catheter management of stenotic Fontan baffles and conduits. J Am Coll Cardiol 1995: 100A; 921-72 (abstract).

21. Chung AM, Perry SB, Keane JF, Lock JE. Late hemodynamic and anatomic results of balloon-expandable stent implantation for coarctation of the aorta. Circulation 1997;8:I 566 (abstract).

22. Suarez de Lezo J, Pan M, Romero M, Medina A, et.al. Balloon-expandable stent repair of severe coarctation of the aorta. Am Heart J 1995;129:1002-8.

23. Morrow WR, Smith VC, Ehler WJ, VanDellen AF, Mullins CE. Balloon angioplasty with stent implantation in experimental coarctation of the aorta. Circulation 1994;89:2677-2683.

24. Mc Leold K, Blackburn M, Gibbs J: Stenting of stenosed aortopulmonary collaterals: A new approach to palliation in pulmonary atresia with multifocal aortopulmonary blood supply. Br Heart J 1994; 71:487-489.

25. Preminger TJ, Lock JE, Perry SB. Traumatic aortopulmonary window as a complication of pulmonary artery balloon angioplasty: Transcatheter occlusion with a covered stent. A case report. Cath and Cardiovasc Diagn 1994;31:286-289.

10. OTHER CATHETERIZATION LABORATORY TECHNIQUES AND INTERVENTIONS: ATRIAL SEPTAL DEFECT CREATION, TRANSSEPTAL PERICARDIAL DRAINAGE, FOREIGN BODY RETRIEVAL, EXERCISE AND DRUG TESTING.

Peter Lang, M.D.

CREATION OR ENLARGEMENT OF AN ATRIAL SEPTAL DEFECT

Rashkind and Miller reported the "Creation of an Atrial Septal Defect without Thoracotomy: a palliative approach to complete transposition of the great vessels" in 1966 [1]. Although a transcatheter technique to treat congenital heart disease had been reported more than ten years earlier [2], the impact of Rashkind and Miller's report on patients with d-transposition of the great arteries and on interventional cardiology in general cannot be overstated. Balloon atrial septostomy (BAS) offered effective palliation for d-transposition of the great arteries and it is still used routinely in these patients.

Balloon atrial septostomy is ideal for a patient with a thin septum primum and a left atrium large enough to accommodate a relatively large balloon. Unfortunately, many patients who would benefit from an atrial level defect do not fit these criteria. Other techniques and procedures including blade atrial septostomy, balloon septoplasty (balloon dilation of the interatrial septum using static balloons) and stenting the interatrial septum, have emerged to manage these patients.

Balloon Atrial Septostomy (BAS)
The most common indication for BAS (Fig. 10-1) is the newborn with d-transposition of the great arteries. We continue to perform BAS "routinely" on patients with d-transposition of the great arteries and an intact ventricular septum, even though the majority could be managed with PGE1 prior to neonatal surgery. Following BAS, PGE1 is discontinued. Despite the use of PGE1, an occasional patient will not mix well and can only be resuscitated with an emergent BAS [3]. Infants with d-transposition of the great arteries and ventricular septal defect may also have some improvement in systemic oxygenation following BAS and they may also benefit from left atrial decompression.
We do not routinely perform BAS in newborns with obligatory interatrial shunts: patients with obligatory right-to-left shunts, those with pulmonary atresia and intact ventricular septum (PA/IVS) and those with tricuspid atresia, rarely develop a restrictive atrial defect. Furthermore, the goal in most patients with PA/IVS is to promote blood flow through the right ventricle; BAS would be counterproductive. Although BAS has been used in the past for patients with obligatory left-to-right shunts, e.g. left atrio-ventricular valvar atresia, we currently prefer to use other techniques.

246

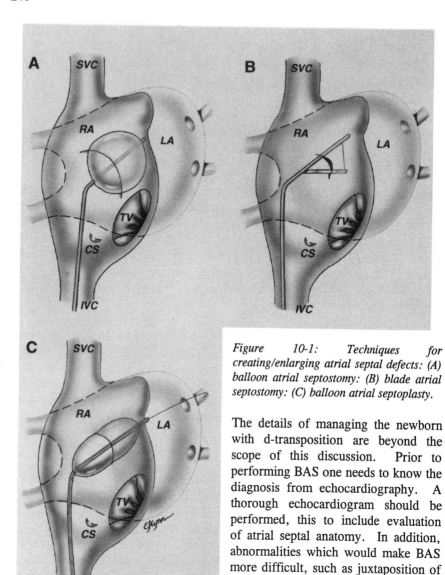

Figure 10-1: Techniques for creating/enlarging atrial septal defects: (A) balloon atrial septostomy: (B) blade atrial septostomy: (C) balloon atrial septoplasty.

The details of managing the newborn with d-transposition are beyond the scope of this discussion. Prior to performing BAS one needs to know the diagnosis from echocardiography. A thorough echocardiogram should be performed, this to include evaluation of atrial septal anatomy. In addition, abnormalities which would make BAS more difficult, such as juxtaposition of the atrial appendages or a left superior vena cava with a large coronary sinus, should be identified. In the occasional patient with a large true ASD, BAS will not be necessary. For the rare patient who is markedly cyanotic and unstable despite PGE1, an abbreviated echo can be performed while arrangements are being made for an immediate BAS. Remember to type and cross-match blood.

The basic technique for BAS has not changed since described in 1966 and is performed from either the femoral or umbilical vein using a 6 or 7F sheath depending on which balloon is used. The balloon catheter can be introduced directly through the umbilical vein without a sheath, but we prefer a sheath with a back-bleed valve long enough to reach the IVC or RA to avoid losing access and to prevent air embolism. Care must be taken to assure that air is removed from the sheath before and after BAS because the balloon, acting as a plunger, can introduce air into the sheath. We do not heparinize the patient if the procedure is to be limited to BAS (Baxter Health Care Corp. Irvine, CA 92714).

The Miller Edwards septostomy catheter, the one we most commonly use has a 5 F shaft, but requires a 7F introducer sheath because of the non-recessed balloon. The distal 2 cm has a 35° angle, which facilitates entry into the left atrium. When inflated with 1 cc (we use dilute contrast in the cath lab and saline for echo guided procedure) the balloon is 13 mm in diameter, with 2 cc it is 16 mm and with 4 cc it is 18 mm. Several other balloons are available. The "Rashkind" balloon (Bard, Billerica, MA 01821) and the Braun balloon (B. Braun, Bethlehem, PA 18018) have end-holes, which can be useful in documenting location and for exchanges over guidewires. Both of these balloons will fit through a 6 F sheath but their maximal inflated diameters are less than the Miller-Edwards balloon.

BAS has traditionally been performed in the cath lab using fluoroscopic guidance but has in recent years been performed in the intensive care unit using echocardiographic guidance[4]. When the ductus venosus is stenotic and difficult to cross, fluoroscopy is invaluable. Without echocardiography, the left atrial position of the Miller-Edwards balloon, which has no end-hole, is determined entirely by the fluoroscopic appearance. To the inexperienced, the difference between the left atrium, right ventricle, coronary sinus, central pulmonary vein, or right atrial appendage is not obvious. Advancing the catheter into a distal pulmonary vein is one way to document location. Echo will clearly show the catheter shaft in the left atrium although it may be somewhat more difficult to locate the tip of the catheter. Needless to say, it is critical to be sure the balloon is in the left atrium before inflating it. If the umbilical vein is used, one has to remember to pull the tip of the sheath into the ductus venosus to avoid its interfering with the balloon when the septostomy is performed.

The balloon is inflated to the desired volume (we commonly start with 2.5-3 cc) in the mid-left atrium. The balloon should be watched continuously and gradually pulled back against the septum during the inflation. An asymmetric balloon suggests entrapment in a pulmonary vein, atrial appendage or small left atrium. A sudden change in position could be due to the balloon popping across the mitral valve. The large balloon in the left atrium can cause hemodynamic compromise especially when the left atrium is small. Therefore, this part of the procedure should be performed in a rapid, yet controlled, manner.

The purpose of BAS is to tear the septum primum. Jerking the balloon through the atrial septum does this, whereas a slow pull or tug will commonly stretch the mobile septum down to the IVC/RA junction. The trick is to produce a rather violent jerk and at the same time, be ready to stop or even reverse the motion before the balloon is pulled into the IVC. There are several ways of doing this. One common method is to place the heel of the right hand on the table while holding the catheter shaft taut between the thumb and index finger. Rolling the hand away from the patient jerks the balloon through the septum without going too far. After each jerk the balloon should be sitting at the mouth of the IVC. The only way to be sure the balloon has come through the septum is to readvance it. If it has crossed the septum, it will move superiorly and to the right border of the heart on fluoro. Failure to cross the septum is almost always due to an inadequate jerk, but if repeated attempts fail, a smaller balloon can be tried. We frequently record the withdrawal on cine film: frame-by-frame analysis of the balloon going through the septum will graphically illustrate the difference between a brisk jerk and a diffident tug. There is a common tendency to advance the balloon just before jerking it. Advancing it 1-2 mm will not present problems but advancing it more risks having the balloon pop across the mitral valve. We commonly repeat the septostomy 2 or 3 times with slightly larger balloons.

Assessing results is not always straightforward. The systemic oxygen saturation in a patient with severe cyanosis will increase within a few minutes if successful whereas the increase in a newborn with a value >80% may be minimal. Echo is the best method to assess the defect in these patients. Following BAS, the prostaglandin infusion is stopped. Numerous complications have been reported over the years. Most are the result of inflating the balloon outside the left atrium or pulling the balloon well down the IVC.

Blade Atrial Septostomy

Based on animal studies, Park and his colleague developed a blade atrial septostomy catheter, which proved effective in a collaborative multi-institutional study [5]. The technique was introduced for the creation or enlargement of interatrial defects in children beyond the first month of life, in whom the atrial septum is no longer pliable and amenable to BAS. When initially introduced, the procedure was employed predominantly for infants and older children with transposition of the great arteries who required improved interatrial mixing. Our own experience was mainly in children with left atrial outlet obstruction, i.e. left AV valve stenosis or atresia and an intact or restrictive interatrial communication[6]. With the advent of balloon atrial septoplasty, we rarely now employ this technique.

Careful precatheterization echocardiographic evaluation is necessary to determine left atrial size, septal thickness, atrial anatomy, and the relationship of any preexisting atrial defect to pulmonary veins or AV valves. After hemodynamic assessment including left atrial pressure and the transatrial gradient, access to the left atrium is gained from the femoral vein either through a pre-existing interatrial communication or using a transseptal needle (see below). Imaging the left atrium on the levo-phase of a pulmonary angiogram facilitates passage of the transseptal needle into small and abnormally shaped left atria. For the same reason, a left atrial angiogram is performed once in the left atrium.

The blade catheter (Cook, Bloomington, IN 47402) has a 6 F shaft and two blade sizes, 9.5 and 13 mm. The blade is opened and closed by pushing and pulling, respectively, the control wire at the proximal end of the catheter. A side port is available to flush the catheter with saline (or contrast); the direction of the side port is similar to the direction of the opened blade. Make sure the blade opens and closes properly prior to insertion.

The blade catheter can be advanced directly to the left atrium but we prefer a long sheath previously positioned in the left atrium. Once the blade catheter is in position, the long sheath is withdrawn to the inferior vena cava. Under fluoroscopic guidance the blade is opened; resistance to opening suggests the blade is trapped in either a pulmonary vein, the left atrial appendage or a small left atrium. In general, the blade is directed antero-leftward for the initial slice (the exact orientation depends on the patient's anatomy), avoiding vital structures such as pulmonary veins, AV valves, or the aorta. The blade orientation is adjusted by rotating the catheter. As opposed to BAS, the blade catheter is pulled slowly across the interatrial septum. Resistance may be considerable and, as with BAS, one must avoid pulling the blade down the IVC when it pops through the septum. If the septum cannot be crossed with a fully opened blade, it can be partially closed. Once across the septum, the blade should be immediately closed. We commonly make several passes through the septum, varying the angle of the blade within a 90° anteroleftward range. Following blade septostomy, a balloon septostomy or balloon septoplasty is performed to further enlarge the hole.

In patients with left atrial outlet obstruction, we attempt to get the gradient below 3 mm Hg. Relieving the left atrial hypertension may increase pulmonary blood flow, depending on the patient's cardiac defect, partially offsetting the decrease in gradient, and increasing systemic oxygen saturation. In patients with right-to-left shunts, enlarging a restrictive atrial defect will decrease the gradient across the defect and may decrease systemic oxygen saturation. If the defect remains inadequate, a second hole can be created with a transseptal needle. Ideally, subsequent blading or ballooning of that hole will create a tear into the first hole and create one large defect.

Atrial Septoplasty
Atrial septoplasty involves dilating defects in the atrial septum using static balloons [7]. The indications are the same as for blade atrial septostomy, which it has replaced at our institution, but atrial septoplasty can be used in patients whose atria are too small to accommodate the blade. We have also used this technique to create atrial defects in patients with pulmonary hypertension [8,9,10].

Dilation of the atrial septum is relatively simple. Since existing defects are more likely to stretch than tear, we prefer to dilate a defect created with a transseptal needle. An exchange-length guidewire is positioned with the distal tip in a left pulmonary vein or in a tight loop on the distal end of the wire within the left atrium. The balloon is then advanced over the wire and positioned across the atrial septum. Staining the septum with contrast during the transseptal puncture makes location of the septum easy, at least for a few minutes. A left atrial angiogram, or injecting contrast though the sheath as it is withdrawn from the left atrium to uncover the balloon can also be used to localize the septum. Finally, one can simply inflate the balloon slightly. The septum, if a transseptal puncture was used, will create a tight waist in the balloon. The waist is then centered and the balloon inflated.

The diameter and length of the angioplasty balloon is determined by the size of the atria and the indications for the defect. In patients with obligatory left-to-right atrial shunts the goal is to create as large a defect as possible. In newborns we would commonly start with a 4 or 5 mm balloon and end with a 10 or 12 mm balloon. In older patients we have used up to a 20 mm balloon. In patients with discretionary right-to-left shunts the goal is to decrease the right atrial pressure; but this must be balanced against excessive decreases in systemic oxygen saturations due to the increased right-to-left shunting. In these patients, we start with a 4 mm balloon and increase the balloon size in increments of 1 mm with frequent hemodynamic measurements until the desired effect is achieved. We rarely use a balloon larger than 8 to 10 mm.

This technique allows one to monitor the effect of graduated dilations and proceed in a stepwise fashion. It is not, however, foolproof. For example, in a patient with obligatory right-to-left shunting, increasing balloon size 1 mm at a time for several balloons had resulted in only mild cyanosis. The next balloon, 1 mm larger than the previous, resulted in severe cyanosis. This is not surprising, because we are not creating round holes similar in size to the balloon but rather irregular tears and slits and the net size created by any single balloon is unpredictable. The same thing happens with BAS and blade septostomy. The only currently available transcatheter technique that overcomes this problem is stenting the atrial septum (Chapter 9).

The newborn with HLHS and a highly restrictive atrial defect, unlike most other newborns with critical heart disease, cannot be stabilized with medical management and will continue to deteriorate until the atrial septum is opened. When arterial pO_2 remains in the low 20's despite maximum medical therapy, we have adopted the approach that the septum should be opened in the cath lab allowing the patient to be sent to surgery after several days of medical management during which time the pulmonary vascular resistance will drop. These patients often have very small left atria, thick atrial septa and abnormally located foramens. For these reasons, BAS is often difficult, complicated and unsuccessful. As the left atrium is too small for the blade, effective palliation requires a transseptal puncture with a Brockenbrough needle followed by atrial septoplasty.

The femoral vein is cannulated and a small catheter placed in the artery for pressure monitoring. A pulmonary artery or wedge angiogram with levo-phase opacifies the left atrium. A transseptal puncture (see below) is then performed, intentionally avoiding the existing atrial defect by overbending the needle tip, creating a more horizontal passage. Because the atrial septum is thick and the left atrium small, pushing with the needle compresses the septum against the back wall of the atrium and occasionally the needle will pop through both structures at the same time. Contrast, injected through the needle, will enter the pericardial space when this happens. If withdrawn slowly the needle can usually be positioned in the left atrium. One option at this point is to advance an 0.014" wire, which most transseptal needles will accept, through the needle and use this wire for balloon dilations.

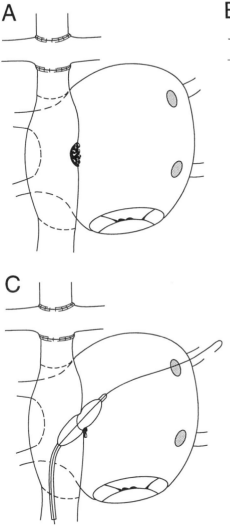

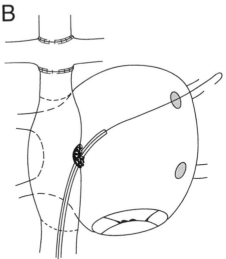

Figure 10-2: Reopening occluded baffle fenestration: (A) clot occluding fenestration: (B) catheter traversing clot with guidewire in left upper pulmonary vein: (C) balloon dilation of fenestration.

We prefer to advance the dilator from the transseptal sheath through the septum over the needle. One can attempt to advance the sheath into the left atrium, but this is usually much more difficult so that we usually advance an 0.018" torque-controlled wire with a short floppy end fashioned into multiple tight loops through the dilator once the needle has been removed. Balloon dilations are performed over this wire. Gradually larger balloons are used, the largest determined primarily by the size of the left atrium but usually 6 to 8 mm. We have occasionally created a second hole in these patients if the first is inadequate.

The observation that a fenestration in a Fontan baffle reduces post-operative effusions has led to the widespread use of this technique. The usual surgical technique is the creation of a 4 mm fenestration with a punch. When an extra-cardiac conduit is employed to direct inferior vena caval flow to the pulmonary

252

arteries, the fenestration is more complex, passing both through the conduit and the lateral wall of the atrium. When fenestrations become partially or completely occluded in the immediate post-operative period, patients may develop a rapidly progressive downward spiral of decreasing cardiac output, metabolic acidosis, and increasing pulmonary vascular resistance [11]. This spiral is commonly heralded by an increase in systemic oxygen saturation as the fenestration closes. Echocardiograms document the lack of a fenestration, indicating that the patient should be taken to the cath lab to have the fenestration opened and to look for associated problems [11] (Fig. 10-2).

Fenestration closure may rarely be due to essentially complete thrombosis of the right atrial baffle in association with kinking or stenosis of the baffle. In others, a thin layer of clot on the baffle will close the fenestration without obstructing baffle flow. Finally, the atrial free wall or native atrial septum occasionally covers the fenestration.

To avoid dislodging an unrecognized clot, we start with an angiogram through a Berman catheter positioned at the IVC/RA junction. This will show if the fenestration is patent, the anatomy of the atrial baffle, including the presence of clot, and give some idea of flow to and through the pulmonary arteries. If the baffle appears unobstructed without thrombi, we proceed directly to opening or enlarging the fenestration. Fenestrations with residual flow are easy to cross and dilate. If completely occluded, one probes the baffle with a catheter and wire, focusing on the mid antero-lateral surface where most fenestrations are located. Even if completely occluded, a slight defect in the baffle surface is commonly seen on the angiograms. Only rarely will one need a transseptal needle. Once across the baffle, an angiogram is performed using a cut-off pigtail over a wire with the side holes straddling the fenestration. A 5 mm balloon is used for the initial dilation and, rarely progressing to using baffle pressure, angiographic patency and systemic saturation value as guides, if the problem was a small, localized clot, these small balloons usually open the fenestration. Success is much less likely if the fenestration is covered by atrial tissue, which may occasionally be seen on the angiograms. A second hole is a better option in these patients. Dealing with a baffle full of thrombus is a more difficult problem. In one patient, the clot and stenosis in the baffle were stented and the fenestration was dilated and stented through the interstices of the first stent. The risk, of course, is a pulmonary embolus. Another patient, with a similar problem was taken immediately to the operating room for revision of the baffle.

TRANSSEPTAL PUNCTURE

Brockenbrough and Braunwald described "A new technique for left ventricular angiography and transseptal left heart catheterization" [12] forty years ago. Due to the presence of inter-atrial communications in many pediatric patients and the ability to perform retrograde left heart catheterization it was not widely used among pediatric cardiologists until recently, when interventions requiring access to the left atrium made transseptal puncture necessary [13,14]. We currently use this technique (Fig. 10-3) for a variety of indications including balloon mitral valvuloplasty, access to the left atrium for electrophysiologic mapping and ablation, creation of inter-atrial communications, access to the pulmonary veins, aortic valvuloplasty in smaller infants, and VSD closure.

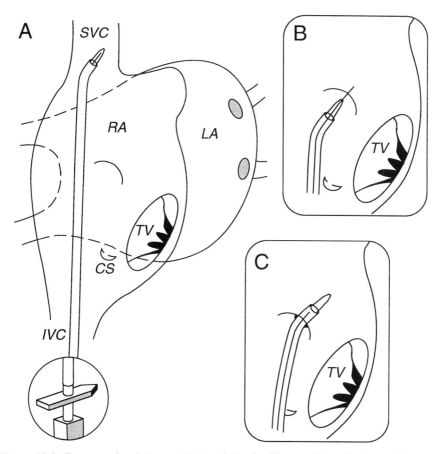

Figure 10-3: Transseptal technique: (A) tips of sheath, dilator and needle in superior vena cava (SVC): (B) dilator tip following withdrawal into fossa ovalis with needle tip protruding into septum: (C) dilator and sheath advanced into left atrium with supporting needle in lumen just proximal to dilator tip.

The equipment required for transseptal puncture includes the needle (available in the short "pediatric" and long "adult" sizes) and a long sheath and dilator (available in 6 and 7F) (Cook, Bloomington IN 47402). To insure that everything fits we advance the needle through the dilator and sheath before insertion. The hubs of the dilator and sheath lock and these need to be separated to allow insertion of the needle into the dilator lumen. The tapered tip of the needle (approximately 4 mm) should extend beyond the tip of the dilator. The needle lumen, which can be closed with a proximal stopcock, allows for pressure measurement, blood sampling and contrast injections to determine location of the tip. We prefer to use contrast injections and attach a 5 cc syringe filled with contrast to the hub. The arrow on the proximal end of the needle points in the same direction as the curve on the distal end.

Many patients with congenital heart disease have anomalies, which make transseptal puncture more difficult. These include a small left atrium, an abnormally oriented atrial septum, an enlarged coronary sinus with LSVC, prominent venous valves, juxtaposition of the atria appendages, a markedly enlarged aorta or situs inversus. These should be identified on precatheterization echocardiograms. If the anatomy is abnormal, we perform a pulmonary angiogram to outline the left atrium.

The curve on the end of the needle is optimal for transseptal puncture from the right femoral vein. If the left femoral vein is used, the radius of curvature should be increased by manually overbending the needle 5-20 cm back from the tip. From the hepatic vein, the needle needs to be straightened slightly. As transseptal puncture is usually a small part of the catheterization, most patients are heparinized at the time it is performed.

The transseptal sheath and dilator are advanced over a previously positioned 0.025" wire to the superior vena cava. The guide wire is removed and the hubs of the sheath and dilator are separated to allow introduction of the needle. If the hubs are separated by pulling the dilator, position in the SVC may be lost, especially in infants. The needle should advance smoothly and usually needs to be rotated to get it through the curves in the pelvis. If one is not careful, the needle can perforate the side of the sheath and dilator. The sheath and dilator hubs should be locked and the needle positioned with its tip 2-5 mm inside the tip of the dilator.

The needle, dilator, and sheath are withdrawn slowly as a unit with the needle aimed to the left and posteriorly. When the anatomy is normal, the needle should point slightly more posteriorly than leftward. We prefer to use biplane fluoro during this part of the procedure. One continues to pull in a slow but steady fashion watching for a slight jump to the left on the AP view as the dilator passes over the superior limbic band and enters the fossa ovalis. This is usually 2/3 of the way from the RA/SVC junction to the diaphragm and almost always lower than the inexperienced expect. The apparatus is then advanced as a unit against the wall of the fossa ovales. When the dilator "engages" the septum the needle is "jabbed" out of the tip of the dilator. If the septum is thin, the needle and occasionally the dilator will pop through the septum but if it doesn't, a small amount of contrast is injected to "tag" the septum. A lot more pushing is required when the septum is thick. In these cases, the entire apparatus is advanced by pushing the sheath with the left hand near the skin. This tents the septum and one has to be prepared to stop pushing and even to pull back a little when the needle finally pops through. Intermittent contrast injections are performed through the needle to determine location. When the needle tip is buried in the septum, it is difficult to inject contrast, but staining the septum is very helpful to determine location and if it is necessary to start over, it is easy to see where the previous attempt was made. When the needle pops through, injecting contrast will demonstrate if it is in the left atrium, the pericardial space, the aorta, the coronary sinus, the pulmonary vein, or the left ventricle. We have found contrast injections much more reliable than pressure measurements in determining position and have abandoned the latter technique. The needle, by itself, is unlikely to do much damage to the atrial or aortic wall, but advancing the sheath and dilator can be very traumatic. If it is necessary to start again, one should usually start from the SVC.

Once in the left atrium, the needle is held firmly while advancing the sheath and dilator until the tip of the dilator is just beyond the tip of the needle. After unlocking the hubs, the sheath is then advanced while holding the dilator and needle as a unit. The sheath commonly catches on the septum. If the septum has been stained one can watch the septum tent up as the sheath is pushed. One has to be careful not to push the septum over the end of the dilator although usually the sheath will pop through before this happens. Occasionally it is necessary to advance the needle and dilator out a left pulmonary vein to get the sheath through, confirming an intravascular position with intermittent contrast injections. Leaving the needle near the tip of the dilator during these maneuvers provides support for the system. Once the sheath is in the left atrium the needle and then the dilator are removed. Pulling the curved needle and dilator can change the orientation of the sheath and cause it to flip out of the left atrium. If the sheath cannot be aspirated it could be kinked but more likely the tip is against the atrial wall. A side-arm adaptor should be inserted into the hub of the sheath to prevent air embolism.

If it is not possible to get the sheath into the left atrium, a guidewire (up to 0.025") can be advanced through the dilator. One can try to use a larger dilator or a small angioplasty balloon (4 mm) to ease entry of the sheath.

The Brockenbrough needle has been used to puncture structures other than the atrial septum. In several patients with d-transposition who had undergone atrial switches, the needle was used to puncture atretic segments between the IVC or SVC and neo-right atrium. These segment were then dilated and stented. We have also reopened the RA/SVC junction following a Glenn anastomosis. These techniques only provide long-term vascular patency when the distance to be bridged is short. In these cases, the basic techniques are the same and success depends on detailed knowledge of the anatomy. In many cases a catheter can be positioned in the chamber or vessel on the other side and the needle aimed at the catheter. In most cases, the curve on the needle needs to be modified.

It is not hard to imagine the complications that can occur from sticking a stiff metal rod with a sharp tip through the heart. When this is kept in mind, fewer complications will occur. We have occasionally perforated the back wall of the atrium with the needle, especially in newborns, without advancing the dilator or sheath into the pericardium. Most of the patients developed small effusions, which can be easily monitored with the small amount of contrast injected into the pericardium at the time of the puncture. Only rarely do these require drainage.

Nevertheless, before performing your first transseptal puncture, we recommend reading the section on pericardiocentesis.

PERICARDIOCENTESIS AND PERICARDIAL DRAINAGE

Pericardial effusions can be post-operative, traumatic, inflammatory, infectious, and malignant. The two basic indications for pericardiocentesis are removal of fluid to establish a diagnosis and treatment of cardiac tamponade [15]. Transcatheter techniques have also been developed to create pericardial windows.

Although a complete description of the hemodynamics and management of cardiac tamponade is beyond the scope of this discussion, several key points should be emphasized. First, fluid administration helps and diuretics hurt. Second, positive pressure ventilation may impair cardiac output. Finally, Isuprel and Epinephrine have been shown to augment cardiac output in the setting of cardiac tampanode, while vasodilators exacerbate the situation. If time permits, coagulation studies should be performed and a type and cross-match sent.

In almost all cases there is time to perform an echocardiogram. The echo confirms the diagnosis of a pericardial effusion, and, more importantly, demonstrates the amount and location of the fluid, and helps identify the safest approach to the fluid. The subxyphoid approach is most commonly used and recommended, even with an asymmetrical collection of fluid, if the pericardial-epicardial separation is at least 5mm from a subxyphoid view. Placing the patient in a 45° sitting position may increase the amount of fluid at the diaphragm. If there is less than 5mm of fluid from this view, apical or parasternal images may demonstrate a safer approach to the fluid. If the image from the apical view demonstrates fluid "en route" to the cardiac apex, there is unlikely to be lung tissue between the probe and the apex of the heart. Thus, a needle can be safely advanced into the pericardium along the same course as the echo beam. The same is true for parasternal views. Pericardiocentesis is routinely performed in the intensive care unit with echo guidance. When unconventional approaches are needed, we recommend bringing the patient to the cath lab where the combination of echo and fluoro are used to guide the procedure.

We generally use a pericardiocentesis kit (Cook, Bloomington, IN 47402) for both pericardiocentesis and long-term drainage. The kit includes an 18 gauge, 6cm long introducing needle, a 50cm, 0.038" J-tipped guidewire, an 8F dilator, and a short flexible 8F pigtail catheter with oversized holes. For infants, we usually use a 4 or 5F pigtail catheter.

Once echocardiography has determined the optimal needle course and the distance the needle must be advanced, the site is prepped and draped and local anesthesia is given. Sedation is given as needed. Using the subxyphoid approach, the 18 gauge needle is introduced just below and slightly to the left of the xyphoid process (Fig. 10-4A). The needle is angled exactly along the course previously determined by the echocardiography probe and advanced with continuous suction until pericardial fluid is obtained. If no fluid is obtained at the predetermined distance (e.g. 6cm), the needle is withdrawn and readvanced at a slightly different

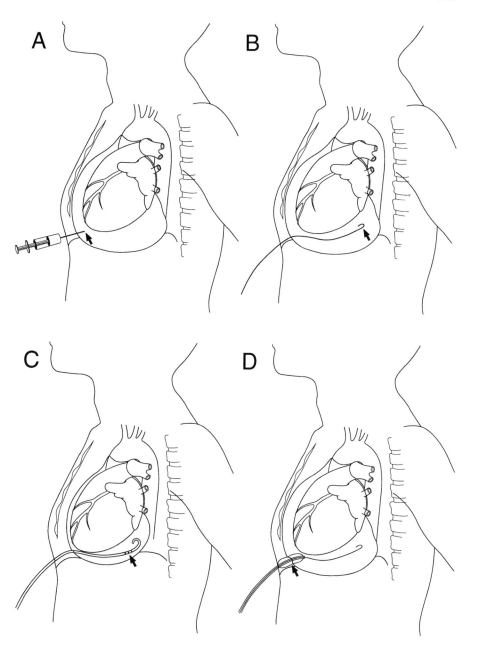

Figure 10-4: Pericardiocentesis technique A= introduction of needle (arrow): B= guidewire introduced (arrow): C= pigtail catheter (arrow) in pericardial space: D = balloon inflation (arrow) to create pericardial – left pleural space window.

angle. If fluid is obtained before it was predicted by the echocardiogram, one can pass the catheter and thereby drain peritoneal fluid. Once pericardial fluid is obtained the guidewire is introduced well into the pericardial space (Fig. 10-4B). After removing the needle, first the dilator and then the catheter are advanced over the wire into the pericardial space (Fig. 10-4C). A stopcock is placed on the pigtail catheter and the fluid is removed.

We no longer use electrocardiographic monitoring of the needle. The appearance a ventricular premature beat may indicate that the myocardium has been touched. If the initial needle aspirate is bloody, it could be from a bloody effusion or because the needle has injured or perforated the heart or a coronary artery. It is often very difficult to differentiate these possibilities: the safest approach is to advance a soft wire well inside the body and demonstrate its location in the pericardial sac. Squirting some of the fluid on a piece of gauze may help. Whole blood tends to sit on top of the gauze whereas a bloody effusion soaks rapidly into the gauze. The hematocrit should be checked, but a decision needs to be made before the result is available. In most instances we leave the pigtail catheter in place for at least several hours. In this manner the pericardium can be completely drained and, perhaps more importantly, the rate at which the fluid is accumulating can be assessed.

The most feared complication of the procedure is coronary artery injury during needle placement. The subxyphoid approach minimizes the risk of coronary artery injury. Catheter placement into the left hemithorax or abdomen has occurred; neither caused significant complications.

A recent extension of percutaneous pericardial drainage has been the description of percutaneous balloon pericardiotomy [16]. This technique uses balloon dilation of the pericardium to create a non-surgical pericardial window (Fig 10-4D). Briefly, once wire access to the pericardial space has been obtained, a standard 15-20 mm angioplasty balloon is introduced. Dilation of the pericardium creates a communication between the pericardium and left pleural space, resulting in effective long-term pericardial decompression. This technique was originally described in adult patients, most with a malignancy. We have used it successfully in patients with post-pericardiotomy syndrome with encouraging results.

ENDOMYOCARDIAL BIOPSY

The use of endomyocardial biopsy in pediatric patients was virtually non-existent until Lurie reported his technique in 1978 [17]. Even following this report, biopsies were rare until the emergence of pediatric heart transplantation. Despite improvements in non-invasive evaluation, the biopsy remains the gold standard for detection of cardiac rejection. The indications for biopsy in non-transplant patients remain uncertain in part, no doubt, due to the inconsistent use of biopsy in evaluating these patients. The availability of smaller bioptomes and sheaths combined with increased experience and the use of echo-guidance [18, 19] have made the procedure (Fig. 10-5) safe, even in small infants [20].

259

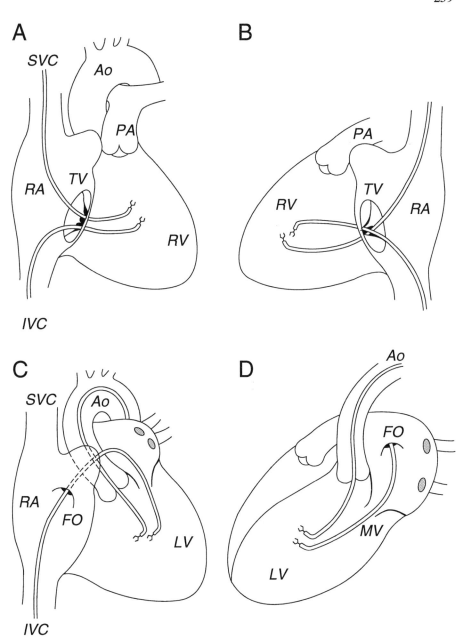

Figure 10-5: Course of sheaths and bioptomes to (1) right ventricular (RV) septal surface from superior (SVC) and inferior (IVC) vena caval approaches (A=Frontal, B= Lateral) and, (2) left ventricular (LV) septal surface from IVC transatrial and retrograde aortic approaches (C=Frontal, D= Lateral).

Transplant Patients

Our current protocol calls for weekly surveillance biopsies for the first 6 to 8 weeks. They are then gradually spaced depending on the clinical course to a minimum of 2 biopsies per year. Routine biopsies are performed on an outpatient basis and we do not type and cross the patients. We use a 5F long sheath (Cook, Bloomington, IN 47401) and a variety of forceps (Argon Division, Athens, TX 7551, Cook, Bloomington, IA 47402, Cordis Corp., Miami, FL 33102). Cooperative patients commonly receive no premedication and we prefer to use the internal jugular vein, which allows the patients to ambulate immediately following the procedure. Uncooperative patients are sedated or, more commonly, given ketamine, which, at our institution requires the presence of an anesthesiologist. In this group of younger patients we tend to rotate venous access between the femoral, internal jugular and occasionally the subclavian veins. We do not heparinize these patients.

In all cases a long sheath is positioned in the right ventricle after shaping the curve to direct the tip towards the right ventricular septal surface. The sheath comes with the distal 1-2 cm angled at 45 to 90°. A second, longer and more proximal curve is produced so that the planes of the proximal and distal curves are perpendicular. The proximal curve directs the sheath from the right atrium through the tricuspid valve and to the body of the right ventricle. This curve is formed by either heat or gently pulling or stripping the sheath and dilator over the thumb. Because the sheath tends to straighten during insertion, we exaggerate the curve. The distal curve directs the tip posteriorly towards the septum. The appropriate curves from the internal jugular and the femoral vein are mirror images of each other. The sheath and dilator can usually be advanced directly into the right ventricle over a wire, but occasionally the sheath is advanced over a balloon-tipped catheter. The sheath is transduced to confirm that it is in the right ventricle. The bioptome is advanced to the end of the sheath and then rotated half a turn towards the septal surface (clockwise for femoral access and counter-clockwise for internal jugular access): of the distal some preshaping is possible and helpful. The handle is then opened and the forceps advanced so that the jaws open as soon as they exit the sheath. They are then advanced against the septum and closed. Squeezing the handle to close the jaws markedly increases the stiffness of the shaft. Therefore, one should pull the forceps into the sheath as soon as the jaws are closed to decrease the risk of perforation. Not infrequently the jaws do not open when advanced out of the sheath. This is most commonly due to malfunction of the forceps but it could be because the bioptome is buried in the myocardium. One should be sure they are free.

We take 5 pieces, all for light microscopy. Following biopsy we perform right-sided hemodynamics. Most patients are in the lab approximately 30 minutes.

Non-transplant Patients

Endomyocardial biopsies in non-transplant patients tend to be performed in conjunction with a complete diagnostic catheterization. Early in our experience, we biopsied both the right and left ventricles in patients with cardiomyopathy. In the first 100 cases there were only 2 patients in whom the 2 ventricles gave different diagnoses. In both cases, 1 ventricle showed endocardial fibroelastosis. Because of this, we no longer biopsy the left ventricle. The femoral vein is usually used in these patients because this site also allows access to the artery. The biopsies are performed using the technique described for transplant patients. In non-transplant patients less than a year of age, we sometimes use echo guidance to insure that the jaws are in contact with the septal surface of the right ventricle for each piece. We usually take 8 to 10 pieces, 5 for light microscopy (especially if myocarditis is suspected), 2 for electron microscopy and the rest for freezing and saving. They are placed in normal saline and taken directly to the pathology department. Following the biopsies, the femoral artery is accessed and the patient is heparinized.

Complications of endomyocardial biopsy are rare [21,22]. In our experience of approximately 2,000 procedures, perforation occurred in 6 patients and only 2 required pericardial drainage.

FOREIGN BODY RETREIVAL

This section will focus on the general principles of retrieval including equipment and technique and retrieval of catheter fragments. Retrieval of devices such as stents, coils, double umbrellas and other closure devices are discussed in the chapters describing these devices. Retrieval techniques are employed in many interventions in which guidewires are snared and these are described in the appropriate sections.

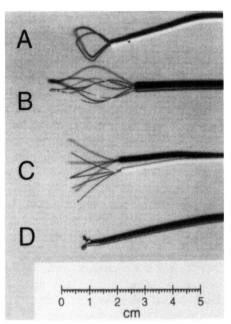

A variety of catheters or devices including snares, baskets, grasping forceps, biopsy and modified forceps can be used for retrieval (Fig. 10-6).

Of these, snares are the most commonly used. They are flexible and can be advanced through a variety of catheters as small as 4F. In the past, we made our own snares by doubling over an 0.018" exchange length guidewire and advancing it through a catheter that would accept an 0.038" wire. We still use this technique when we are focussed on the cath lab supply budget. More often, we use commercially available Amplatz snares

Figure 10-6: Retrieval devices A=homemade snares, B=basket, C=grabber, D=forceps/bioplane.

262

from Microvena, which come in a variety of diameters (Microvena Corp., White Bear Lake, MN 5510; Fig. 10-7).

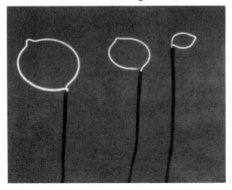

0 1 2 3 4 5
cm

Figure 10-7: Retrieval devices: Amplatz snares of various sizes.

To use the snare, the catheter through which the snare is to be advanced is positioned next to the foreign body either directly or over an exchange wire. The snare is advanced through the catheter and opens as it emerges from the tip of the catheter. The open snare is manipulated around the foreign body by pushing, pulling and/or rotating the snare and/or catheter. Once around the foreign body, the catheter is advanced to close the snare around the foreign body. Constant tension is maintained to insure the snare remains closed.

Functionally, the basket is very similar to the snare. Catching the foreign body is usually relatively easy with a basket. The drawback is that baskets are less flexible and more difficult to position than snares. The problem with grabbers is that, as the name implies, they will grab anything including valves, myocardium and vessel walls. Forceps often seem like a good idea, but, in practice, they are relatively difficult to position. It is also difficult to grasp and hold most foreign bodies with forceps.

Other than devices, the most common indication for retrieval is a catheter fragment. Intracardiac lines placed at cardiac surgery will occasionally get stuck or break during attempted removal. Broviac or similar central lines can break or become disconnected from the hub and embolize to the heart or pulmonary arteries. A sheath large enough to accommodate the doubled-over catheter fragment should be used. The vascular access site depends, of course, on where the fragment is. The snare catheter is positioned alongside the fragment and the snare is opened and maneuvered around one end of the fragment. The snare should be firmly closed but avoid breaking or cutting the fragment in two with the snare. Catheter fragments can be easily and safely pulled through valves. If retrieving an object from the pulmonary artery that you do not want to pull across the tricuspid valve, it can be pulled into a long sheath positioned in the pulmonary artery.

Needless to say, it is much easier, though perhaps not as rewarding, to retrieve objects that are visible or radio-opaque. Over the years, we have lost a number of fragments from broken angioplasty balloons, some quite large. They are not visible on fluoro except as a filling defect on contrast injections. In one case, a large fragment could not be found despite numerous contrast injections. It was eventually found and removed from the left ventricular outflow tract using echocardiography.

For objects too large to fit into a sheath it is usually less traumatic to pull them to the femoral vein and then perform a cut-down. Occasionally a foreign body can be pulled into but not out of a sheath. If the sheath is removed, access is lost. To avoid this problem a guidewire can be advanced through the sheath before pulling the foreign body into the sheath. If it is necessary to remove the sheath, the wire is still in position preserving vascular access.

EXERCISE TESTING

For decades, prior to the evolution of objective non-invasive measures of cardiac performance, exercise testing provided an independent assessment of ventricular function. The use of exercise testing became popular when Master and colleagues reported electrocardiographic recordings during a standardized 2-step fitness test [23]. A variety of testing modalities have been subsequently introduced, including treadmills and bicycle ergometers, as well as applications that allow exercise performance to be monitored by electrocardiography, echocardiography, and hemodynamic monitoring as part of a cardiac catheterization. The introduction of increasingly sensitive non-invasive measures of cardiac performance has resulted in a marked decrease in the number of exercise tests performed in the catheterization laboratory. Despite this, it is clear that exercise testing in the cath lab has been useful in predicting the onset of ventricular dysfunction and testing the degree of hemodynamic normalization following repair of congenital heart disease. Some of the information acquired in the cath lab cannot be duplicated by other means.

Three forms of exercise testing have been used in the cath lab: isometric, upright isotonic and supine isotonic. Each has its advantages and disadvantages (table).

Table: Hemodynamic Responses To Exercise.

Type of exercise	Change in RA pressure	Change in C.O.	Change in Ao pressure	Change in O_2 consumption
Isometric	Increase	Small Increase	Marked Increase	Small Increase
Supine Isotonic	Decrease	Moderate Increase	Small Increase	Moderate Increase
Upright Isotonic	No Change	Marked Increase	Small Increase	Marked Increase

264

Isometric exercise is easy to perform and requires little equipment; unfortunately, it has little physiologic effect other than to raise afterload. Upright exercise testing places the largest demand on the cardiovascular system, resulting in the highest cardiac output and oxygen consumption; unfortunately, it is difficult to perform in the cath lab. For those reasons, most exercise testing in the cath lab has been done with supine isotonic exercise. For supine bicycle ergometry, the feet are strapped to the pedals of the bicycle ergometer, which is attached to the cath table or suspended from a ceiling rack. For most patients, we aim for an exercise load of 50 watts/meter^2. A bicycle ergometer with a variable resistance program is used, so that the amount of work done is constant irrespective of the cycling rate. Once the patient begins, 2-3 minutes are needed to achieve a steady work load and steady state hemodynamics. At this time, oxygen consumption, pressures and oxygen saturations are quickly measured. We have found it possible to use the bicycle even with catheters in the femoral artery and vein. The use of a double-lumen, balloon-tipped catheter in the vein allows simultaneous measurements of pulmonary artery and right atrial pressures and intermittent measurements of the pulmonary capillary wedge pressure. Similarly, the use of an arterial sheath and a pigtail catheter 1 F size smaller than the sheath allows simultaneous monitoring of left ventricular and arterial pressures in patients with left ventricular outflow obstruction.

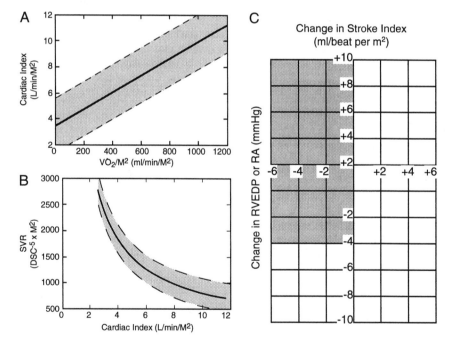

Figure 10-8: Relationships in 23 normal children (age 4-15) undergoing supine bicycle exercise: A=oxygen consumption and cardiac index: B=cardiac index and systemic vascular resistance (SVR): C=stroke index and right ventricular end diastolic (RVEDP) or right atrial (RA) pressure.

Although not impossible, it is quite difficult to perform an exercise test in a patient with an intracardiac shunt. During leg exercise, IVC blood becomes markedly desaturated compared to the SVC blood and it is, therefore, difficult to determine the mixed venous oxygen saturation. Thus, cardiac output can not be measured using the Fick technique and thermodilution outputs are equally misleading.

Upright isotonic exercise with the bicycle or the treadmill can be performed using radial artery lines and brachial, internal jugular, or subclavian venous lines. Exercise gradients across left heart structures cannot be measured, but these studies may be a more physiologic test of conditions such as pulmonary artery hypertension. Normalized data of exercise response allow for comparison of patient data (Fig. 10-8).

DRUG TESTING

Despite advancements in non-invasive diagnostic modalities, there is still an important role for invasive monitoring to assess the effects of drugs. Drug testing may be undertaken as part of clinical trials to evaluate a particular drug or to test one or more drugs in a particular patient. The most common indications for drug testing are to optimize therapy in patients with congestive heart failure and to manipulate pulmonary vascular resistance (PVR) in patients with pulmonary artery hypertension. If the necessary data can be obtained with 1 or 2 catheters and does not require catheter manipulation, these studies can be performed in the intensive care unit. Studies requiring more catheter manipulation are more easily conducted in the cath lab. These catheterizations can be complex and time consuming, especially in patients with structural heart disease. It is important to decide what information is needed and how to most efficiently collect it prior to starting.

The common indication for drug testing a patient with congestive heart failure is to attempt to optimize medical management. These patients are commonly on ionotropes, diuretics, after-load reducing agents or perhaps other drugs such as beta-blockers. The clinical status can often be improved by changing the regimen while monitoring the hemodynamics. Specifically, at a minimum, one would like to monitor changes in right and left atrial (pulmonary capillary wedge) pressures, systemic and pulmonary artery pressures and resistances and cardiac output. In the absence of structural heart disease this can be done relatively easily with an arterial line and a thermodilution catheter in the pulmonary artery. The distal port on the thermodilution catheter is used for pulmonary artery and wedge pressures and the proximal port for right atrial pressures. Once in place no catheter manipulation is required and these patients are commonly studied in the ICU. The presence of structural heart disease would necessitate more catheter manipulation to, for example, account for shunts. On the other hand, if previously unrecognized structural heart disease is diagnosed at the catheterization, the need for drug testing may be eliminated.

The most common indication for drug testing, in our experience, is pulmonary artery hypertension. The minimum measurement that is required for assessing a drug is the pulmonary vascular resistance. Thus, one needs pulmonary artery and pulmonary capillary wedge pressures and cardiac output. In the absence of structural heart disease this information can be obtained with a thermodilution catheter in the pulmonary artery. The presence of structural heart disease, especially intra- and extracardiac shunts, necessitates a more involved study. Consider the patient with an unrestrictive ventricular septal defect, a bi-directional shunt and pulmonary hypertension. An agent which lowers PVR will not change the pulmonary artery systolic pressure in the presence of an unrestrictive VSD, but will increase the pulmonary blood flow. In the presence of shunts, the Fick method is used to calculate systemic and pulmonary blood flow. Thus, one needs to measure oxygen comsumption and oxygen saturations in the SVC (mixed venous), pulmonary artery, pulmonary vein, and systemic artery. In the presence of a right-to-left shunt, the pulmonary vein and systemic arterial saturations are not equal. The complexity of the case increases if there is no patent foramen ovale and one has to perform a transseptal puncture to gain access to the pulmonary veins. It is further complicated by the knowledge that many pulmonary vasodilators alter pulmonary venous saturation. Oxygen is an obvious example, but many drugs can increase pulmonary arterio-venous shunting (this is rarely uniform throughout the lung) and lower pulmonary venous saturations. In some cases it may be necessary to leave a catheter in the left atrium and add a second venous line. In other cases it may be reasonable to make some assumptions. The same patient with a large VSD is given nitric oxide following baseline studies, increasing the systemic saturation from 90 to 95%. It is unclear whether the residual systemic desaturation is due to residual right-to-left shunting or pulmonary venous desaturation in the absence of a right-to-left shunt. In either case, the pulmonary venous saturation is between 95 and 100%. If the PVR is 18 Woods units using 95% and 21 Woods units using 100%, the uncertainty is unlikely to be important.

Creativity in the types and number of catheters used, based on the patient's anatomy and information needed, can greatly simplify these studies. Patients with hypertrophic cardiomyopathy are frequent subjects of drug trials. One parameter commonly monitored is the left ventricular outflow tract gradient. This can be done using a single catheter and a pullback for each dose or drug. Alternatively, a sheath can be placed the femoral artery and a pigtail catheter, 1 F size smaller than the sheath, in the left ventricle. This allows for continuous monitoring of the gradient.

Finally, catheterizing patients with pulmonary hypertension can be associated with significant morbidity and even mortality secondary to sedation, blood loss or during pulmonary angiography. Patients with no intra-cardiac communications are particularly susceptible to a pulmonary hypertensive crisis. The use of a relatively safe agent such as inhaled nitric oxide in the setting of pulmonary artery hypertension and restrictive cardiomyopathy can lead to the development of pulmonary edema when the increased pulmonary blood flow returns to a non-compliant left ventricle. Even oxygen, which routinely elevates systemic vascular resistance, can cause problems in patients with borderline left ventricular function. While this chapter lists some of the less common diagnostic and interventional procedures performed in the cath lab, other procedures will emerge as some listed here will disappear. Even for standard procedures, we anticipate that innovation will continue to make them safer and more effective.

REFERENCES

1. Rashkind W.J. and Miller W.W. Creation of an atrial septal defect without thoracotomy: A palliative approach to complete transposition of the great vessels. J. Am Med Assoc. 196:991-992, 1966.
2. Rubio V., Limon-Larson R. Treatment of pulmonary valve stenosis and of tricuspid stenosis using a modified catheter. Second World Congress of Cardiology 1955;2:205-10.
3. Lang P, Freed M.D., Bierman F.Z. et al. The use of Prostaglandins E1 in infants with d-transposition of the great arteries and intact ventricular septum. Am J. Cardiol. 1979;44:76.
4. Allan L.D. Leanaje R., Wainwright R., et al. Balloon septostomy under two dimensional echocardiographic control. Br. Heart J 1982;47:41-43.
5. Park S.C., Neches W.H., Mullins C.E., et al. Blade atrial septostomy: Collaborative Study. Circulation 1982, 66:258-266.
6. Perry S.B., Lang P., Keane J.F., et al. Creation and maintenance of an adequate interatrial communication in patients with left atrioventricular valve atresia or stenosis. Am J. Cardiol 1986, 58:622-626.
7. Mitchell S.E., Kan J.S., Anderson J.H., et al. Atrial septostomy: stationary angioplasty balloon technique [Abstract]. Pediatr Res 1986, 20;173a.
8. Hausknecht M.J., Sims R.E., Nihill M.R., et al. Successful palliation of primary pulmonary hypertension by atrial septostomy. Am J Cardiol 1978, 42;453-457.
9. Kerstein D., Levy P.S., Hsu D.T., et al. Blade balloon atrial septostomy in patients with severe primary pulmonary hypertension. Circulation 1995, 91;2028-2035.
10. Rothman A., Beltran D., Kreitt J.M., et al. Graded balloon dilation atrial septostomy as a bridge to lung transplantation in pulmonary hypertension. Am Heart J 1993, 6:1763-1766.
11. Nishimoto K, Keane JF, Jonas R.A. Dilation of intra-atrial baffle fenestrations: Results in veno and in vitro. Cath and Cardiovasc Diag 1994, 31:73-78.
12. Brockenbrough E.C., and Braunwald E. A new technique for left ventricular angiocardiography and transseptal left heart catheterization. Am J. Cardiol 1960, 6:1062-1064.
13. Duff D.E. and Mullins C.E. Transseptal left heart catheterization in infants and children. Cath. Cardiovasc Diagn. 1978, 4:213-223.
14. Mullins C.E. Transseptal left heart catheterization: Experience with a new technique in 520 pediatric and adult patients. Pediat. Cardiol. 1983, 4:239-246.

15. Zahn E.M., Houde C., Benson L., et al. Percutaneous pericardial catheter drainage in childhood. Am J. Cardiol 1992, 70:678-680.

16. Ziskind A.A., Pearce A.C., Lemmon C.C., et al. Percutaneous balloon pericardiotomy for the treatment of cardiac tamponade and large pericardial effusions: Description of technique and report of the first 50 cases. J Am Coll Cardiol 1993, 21:1-5.

17. Lurie P.R., Fujita M. and Neustein H.B. Transvascular endomyocardial biopsy in infants and small children: Description of a new technique. Am J Cardiol 1978, 42;453-457.

18. Salka S., Siefel R. and Sagar K.B. Transvenous biopsy of intracardiac tumor under transesophageal echocardiographic guidance. A Heart J 1993, 125:1782-1784.

19. Miller L.W., Labovitz A.J., McBride L.A., et al. Echocardiography-guided endomyocardial biopsy. A 5 year experience. Circulation 1988, 78(suppl III):III-99-102.

20. Billingham M.E. The safety and utility of endomyocardial biopsy in infants, children and adolescents. Editorial comment. J Am Coll Cardiol 1990, 15;443-445.

21. Deckers J.W., Hare J.M., and Baughman K.L. Complications of transvenous right ventricular endomyocardial biopsy in adult patients with cardiomyopathy: A second-year survey of 546 consecutive diagnostic procedures in a tertiary referral center. J Am Coll Cardiol 1992, 19:43-47.

22. Yoshizato T., Edwards W.D., Alboliras E.T. et al. Safety and utility of endomyocardial biopsy in infants, children and adolescents: A review of 66 procedures in 53 patients. J Am Coll Cardiol 1990, 15;436-42.

23. Master A.M, Oppenheimer E.T. A simple exercise tolerance test for circulatory efficiency with standard tables for normal individuals. Am J Med Sci. 1929, 177;223.

11. CATHETERIZATION OF THE ADULT PATIENT WITH CONGENITAL HEART DISEASE

Michael J. Landzberg, M.D.

Adult patients with congenital heart (ACH) disease are a product of medical and surgical advances of the second half of the twentieth century. A review at our own institution revealed that the 17-year survival of those born with all types of congenital heart disease was 84%. Despite the achievements of pediatric caregivers, many of these patients, particularly those with complex lesions, face a world not yet fully prepared for their adult care. Throughout the stages of their adolescent and adult years, congenital heart disease "survivors" present with problems often different from those encountered in their pediatric lives. Novel medical, surgical and catheter-based diagnostics and therapeutics have led to an increased use of the catheterization laboratory in the management of these patients. While simple defects predominated in the catheterization laboratory three decades ago, a marked shift toward more complex lesions was evident 20 years later [1]. In the past decade however, with the advent of interventional procedures, simple lesions such as pulmonary stenosis, patent ductus arteriosus and atrial septal defect are once again being catheterized.

In this chapter we will:
1. Review the primary differences in presentation of the ACH patient for the catheterizing physician trained in the management of congenital heart disease patients.
2. Review the general principles of catheterization of ACH patients.
3. Outline the risks and needs for specific groups of ACH patients.
4. Briefly describe techniques, indications and results of catheterization-based management of particular lesions in the ACH patient.

1. THE ACH PATIENT

The ACH patients will, in general, manifest increasing and cumulative effects from complex palliative procedures such as modified Fontan operations, surgical scarring, insufficient myocardial preservation during prior surgery, uncorrected abnormalities in ventricular pre-load and after-load, alteration in red blood cell mass and tissue perfusion, and progressive tendency to decreased myocardial compliance with aging. These effects contribute to increasing systolic and diastolic ventricular dysfunction, and to the progressive incidence of arrhythmia seen in these patients, atrial enlargement, sluggish atrial flow and thrombosis, and development of atrial arrhythmia (see Chapter 14). In some patients, inadequately controlled pulmonary blood flow may lead to pulmonary vascular disease, in situ thrombosis, and after-load effects on pulmonary ventricular function.

Prior to, and during catheterization of ACH patients, one must consider coexisting morbidity that may be rarely seen in pediatric patients with congenital heart disease. Diabetes mellitus, obesity, systemic hypertension, hypercholesterolemia, peripheral- and cerebro-vascular disease, coronary atherosclerosis, chronic lung disease, chronic erythrocytosis, spinal disease, alcohol and drug use, and potential for pregnancy, all can influence patient well-being and safety during catheterization. A review of the potentials of these illnesses at the time of catheterization is beyond the scope of this text, though a few general principles are offered:

1. Catheterization of the ACH patient may reveal previously unrecognized anatomic or physiologic abnormalities, which will require intervention. Recognition of the catheterization laboratory as an "operating theater", with commensurate institutional support and generalized, yet appropriate, patient consent is requisite.

2. Variation in systemic blood pressure is generally less well tolerated in the adult patient, and volume resuscitation or pressor support should be contemplated for either SBP ≤ 90 mm Hg or a significant deviation from baseline. In particular, adequate hydration prior to study is very important in cyanotic polycythemic ACH patients. Support for acute hemodynamic compromise must be available, including appropriately sized mechanical ventricular and ventilatory support, and inhaled and intravenous pulmonary vasodilators.

3. Recent pre-catheterization assessment of lower extremity venous thrombosis in patients at increased risk (presumed paradoxical embolization, obesity, cigarette smoking, oral contraceptive use, peripheral vascular disease, raised systemic venous pressures or non-pulsatile systemic venous flow) may reduce potential for dislodgment and embolization, especially with use of large caliber sheaths and catheters. At the beginning of the catheterization an initial femoral – iliac – vena caval angiogram is recommended in all such patients.

4. When a transseptal study is performed, particular caution should be taken to avoid manipulation in the atrial appendage due to increasing risk of left atrial thrombus.

5. Long-standing erythrocytosis reduces glomerular filtration rate and increases viscosity, raising risk for contrast-induced acute tubular necrosis and vascular thrombosis.[2]

6. Prior to catheterization, a measurement of beta-HCG and a discussion of teratogenic risks of radiation is mandatory for ALL women.

2. GENERAL PRINCIPLES FOR CATHETERIZATION OF THE ACH PATIENT

Patient size, chamber dilation and vessel distortion present additional technical challenges that can be overcome with increased experience. Options for vascular access may be more varied (radial, brachial, axillary, internal jugular, subclavian), though direct femoral puncture remains the most widely utilized approach. Obesity may make vessel localization for access and hemostasis more difficult, and fluoroscopic confirmation of puncture over the femoral head allows appropriate vessel tamponade with compression after catheter removal. Manual dissection of the entry site prior to puncture allows outward "tracking" of bleeding in the event of unsuccessful compression. Appropriately prolonged and increased manual or mechanical tension is required to adequately ensure hemostasis in these patients.

The use of "J"- or floppy-tipped guidewires for systemic arterial access is often recommended due to the increased incidence of systemic arterial atherosclerosis and decreased arterial compliance in an aging population. Appropriate catheter positioning may be facilitated by use of torque-controllable, extendible, tip-deflecting, stiff, extra-stiff, 0.035" and 0.038" guidewires, as well as by increased use of shaped catheters designed for peripheral or coronary use. Stiff "coronary-guide" catheters may be utilized as an outer sleeve to increase catheter stability over a long or tortuous pathway.

3. SPECIAL CIRCUMSTANCES

Pregnancy
The increased pre-load, heart rate and cardiac output of pregnancy, coupled with decreased, though usually normal, systolic function, may exacerbate pre-existing hemodynamic compromise. Catheterization is safe to mother and fetus when limited to those circumstances (usually mitral or ventricular outflow obstruction) when catheter-based intervention is recommended by a combined cardiology and high-risk obstetrics team. Regardless of alimentation, the pregnant woman is considered to have a "full-stomach", and thus increased risk of reflux and aspiration. Radiation exposure should be minimized and the uterus should be appropriately shielded. In such circumstances, the unknown long-term teratogenic risks of low-dose radiation exposure to fetus in modern laboratories is outweighed by fetal benefit from improved hemodynamics. Availability of fetal monitoring and urgent access to the delivery room should be arranged by the obstetrical staff prior to catheterization.

Down Syndrome
The adult patient with Down syndrome frequently has increasing medical co-morbidity (thyroid disease, upper and lower airway disease, gastrointestinal reflux, aspiration, limited communication skills and dementia). Despite alimentation, the patient should be considered to be at increased risk of aspiration. Assessment of pulmonary vascular resistance should take into account alterations in ventilation and increased incidence of pulmonary vascular disease. Mechanical ventilation to ensure adequate ventilation or to enable assessment of pulmonary vascular resistance may be necessary.

Diabetes mellitus
Planning for, and monitoring of, the diabetic patient should be similar to that in pediatric patients. Increased use of Metformin in adult diabetic patients should be recognized and may result in profound uncontrollable acidemia with iodine contrast administration in patients with reduced glomerular filtration. Thus Metformin use should be discontinued > 48 hours prior to catheterization in patients with abnormal glomerular filtration, and should be held after catheterization until renal function has returned to baseline. Regardless of age, these patients have an increased potential for renovascular and diffuse atherosclerotic disease.

Systemic ventricular failure
Catheterization may assist in "tailoring" of ongoing medical or surgical therapies, or may assess candidacy for additional options such as organ transplantation. These patients should be on optimal therapy prior to catheterization to improve assessment of the potential for future treatments.

Pulmonary ventricular failure/pulmonary vascular disease
In the adult, the failing right (pulmonary) ventricle appears to tolerate acute compromise poorly, and rapid uncorrectable hemodynamic collapse may ensue. Avoidance of large shifts in preload and afterload are important. Recent therapeutic advances for patients with acquired or congenital pulmonary vascular disease have improved survival and improved quality of life. Assessment of pulmonary vascular reactivity as a marker for further surgical or medical therapy has taken an increasingly larger role in the ACH catheterization laboratory. The response to intravenous (prostacyclin) or inhaled (nitric oxide) pulmonary vasodilators is a necessary part of the hemodynamic assessment in such patients.

Right ventricular outflow enlargement
A transannular patch repair, persistent or recurrent right ventricular outflow obstruction, or elevated distal pulmonary artery pressure in patients with tetralogy of Fallot will increase the incidence of right ventricular or pulmonary arterial dilation. Criteria for timing of right ventricular outflow reconstruction in this setting remain unknown. Catheterization of such patients may help define hemodynamics in the setting of changing exercise capacity or worsening arrhythmia, or to define anatomy in the setting of chest pain or cyanosis with suspected pulmonary arterial dissection, or compression of contiguous structures. Catheter entry to the main or right pulmonary artery may be difficult with marked right ventricular and main pulmonary artery enlargement, even in the setting of an internal jugular or subclavian venous approach. A balloon end-hole catheter stiffened at its distal end with a sharp "S"-shaped bend to the stiff end of a 0.035" wire may be directed out the main pulmonary artery from a dilated right ventricle with increased ease. A Judkins left coronary catheter withdrawn from the left pulmonary artery and while in the main pulmonary artery, angled towards the right will facilitate guidewire passage into the right pulmonary artery.

Coronary ischemia

Coronary ischemia and infarction may occur in the ACH patient secondary to prior procedures or due to coronary atherosclerosis, although it is rare. The ability to dilate and/or stent such lesions can be lifesaving.

Cyanosis

While the ACH patient may have pulmonary parenchymal and ventilatory causes for cyanosis (e.g. cigarette use, obesity, scoliosis), congenital or acquired vascular causes for cyanosis should be sought with vigor due to the long-term multiple organ system ravages of chronic cyanosis and erythrocytosis. Right to left shunting may occur from systemic veins to pulmonary veins, atrial baffle leaks, patent foramen ovale, and right ventricular shunting due to obstructed pulmonary arteries should be explored and often corrected in the catheterization laboratory. Similarly, pulmonary venous desaturation in the setting of pulmonary venous hypertension due to intravascular obstruction or extravascular compression by an enlarging right atrium or pulmonary artery should be excluded [3].

4. CARE OF THE ACH PATIENTS WITH SPECIFIC LESIONS

Secundum-type atrial septal defects (ASD-2)

ASD is the second most common cause of congenital heart disease in the adult patient. Patients with unoperated or previously unrecognized ASDs are, therefore, not infrequent in the general internist's or cardiologist's practice. We rely primarily upon physiologic confirmation of excessive right ventricular volume loading by echocardiography, rather than primary catheterization-based documentation of significant shunting (pulmonary/systemic flow$\geq$1.5) as evidence of a hemodynamically "significant" shunt, although the superiority of this assessment in predicting clinical morbidity is unproven. We therefore do not perform "routine" catheterization of patients with ASD for determination of intracardiac shunting. Large shunts increase the risks from dyspnea, congestive failure, atrial arrhythmias, and, less commonly, pulmonary hypertension or paradoxical embolization. While surgical patch closure of ASD-2 remains one of the safest and most effective adult cardiac surgical procedures, significant perioperative morbidity may ensue. Increasing age (with medical co-morbidities) and the presence of pulmonary hypertension are independent risk factors for increased surgical mortality. Surgical success is generally uniform, yet may be accompanied by minor, but persistent, shunting detectable by Doppler echocardiography (reported to occur in 7-8% of surgically treated patients). The incidence of major or minor neuropsychiatric complications after cardiopulmonary bypass in this population has refocused attention on transcatheter closure techniques.

Closure devices, currently investigational, for adults with ASD-2 are reviewed extensively in Chapter 7. Clinical experience in ACH patients has been greatest with the Bard clamshell septal occluder and the Sideris standard buttoned device, and to date remains limited for the other devices [4-6]. The technique of deployment in the adult is similar to that utilized for the pediatric patient (Chapter 7).

Among our initial 35 adult patients (aged 18-76 years) undergoing transcatheter ASD-2 closure with a Bard clamshell septal occluder, 21 (60%) had either a significantly increased risk of operative morbidity or mortality, reflecting our bias toward offering this technique to higher risk patients. All 32 patients with appropriately sized defects (≤ 24 mm maximal stretched diameter) had stable device implantation in the atrial septum. Significant residual leaks occurred in 5 patients (device arm herniation across the atrial septum at time of deployment in 3, and implantation of an inappropriately small device in 2). Defects were subsequently closed by either implantation of a second device (3) or via surgery (2). No embolic events, arrhythmias, or bouts of bacterial endocarditis have occurred in 42-67 months of follow up. Minimal residual shunting detected by Doppler echocardiography was present in 32% of patients at 1 year of follow-up. In general, late morbidity has been extremely rare. There are, as yet, few reports of other devices used exclusively in adults.

Patent foramen ovale (PFO)-Presumed paradoxical embolism

Therapeutic closure of PFOs in patients with stroke and presumed paradoxical embolism (PPE) remains controversial since the cause and natural history of these embolic events are unclear.[7-9] A recent study in 140 consecutive patients suggests an infarct or transient ischemic recurrence rate of approximately 4% per year, even with antiplatelet or anticoagulant therapy[8]. The ability of clinical (multiple prior embolic events or silent events by brain scanning, occurrence with Valsalva straining) or echocardiographic ("large volume" right to left shunting, atrial septal aneurysm) features to identify patients at high risk for recurrence is unknown, though several lines of evidence suggested that patients with larger holes are at increased risk. Although a recent study recommends PFO closure (10), the data are not yet compelling.

Our experience with PFO ± atrial septal aneurysm closure in 38 patients with PPE revealed successful implantation in all patients, tiny residual Doppler echocardiography-detectable shunting in 21%, and no recurrent cerebral infarcts at a mean follow-up of 37 months[11]. Two patients (one with residual shunting, one with left atrial granulation tissue near a broken device arm) had transient neurologic ischemia. Both underwent surgical device removal and PFO closure without complication. The decision to close PFOs associated with cryptogenic stroke is complicated by the high frequency of PFOs in the normal population (at least 10%), and the common occurrence of idiopathic strokes in adult populations. It is likely that most PFO/stroke patients have two diseases (a PFO and a thrombotic propensity); In these patients, PFO closure will successfully treat the potential for embolization of venous thrombus to the systemic and cerebral circulations. However, in every large series of PFO/stroke patients, the PFO may be an "innocent bystander" unrelated to the stroke. In a relatively small number of such patients, recurrent strokes may occur despite successful PFO closure (Fig. 11-1).

Younger (< 40 years old) patients, and those with a relative contraindication to anticoagulation appear to be best candidates for transcatheter PFO closure in the setting of cryptogenic stroke. For others, oral anticoagulation appears reasonable.

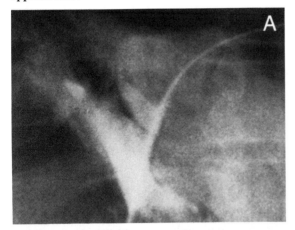

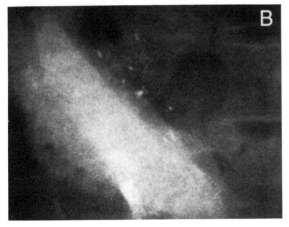

Figure 11-1: (A) Intracardiac passage of contrast across the foramen ovale (orthodeoxia-platypnea) after an injection into the right atrium. A guidewire is anchored in the left upper pulmonary vein. The patient, status post thoracotomy, was unable to work given resting aortic oxygen saturation: supine: 100%, standing: 82% (B) Right atrial angiogram demonstrates elimination of shunt flow after implantation of a clamshell occluder on the atrial septum. After PFO closure the patient returned to work with finger oxymetry: supine 100%, standing 100%.

Only a randomized prospective trial will successfully address these issues. At this time, "compassionate" device implantation should be reserved for patients with absolute contraindication to medical therapy or with recurrences of embolic phenomenon.

Patent foramen ovale (PFO)-Hypoxemia

Pressure loaded right atria may lead to right-to-left shunting in patients with a PFO. This may accompany chronic alteration of right-sided filling or capacitance (right ventricular infarction, pulmonary embolism, Ebstein anomaly), or transient alteration in right ventricular filling seen with changing from a supine to an upright position (orthodeoxia-platypnea syndrome).

We have closed PFOs in 32 adults with right ventricular infarctions, Ebstein anomaly, and the orthodeoxia-platypnea syndrome[12]. In all but two patients, both with Ebstein anomaly, catheter closure has relieved cyanosis and symptoms, and eliminated the need for open heart surgery. The long-term benefit of PFO closure in patients with Ebstein anomaly requires further study.

Patent Ductus Arteriosus-PDA

In adults, an audible PDA may increase the risk for developing bacterial endocarditis or left ventricular dysfunction. Surgical PDA closure in the adult is more complicated than in children because of ductal calcification, friability and aneurysmal dilation, as well as the increased risk of multiple organ system comorbidity. Transcatheter techniques utilizing the Ivalon plug, the Botallo occluder, the Rashkind and Bard double umbrella occluders, the buttoned device, and embolization coils (routine, screw-apart, bagged) have been attempted to offset this increased adult surgical risk [13-18].

Our initial experience with the Bard patent ductus occluders for attempted PDA closure in 21 adults revealed safe implantation in adults regardless of shape or calcification of the PDA, or the presence of pulmonary hypertension or congestive heart failure, although residual leaks were not rare. A 50% incidence of an echocardiographically-detectable residual shunt can be detected immediately after device implantation, decreasing to approximately 20-25% at 6 months after device implantation. Nearly 100% occlusion can be accomplished in all patients with implantation of additional devices or embolization coils, as necessary. More recently, coils have been more widely used, even in the adult PDA.

At present, until there is definitive resolution of the long-term endarteritis risk [19,20], we close all audible PDA's in adult patients via a transcatheter approach. Patients should not leave the catheterization laboratory with more than minimal residual ductal flow. Bacterial endarteritis precautions are maintained until no residual echocardiographic shunt is detectable. Repeat transcatheter PDA closure should be performed as needed.

Ventricular septal defects (VSD)

Transcatheter closure techniques have been applied to the treatment of congenital and acquired forms of VSDs in adult patients in an attempt to eliminate the need for, or reduce the risk and complexity of surgical repair[21]. In what is perhaps the most technically demanding of interventional catheter procedures performed in our laboratory, we have successfully offered closure to adults with acquired ventricular septal rupture (VSR) after myocardial infarction (MI) or with congenital or post-operative residual muscular VSDs anatomically distant from the aortic and atrioventricular valves. Although closure of congenital VSDs is reviewed in Chapter 7, the adult with a post-MI VSD represents a special challenge.

While recent advances in surgical strategies have dramatically improved the short and intermediate term survival of adults with VSD after MI, operative risk remains substantial and may be compounded by the location of the VSD, the presence of right or left ventricular dysfunction or multiple organ system failure and medical co-morbidities, or prior incomplete surgical attempt at repair. From February 1990 to the present, we have utilized either the Bard septal clamshell occluder or the CardioSEAL device to limit VSD after MI in patients without prior surgical repair who were felt to have prohibitive surgical risk (n=7) or patients who had significant residual shunting after attempted surgical VSD closure (n=11). Septal rupture was often associated with a wide (18-21 mm) necrotic "lake" within the septum, while defects in the patch margin ranged from 8-25 mm by maximal balloon stretching (Fig. 11-2).

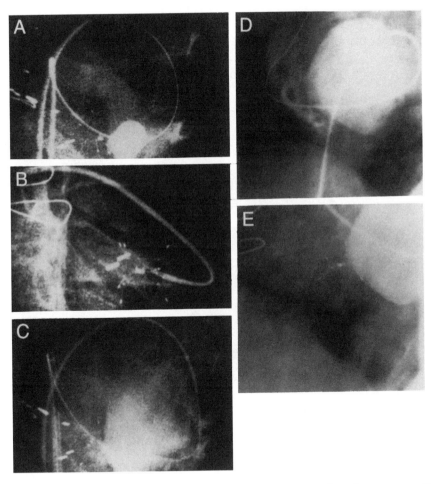

Figure 11-2: Balloon stretch sizing (A) of the central necrotic portion of a post-operative residual patch margin defect after primary surgical repair of ventricular septal rupture (VSR) after myocardial infarction (MI) in a patient requiring mechanical inotropic support. Transseptal deployment of a Clamshell Occluder (B) leads to modest acute decrease in angiographic shunt (C), but patient markedly improves to NYHA II symptoms.
Shunt flow (D) can be totally eliminated (E) in some patients with postoperative residual shunting after VSR after MI.

278

To date, at catheterization we have not encountered a defect that was not anatomically or procedurally amenable to device implantation. Of the 11 patients with post-operative residual patch-margin defects, survival in X patients (mean 54 months) has not been limited by procedural success; mortality (n = 2) was due to unrelated sepsis and chronic respiratory failure. Of the 7 patients without prior surgical repair, survival past hospitalization or to the present occurred in only 3 patients, all of whom presented months after initial VSR. All survivors are in NYHA class II or better.

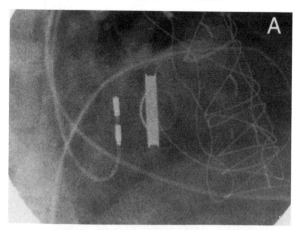

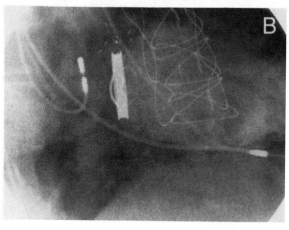

Figure 11-3: Paravalvar mitral regurgitation (A) resulting in left atrial hypertension and dyspnea, is eliminated after placement of an occlusion device (B), with resolution of symptomatology.

Postoperative residual defects, collaterals, and fenestrations

As with children, embolization coils and umbrella-type devices have been utilized in adults with high or prohibitive surgical risk, to successfully eliminate residual central aorta or systemic to pulmonary artery shunts or collaterals, systemic venous to pulmonary venous shunts or collaterals, interatrial baffle communications or iatrogenic Fontan fenestrations, left superior or inferior vena caval connections to the left atrium, coronary artery fistulae, systemic and pulmonary arteriovenous malformations, and paravalvar leaks (Fig. 11-3). The role of combined surgically-fenestrated repair of intracardiac defects associated with pulmonary vascular disease in concert with subsequent long-term pulmonary vasodilator therapy and ultimate transcatheter fenestration closure, remains to be defined.

Valvar aortic stenosis (VAS)

The acceptance of balloon aortic valvuloplasty (BAV) as palliation for children with congenital VAS is in contradistinction to treatment of elderly patients with calcific VAS. Two recent reports have underscored the utility of BAV in selected young and intermediate-aged adults.[22, 23]

At Boston Children's Hospital, 18 young adults (aged 17-40 years) with congenital VAS (15 with identified valvular dysmorphology-12 bicuspid valves, 3 unicuspid valves) underwent BAV with balloons chosen to be 90-100% the diameter of the aortic annulus.[22] Immediate procedural success, achieved in 16/18 patients, yielded a decrease in peak systolic ejection gradient from 85 to 38 mm Hg, without periprocedural death, MI, or recognized embolization. Only 1/11 had increase in degree of aortic insufficiency after BAV classified as ≥ mild-moderate. During a mean follow-up of 38 months, 5 patients required aortic valve surgery (two for initially ineffective dilation, two for increasing transvalvar gradient and one for bacterial endocarditis late after BAV). Patients with increased valvular calcification demonstrated a trend toward higher gradients both before and after BAV, and decreased incident-free survival compared to patients without calcified valves (Fig. 11-4).

A

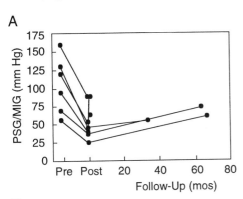

B

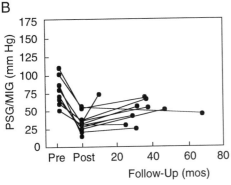

Figure 11-4: Peak systolic ejection gradient (PSG) before and after aortic valvuloplasty as assessed at catheterization, and maximal instantaneous gradient (MIG) as assessed by Doppler echocardiogram at most recent follow-up. (A), patients with calcified aortic valves, (B), patients with noncalcified aortic valves.

Sandhu and colleagues reported similar short- and intermediate-term transvalvar gradient reduction with BAV (from 73 mmHg before BAV to 35 mm Hg immediately after dilation) in 15 younger (aged 16-24 years) patients with congenital VAS (12 bicuspid).[23] Only 2/6 had increase in degree of aortic insufficiency after BAV classified as ≥ mild-moderate. During a mean follow-up of 18 months, 3 patients required aortic valve surgery (two for initially ineffective dilation, one for severe aortic regurgitation). Correlation of BAV success to degree of valvar calcification in this younger aged population was not examined.

These findings suggest that BAV for non-calcified congenital VAS in the young- and intermediate-aged adult can provide effective palliation and prolong the interval to surgical intervention without significantly increasing cardiac morbidity or serious complications. Risk and success of surgical repair for the uncommon patient sustaining avulsion of a valvular cusp during BAV does not appear compromised by attempted BAS, with timely echocardiographic evaluation and surgical therapy.[24]

Valvar pulmonary stenosis (VPS)

While the First and Second Natural History of Congenital Heart Defects Studies outlined the course and treatment of VPS primarily in infants and children, the natural history of VPS in the older patient is less well defined. Balloon pulmonary valvuloplasty (BPV) has become the treatment of choice for young patients with VPS (see Chapter 6).

Numerous recent single-center reports, each with 4-53 patients, have demonstrated similar immediate gradient reduction with BPV for VPS in young and middle aged adults, aged 13-55 years, utilizing standard single, Inoue, or double balloon techniques to achieve a balloon-annulus dimension ratio between 1.1 and 1.4.[25-29] The mean follow-up in these series has ranged from 0.5-6.9 years, and when compared to results in pediatric-aged individuals, has revealed a decreased incidence of peri-procedural morbidity and restenosis in the adult. Hemodynamically-compromising or therapy-requiring infundibular spasm is uncommon and has not been seen in either our experience or in the largest reported series. Although individual instances of surgically treated pericardial tamponade, severe infundibular obstruction, peri-procedural sepsis, and post-procedural diffuse pulmonary edema have recently been reported. We take particular care to avoid prolonged reductions in cardiac output in the elderly, or those with low output at baseline. Pulmonary regurgitation after BPV is usually mild and without sequelae in the intermediate-term. During follow-up, need for surgical intervention for non-dysplastic valves has not been reported.

Given the low attendant morbidity of this procedure, we currently perform BPV in any adult patient with gradients over 40 mmHg either in the individual with unoperated VPS or with recurrent VPS after initial surgical treatment.

Coarctation of the Aorta (CoA)

Clinically detectable CoA in the adult with a resting gradient ≥ 20 mm Hg between upper and lower extremities carries an increasing risk of progressive left ventricular dysfunction, persistent systemic arterial systolic hypertension, premature cerebrovascular and coronary atherosclerosis and potential (especially during pregnancy, surgery or catheterization) for dissection or rupture of the aorta, coronary and cerebral vessels. Modern surgical success in the adult is excellent, with a perioperative mortality ≤ 2% for native CoA repair. During long-term follow-up, recoarctation likely occurs in < 10-20% of patients (depending upon the type of surgical repair), with the current surgical risk of mortality for reoperation, paraplegia and late aneurysm formation at the site of repair estimated ≤ 2% in appropriate centers. In children, balloon dilation (BD) or stenting of recurrent, or persistent, CoA following surgical correction is now considered the therapy of choice, and BD is considered an effective alternative at some centers to surgical correction as therapy for native CoA.[31-35] Success (defined either as gradient reduction of ≥ 50% and an increase in angiographic luminal diameter ≥ 30%, or, more recently, as a residual gradient ≤ 20 mm Hg) is high (> 80%) and morbidity is low, using balloons chosen to be 3-4 times the diameter of the CoA and not more than 150% the transverse arch diameter. Our previous institutional bias favoring surgical repair versus BD of native CoA in the absence of severe left ventricular dysfunction in adults is changing due to the increasing use of balloon-assisted stenting of CoA.

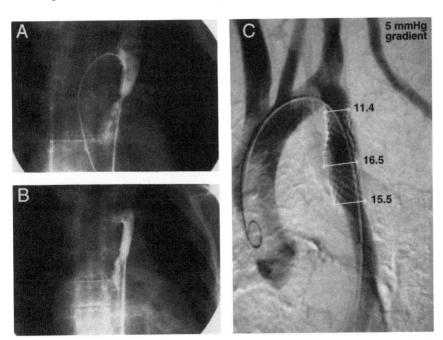

Figure 11-5: Unrecognized coarctation of the aorta (80 mm peak systolic gradient) leading to left heart failure and premature atherosclerosis of the coronary and cerebral arterial vasculature (A). Initial balloon dilation and stent implantation, with small distal dissection (B), later covered with a second stent (C). Residual gradient across the entire segment of < 5 mm Hg was noted.

Dilation of postoperative recurrent stenoses in 548 patients at multiple centers in the Valvuloplasty and Angioplasty of Congenital Anomalies (VACA) Registry was recently reported.[32, 36] While the number of adults was small there were no detectable early differences in risk of success or adversity based upon adult age. Less than a 20 mm Hg gradient was achieved in 75% of patients after BD. Procedure-related death occurred in 0.7%, with peri-procedural stroke in 0.6%. Transmural (0.7%) or intimal dissection (1.6%) has occurred, with rare individual cases requiring immediate surgical repair. Dilation of native CoA in a small number of adolescents and adults was also reported in the Registry data with early results similar to the postoperative group.[32] There have, in addition, been 2 reports from single centers concerning dilation of native CoA in 35 and 43 patients, respectively, in this age group highlighting similar results, with immediate success in 74-93%.[30, 34] The definition of post-procedural aneurysm formation has varied, this complication has been reported in 7-12% of patients, with rare reported instances of enlargement during follow-up. Due to relatively small numbers of patients in these series, the longer-term natural history and impact of aneurysm formation has yet to be sufficiently defined.

Balloon-assisted stenting of the aorta without precedent maximal balloon dilation permits use of smaller, non-"oversized" balloons with less risk of dissection and rupture of the aortic wall.[37] Use of balloon-assisted stenting of native or recurrent CoA in 12 of our adolescents and adults has allowed for graded dilations and near-full relief of gradient, even in tubular stenotic areas (Fig.11-5).

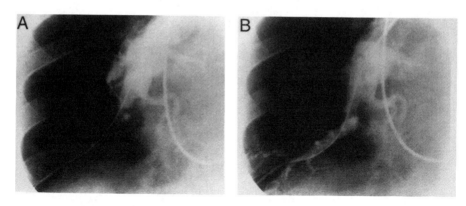

Figure 11-6: High pressure balloon dilation of post-operative proximal RPA stenosis (A) leads to elimination of gradient, increased angiographic vessel caliber (B) and resolution of flow imbalance by nuclear lung scintigraphy.

Thus we currently recommend balloon-assisted stent implantation, or BD alone as therapy of choice for all adults (a) with recurrent CoA defined as resting gradient ≥ 20 mm Hg, and (b) with native CoA and left ventricular dysfunction or significant risk from surgical repair due to medical co-morbidity. The role of stent implantation for relief of CoA gradient ≤ 20 mm Hg, or for women of childbearing age to decrease risk of subsequent rupture during pregnancy has yet to be determined.

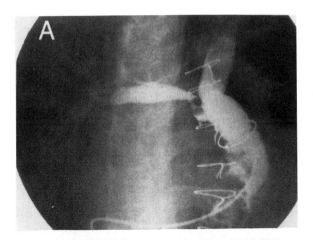

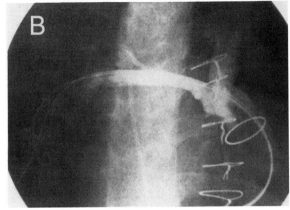

Figure 11-7: Right lower lobe segmental vessel before (A) and after (B) 7 mm balloon dilation. Mean central PA pressure fell from 60 mm Hg to 40 mm Hg. Reperfusion pulmonary edema was recognized 15 minutes after dilation.

Proximal and peripheral pulmonary artery stenosis

In adults, application of balloon dilation and balloon-assisted stent implantation as primary therapy for native and post-operative narrowings in the pulmonary ventricular outflow (tetralogy of Fallot, {Fig. 11-6},Rastelli-type repair, including homograft after the Ross procedure), as well as in the proximal and distal pulmonary vasculature, has success similar to that observed in children. We have dilated 35 adults with isolated peripheral pulmonary artery stenoses or acquired chronic distal thromboembolic pulmonary hypertension (Fig. 11-7).

Most of these patients were profoundly debilitated and referred for organ transplantation. The most frequently encountered complication was development of transient "reperfusion pulmonary edema" in segments of lung with restored pulmonary blood flow after dilation. No living patient in 3-4 years of follow-up has required transplantation, and all have improvement in exercise tolerance.

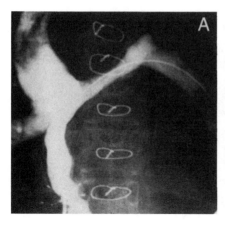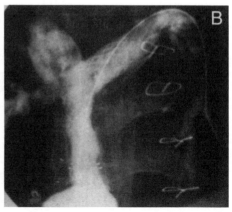

Figure 11-8: Postoperative Fontan baffle to LPA stenosis (A) in a patient presenting with protein losing enteropathy. Ascites and diarrhea eventually resolved after balloon assisted stent implantation and removal of obstruction to flow (B). The patient is chronically anticoagulated

Systemic and pulmonary venous obstruction

Successful application of balloon dilation and balloon-assisted stent implantation as therapy for native, acquired, or post-operative narrowings in the systemic and pulmonary veins, such as after atrial switch repair or the Fontan procedure, has yielded success similar to that achieved in children. (Fig. 11-8)

CONCLUSIONS

Recent ACC/AHA guidelines on interventional catheterization in patients with congenital heart disease underscore the "investigational" nature of most of the techniques outlined in this chapter concerning catheter-based care of the ACH patient. However, these same guidelines recognize an inability to approach these illnesses with large-scale or randomized trials, and, therefore, advocate continued investigation and use of catheter-based diagnostics and therapeutics to either support or supplant surgical procedures in these patients. Currently, we consider the applications of these techniques as 1)procedures of choice, 2)effective alternatives to surgical therapy, or 3) treatments with unproven effects (Table 1).

285

Table 1. Catheter-Based Interventions for the Adult with Congenital Heart Disease

Procedure of Choice	Effective Alternative to Surgery	Unproven Effect
Device closure PDA	**Device closure** ASD-2	**Device closure** PFO (Ebstein disease)
VSD-postoperative residual VSD-congenital muscular Fenestrated Fontan baffle PFO (cyanosis)	PFO (stroke) VSD-post-MI	
Balloon/stent dilation	**Balloon/stent dilation**	**Balloon/stent dilation**
Peripheral pulmonary stenoses Recurrent CoA	Native CoA Conduit/baffle obstruction	Subvalvar AS TOF Pulmonary venous stenosis
Balloon valvulotomy Valvar PS	**Balloon valvotomy** Valvar AS	
Coil embolization Thoracic collaterals/PDA Post-operative residual shunts Coronary artery fistula Pulmonary AVM	**Coil embolization**	

REFERENCES

1. Flanagan MF, Leatherman GF, Carls A, et al. Changing trends of congenital heart disease in adults: A catheterization laboratory perspective. Cath and Cardiovasc Diag. 1986, 12:215-218.
2. Flanagan MF, Hourihan M, Keane JF. Incidence of renal dysfunction in adults with cyanotic congenital heart disease. Am J Cardiol. 1991, 68:403-406.

286

3. Kreutzer J, Keane JF, Lock JE, et al. Conversion of modified Fontan procedure to lateral atrial tunnel. The J of Thorac and Cardiovasc Surg 1996,111: 1169-1176.
4. Prieto LR, Foreman CK, Cheeatham JP, et al. Intermediate-Term Outcome of Transcatheter Secundum Atrial Septal Defect Closure Using the Bard Clamshell Septal Umbrella. Brief Reports 1996, 1310-1312.
5. Sideris EB, Leung M, Yoon JH, et al. Occlusion of large atrial septal defects with a centering buttoned device: Early clinical experience. Am Heart J 1996, 131:356-359.
6. Sievert H, Babic UU, Ensslen R, et al. Transcatheter Closure of Large Atrial Septal Defects With the Babic System. Cathet Cardiovasc Diagn 1995, 36:232-240.
7. Mas JL, Zuber M. Recurrent cerebrovascular events in patients with patent foramen ovale, atrial septal aneurysm, or both, and cryptogenic stroke or transient ischemic attack. Am Heart J 1995, 130:1083-1088.
8. Bogousslavsky J, Garazi S, Jeanrenaud X, et al. Stroke recurrence in patients with patent foramen ovale. Neurology 1996, 46:1301-1305.
9. Mugge A, Daniel WG, Angermann C, et al. Atrial Septal Aneurysm in Adult Patients (A Multicenter Study Using Transthoracic and Transesophageal Echocardiography). Circulation 1995, 91:2785-2792.
10. Nendaz MR, Sarasin FP, Junod AF. Preventing stroke recurrence in patients with patent foramen ovale: Antithrombotic therapy, foramen closure, or therapeutic abstention? A decision analytic perspective. Am Heart J 1997, 135:532-541.
11. Bridges ND, Hellenbrand W, Latson L, et al: Transcatheter closure of patent foramen ovale after presumed paradoxical embolism. Circulation 1992, 86:1902-08.
12. Landzberg MJ, Sloss LJ, Faherty CE, et al. Orthodeoxia-Platypnea Due to Intracardiac Shunting--Relief with Transcatheter Double Umbrella Closure. Cathet Cardiovasc Diagn 1995, 36: 247-250.
13. Harrison DA, Benson LN, Lazzam C, et al. Percutaneous Catheter Closure of the Persistently Patent Ductus Arteriosus in the Adult. Am J Cardiol 1996,77:1094-1097.
14. Sievert H, Ensslen A, Fach H, et al. Transcatheter closure of patent ductus arteriosus with the Rashkind occluder (Acute results and angiographic follow-up in adults). Eur Heart J 1997, 18:1014-1018.
15. Hijazi ZM, Geggel RL. Transcatheter Closure of Patent Ductus Arteriosus Using Coils. Am J Cardiol 1997, 77:1279-80.
16. Podnar T, Masura J. Percutaneous Closure of Patent Ductus Arteriosus Using Special Screwing Detachable Coils. Cathet Cardiovasc Diagn 1997, 41:386-391.
17. Farhouch B, Moore JW. Balloon occlusion delivery technique for closure of patent ductus arteriosus. Am Heart J 1997, 133:601-4.

18. Ing FF, Recto MR, Saidi A, et al. A Method Providing Bidirectional Control of Coil delivery in Occlusions of Patent Ductus Arteriosus With Shallow Ampulla and Potts' Shunts. Am J Cardiol 1997, 79:1561-63.

19. Huggon IC, Qureshi SA. Is the prevention of infective endarteritis a valid reason for closure of the patent arterial duct? Eur Heart J 1997, 18:364-366.

20. Thilen U, Astrom-Olsson K. Does the risk of infective endarteritis justify routine patent ductus arteriosus closure? Eur Heart J 1997, 18:503-506.

21. Landzberg MJ, Lock JE. Transcatheter management of ventricular septal rupture after myocardial infarction. Sem Thorac Cardiovas Surg 1998, 10:128-132.

22. Rosenfeld HM, Landzberg MJ, Perry SB, et al. Balloon Aortic Valvuloplasty in the Young Adult with Congenital Aortic Stenosis. Am J Cardiol 1994, 73:1112-1116.

23. Sandhu SK, Lloyd TR, Crowley DC, et al. Effectiveness of Balloon Valvuloplasty in the Young Adult with Congenital Aortic Stenosis. Cathet Cardiovasc Diagn 1995, 36:122-127.

24. Minich LL, Tani LY, Hawkins JA, et al. Use of Echocardiography for Detecting Aortic Valve Leaflet Avulsion and Predicting Repair Potential After Balloon Valvuloplasty. Am J Cardiol 1995, 75:533-535.

25. Kasab SA, Ribeiro PA, Zailbag MA, et al. Percutaneous Double Balloon Pulmonary Valvotomy in Adults: One-to Two-Year Follow-Up. Am J Cardiol 1988, 62:822-24.

26. Herrmann HC, Hill JA, Krol J, et al. Effectiveness of Percutaneous Balloon Valvuloplasty in Adults with Pulmonic Valve Stenosis. Am J Cardiol 1991, 68:1111-1113

27. Kaul UA, Singh B, Tyagi S, et al. Long-term results after balloon pulmonary valvuloplasty in adults. Am Heart J 1993, 126:1152-55.

28. Teupe CHJ, Burger W, Schrader R, et al. Late (Five to Nine Years) Follow-Up After Balloon Dilation of Valvular Pulmonary Stenosis in Adults.

29. Chen CR, Cheng TO, Huang T, et al. Percutaneous Balloon Valvuloplasty for Pulmonic Stenosis in Adolescents and Adults. N Engl J Med 1996, 335:21-25

30. Tyagi S, Arora R, Kaul UP, et al. Balloon Angioplasty of native coarctation of the aorta in adolescents and young adults. Am Heart J 1992, 123:674-680.

31. Fawzy ME, Dunn B, Galal O, et al. Balloon coarctation and angioplasty in adolescents and adults: Early and intermediate results. Am Heart J 1992, 124:167-171.

32. McCrindle BW, Jones TK, Morrow WR, et al. Acute Results of Balloon Angioplasty of Native Coarctation Versus Recurrent Aortic Obstruction Are Equivalent. JACC 1996,28:1810-1817.

33. de Giovanni JV, Lip GYH, Osman K, et al. Percutaneous Balloon Dilatation of Aortic Coarctation in Adults. AJC 1996,77:435-439.

34. Fawzy ME, Sivanandam V, Galal O, et al. One-to-Ten Year Follow-Up Results of Balloon Angioplasty of Native Coarctation of the Aorta in Adolescents and Adults. JACC 1997,30:1534-41.

35. Shim D, Lloyd TR, Moorehead CP, Bove EL, Mosca RS, Beekman RH. Comparison of Hospital Charges for Balloon Angioplasty and Surgical Repair in Children With Native Coarctation of the Aorta. JACC 1997,79:1143-1146.
36. Rao PS, Galal O, Wilson AD. Feasibility and effectiveness of repeated balloon dilatation of restenosed congenital obstructions after previous balloon valvuloplasty/angioplasty. Am Heart J 1996,132:403-407.
37. Thanopoulos BV, Triposkiadis F, Margetakis A, Mullins CE. Long segment coarctation of the thoracic aorta: Treatment with multiple balloon-expandable stent implantation. Am Heart J 1997,133:470-3.
38. Saidi A, Bezold L, Altman C, Aynes N, Bricker JT. Outcome of pregnancy following intervention for coarctation of the aorta. Am J Cardiol 1998: 82:786-788.

12. ANESTHESIA IN THE CATHETERIZATION LABORATORY

Peter C. Laussen MB.BS
Dolly D. Hansen M.D.

INTRODUCTION

Adequate sedation and anesthesia during cardiac catheterization are essential to facilitate acquisition of meaningful hemodynamic data and to assist during interventional procedures. For the most part, hemodynamic or diagnostic catheterization procedures can be performed under sedation in all age groups. While in many interventional procedures such sedation may be appropriate, in ill patients or those procedures that are lengthy or potentially associated with significant hemodynamic compromise, or are prolonged, general anesthesia is preferable.

Whatever technique is used, it is essential that hemodynamic data be attained in conditions as close to normal as possible. When using sedation, careful monitoring is essential to ensure that respiratory depression is avoided. During anesthesia, the effects of inspired oxygen concentration, mechanical ventilation and hemodynamic side effects of various anesthesia agents must be considered. Post procedure monitoring either in a recovery room or intensive care unit is mandatory.

NORMAL CARDIO-RESPIRATORY PHYSIOLOGY IN NEONATES AND INFANTS

Neonates have a limited respiratory reserve and are prone to ventilatory failure and hypoxemia. The mechanical disadvantage of increased chest wall compliance results in a reduction in functional residual capacity (FRC) and an increase in closing capacity, such that airway closure may occur during normal tidal ventilation. The reliance on the diaphragm as the main muscle of respiration means that distention of the stomach or positioning on the catheterization table could limit diaphragm excursion and significantly reduce lung volumes, leading to impaired ventilation. The metabolic rate of neonates and infants is increased, and oxygen consumption approaches 2-to-3 times the adult level. This increase in consumption in the face of diminished oxygen reserve from a reduction in FRC, means that airway obstruction or respiratory depression will result in rapid arterial oxygen desaturation.

The immature myocardium of a neonate has a diminished contractile mass, a lower velocity of shortening, a diminished length-tension relationship, and a reduced ability to respond to afterload stress.[1] The stroke volume is relatively fixed and an increase in cardiac output is therefore primarily heart rate dependent. Further, the cytoplasmic reticulum and T-tubular system are underdeveloped, and the neonatal heart is dependent on trans-sarcolemmal flux of extracellular calcium to initiate and sustain contraction.

The large surface area to body mass ratio of infants and neonates predisposes them to hypothermia, which may increase metabolic rate and delay recovery from sedation and anesthesia. Hypothermia is a particular concern in the catheterization laboratory because of radiant and convective heat loss; prolonged exposure of the patient after sedation or general anesthesia and during preparation for catheterization may result in significant heat loss. In addition, the use of cold flush solutions and damp towels in contact with the patient will also contribute to hypothermia.

CATHETERIZATION LABORATORY ENVIRONMENT

Cardiac catheterization laboratories are often remote from the operating room, and rarely configured to accommodate anesthetic personnel. Relative to patient size, the lateral and anterior-posterior cameras used for imaging are in close proximity to the patient's head and neck, limiting access to the airway. An anesthetic machine and monitor around the patient will further limit access and confine the space in which the anesthesiologist may work. In addition, the environment is darkened to facilitate viewing of images. Monitoring with capnography and pulse oximetry is mandatory.[2]

Care must also be taken when positioning a patient on the catheterization table to reduce pressure and nerve traction injury. In particular, brachial plexus injury may occur when patients' arms are positioned above their heads for a prolonged time to make room for the lateral camera. To facilitate femoral vein and arterial access, the pelvis is commonly elevated from the catheterization table. This may displace abdominal contents cephalad, restricting diaphragm excursion, and increasing the risk for respiratory depression in a sedated patient. For these reasons, and also because of the effects on cardiac structure displacement for imaging purposes, it is important to remove most elevating towels when lines have been placed.

The majority of diagnostic, non-interventional hemodynamic catheterization studies can be performed with the patient sedated, breathing room air or supplemental oxygen. This permits measurement of meaningful hemodynamic data and accurate calculations of cardiac output, shunt fraction, and vascular resistances. To limit the amount of sedation, sufficient local anesthetic at vascular access sites is crucial.

Many interventional procedures that cause limited hemodynamic stress can be performed using sedation alone, including patent ductus arteriosus closure, coil embolization of collaterals, and balloon dilation of pulmonary valve stenosis. However, each patient needs to be carefully evaluated; high risk patients must be identified prior to catheterization.

Appropriate sedation protocols will enable the majority of hemodynamic and some interventional catheterization procedures to be managed by nurses trained in pediatric sedation and the cardiac catheterization environment. Anesthesia staff must nonetheless be readily available to manage respiratory depression and airway obstruction, or provide additional control if the limits of the sedation protocol have been reached and the patient remains unsettled. The drugs and doses commonly used for sedation usually have minimal hemodynamic effect in a well-compensated patient and the main consideration is airway maintenance and avoidance of respiratory depression. Guidelines for pediatric sedation have been formulated by the American Academy of Pediatrics.[3]

As for any invasive procedure, patients should be fasted according to institutional guidelines. Children often arrive at the catheterization laboratory accompanied by parents, and separation may be a difficult time; sedation in the preoperative holding area is often necessary. Numerous techniques can facilitate this process, including both oral medications (midazolam 0.5-to-0.75 mg/kg or chloral hydrate 50-to-80 mg/kg), and intramuscular agents such as demerol compound (meperidine 25mg, promethazine 6.25mg, and chlorpromazine 6.25mg/ml) at a maximum dose of 0.1 ml/kg or total volume 2.0ml. If a patient has an intravenous line in situ, a small bolus of midazolam 0.05 mg/kg or morphine 0.05 mg/kg will facilitate separation from parents.

Routine patient monitoring should include ECG, non-invasive blood pressure, arterial oxygen saturation, and temperature. Respiratory rate and end-tidal CO_2 can be measured by capnography using nasal prongs in spontaneously breathing patients.[4]

Protocols for maintenance of sedation during the procedure varies between institutions. One method is to use intermittent boluses of morphine and midazolam up to a total dose of 0.3 mg/kg each. Diphenhydramine hydrochloride in a dose of 0.5-to-1 mg/kg may provide additional sedation. Droperidol 0.05-to-0.1 mg/kg may also be given intravenously, although its alpha blocking properties may cause hypotension.

For some patients, continuous intravenous sedation is necessary. In our hospital, this is administered only by an anesthesiologist who is readily available to manage the airway. A combination of ketamine and midazolam infused at 2-to-5 mg/kg/hr and 0.1 mg/kg/hr respectively is often successful in maintaining sedation without respiratory depression or airway compromise. A titrated continuous infusion of propofol 50-to-100 mcg/kg/min may also be used; however, airway protection is usually necessary and it can cause hypotension in patients with congenital heart disease and cardiac failure.

INDICATIONS FOR GENERAL ANESTHESIA

Patient and procedural factors are considerations when planning general anesthesia. Patients who have a limited cardio-respiratory reserve may not tolerate prolonged sedated procedures, particularly if respiratory depression or airway obstruction occurs concurrently. Respiratory distress may occur in supine patients with significant congestive cardiac failure, pulmonary hypertension or limited diaphragm excursion due to an enlarged liver or ascites.

General anesthesia may also be indicated because of the risks and possible complications associated with certain procedures. At critical phases during some interventions such as device and stent placement, patients must remain absolutely still: sudden patient movement may dislodge the device or stent positioning. When hemodynamic compromise is likely to occur during an intervention, such as placement of VSD occlusion devices, dilation of multiple peripheral pulmonary artery stenoses or balloon dilation of a stenotic mitral valve, general anesthesia is usually recommended.

SEDATION FOR CATHETERIZATION PROCEDURES (Table 12-1)
Table 1 Sedation Protocol for Procedures Performed in the Cardiac

Catheterization Laboratory at Children's Hospital, Boston

Premedication

Midazolam	PO	0.5-0.75 mg/kg
Chloral Hydrate	PO	50-80 mg/kg
Demerol Compound	IM	0.05-0.1 mg/kg (max 2cc)

Conscious Sedation

I. Children   10 kg
A. Midazolam   0.025-0.05mg/kg IV, q 5-10 min up to 0.1 mg/kg, then
B. Morphine   0.025-0.05 mg/kg IV.
C. Give alternately q 5-10 min until desired response
D. Total dose of each medication not to exceed 0.4 mg/kg over 4-5 hours

II. Children > 10 kg up to 25 kg
A. Demerol compound as a premedication:
1. Midazolam   0.025-0.05 mg/kg IV, q 5-10 min IV up to 0.3 mg/kg total
2. Morphine   0.025-0.05 mg/kg IV, not to exceed 0.3 mg/kg total

A. No premedication
1. Midazolam   0.025-0.05 mg/kg IV, q 5-10 min up to 0.2 mg/kg, then
2. Morphine   0.025-0.05 mg/kg IV, q 5-10 min alternating
3. Total dose of each medication not to exceed 0.4 mg/kg
4. Benadryl 1 mg/kg IV drip over 20 min

B. Midazolam PO as a premedication
1. Morphine   0.025-0.05 mg/kg IV, q 5-10 min up to 0.2 mg/kg, then
2. Midazolam 0.025-0.05 mg/kg IV, q 5-10 min up to 0.2 mg/kg
3. Total dose of each medication not to exceed 0.4 mg/kg
4. Benadryl 1 mg/kg IV drip over 20 min

III. Children > 25 kg (including adults)
No premedication or Midazolam PO as a premedication
1. Midazolam 0.025-0.05 mg/kg IV, q 5-10 min up to 0.2 mg/kg, then
2. Morphine 0.025-0.05 mg/kg IV, q 5-10 min up to 0.2 mg/kg
3. Total dose of each medication not to exceed 0.4 mg/kg
4. If desired goals are not reached, Droperidol 0.025 mg/kg IV drip over 15-30 min can be repeated up to 2 times.

Patients may breathe spontaneously or have assisted ventilation during general anesthesia. Spontaneous ventilation techniques can be achieved with intravenous anesthesia agents such as ketamine and propofol, or with inhalation anesthetic agents and airway protection using a laryngeal mask. For the most part, however, general anesthesia will require assisted ventilation following paralysis with a neuromuscular blocking drug and endotracheal intubation.

Chloral Hydrate

Chloral hydrate is commonly used for sedating children. It can be administered orally or rectally in doses ranging from 50-to-100 mg/kg (maximum dose 1gm). The onset of action is within 15-to-30 minutes; the duration of action is between 2-to-4 hours. Between 10-to-20% of children will have a dysphoric reaction to chloral hydrate, frequently manifested as excitability and uncooperativeness. Alternatively, some children may become excessively sedated with respiratory depression and potential inability to protect their airway. The American Academy of Pediatrics has published guidelines for the use of chloral hydrate.[5] While they noted that chloral hydrate is often administered in repetitive doses to maintain prolonged sedation in infants and children, they raised significant concerns about this practice. Chloral hydrate is metabolized to trichloroethanol and trichlorocetic acid, both of which are pharmacologically active with long half lives of over 24 hours and will lead to accumulation during repetitive dosing.

Midazolam

Midazolam is a short acting, water soluble benzodiazepine that can be administered intravenously, intramuscularly, orally, and rectally. It is a commonly prescribed premedicant prior to anesthesia and surgical procedures and is an effective sedative. However, if cardiac output and splanchnic perfusion is reduced, hepatic metabolism of midazolam will be reduced and the drug will accumulate. Oral midazolam is useful for anesthesia premedication at a dose of 0.5-to-0.7 mg/kg. The onset time is between 15-30 minutes with a duration of action of 2-to-4 hours. Intravenous midazolam is usually well tolerated; however, significant hypotension may occur in patients with poorly compensated cardiac failure who are dependent on endogenous catecholamines to maintain vascular resistance and blood pressure.

Other benzodiazepines such as diazepam and lorazepam may be administered intravenously but neither is recommended. Diazepam is painful when administered intravenously and Lorazepam has an elimination half life of about 18 hours and is rarely necessary during catheterization procedures.

SPECIFIC ANESTHETIC AGENTS
Table 12-3
Dosages of Drugs Commonly Used for Anesthesia in the Catheterization Laboratory

Drug		Dose
Analgesics		
Morphine	IV bolus	0.1-0.2 mg/kg
	IV infusion	25-50 µg/kg/h
Fentanyl	IV bolus for analgesia	0.5-1 µg/kg (max 4-5 µg/kg)
	IV bolus for intubation	10-15 µg/kg
	IV infusion	2-5 µg/kg
Remifentanil	IV Infusion	0.25-1 µg/kg/min
Ketamine	IV bolus	1-2 mg/kg
	IM bolus	5-10 mg/kg
	IV infusion	2mg/kg/h
Anesthetic Agents		
Thiopental	IV bolus	3-5 mg/kg
Pentobarbital	IV bolus	1-2 mg/kg
Propofol	IV bolus	1.5-3 mg/kg
	IV infusion	50-150 µg/kg/min
Etomidate	IV Bolus	0.2-0.3 mg/kg
Muscle Relaxants		
Succinylcholine	IV bolus (neonates and infants)	2 mg/kg
	IV bolus (children to adults)	1 mg/kg
	IM bolus	3-4 mg/kg
Rocuronium	IV bolus	0.6-1.2 mg/kg
Vecuronium	IV bolus	0.1 mg/kg
	IV infusion	0.05-0.2 mg/kg/h

Atracurium	IV bolus	0.5 mg/kg
Cisatracurium	IV bolus IV infusion	0.2 mg/kg 0.2 mg/kg/h
Pancuronium	IV bolus (intubating dose) IV bolus (maintenance dose)	0.2 mg/kg 0.1 mg/kg

Opioid Analgesics

Opioids provide excellent analgesia, and in very high doses may provide anesthesia. Commonly used opioids include morphine, fentanyl, sufentanil, and alfentanil which are all pure agonists. Morphine has additional sedative properties. The synthetic opioids fentanyl, alfentanil and sufentanil provide intense analgesia without much sedation, and, therefore, need to be used in conjunction with agents such as benzodiazepines. They have a shorter duration of action than morphine and generate less histamine release, causing less vasodilation and hypotension. While synthetic opioids may provide hemodynamic stability, patients with poorly compensated cardiac failure and high endogenous circulating catecholamine levels, may become hypotensive after a bolus dose. Fentanyl is approximately 100 times more potent than morphine with a high degree of lipid solubility allowing rapid penetration of the blood brain barrier. It therefore has a rapid onset and its termination of action is primarily determined by re-distribution rather than metabolism. Its opioid effects last for 30-to-45 minutes, although respiratory depression may last considerably longer. Fentanyl blocks the stress response in a dose related fashion, while maintaining both systemic and pulmonary hemodynamic stability.[6,7] It is therefore a useful agent to use during catheterization procedure.[8] Chest wall rigidity may occur with a rapid bolus, although this is an idiosyncratic and dose related reaction. Remifentanil is a new synthetic ultra-short acting opioid, rapidly metabolized by non-specific tissue esterases.[9] It is unique among the currently available opioids because of its extremely short context-sensitive half time (3-5 minutes), which is largely independent of the duration of infusion. Remifentanil may cause significant respiratory depression and is usually administered to patients who are mechanically ventilated. It may be useful for patients with limited cardio-respiratory reserve because intense analgesia is provided without significant hemodynamic complications. Patients usually emerge quickly once the infusion has been stopped, and opioid side effects are reduced because of the short duration of action. Nevertheless, this is an expensive drug and is not recommended for routine use.

Ketamine

Ketamine is a phencyclidine derivative that effectively dissociates the thalamic and limbic systems and provides intense analgesia. It has a rapid onset, short duration of action between 10-to-15 minutes and an elimination half life between 2 and 3 hours. Effective intravenously or intramuscularly; it provides adequate anesthesia for most catheterization procedures, and produces a type of catalepsy whereby the eyes remain open, usually with nystagmus and intact corneal reflexes. Occasionally, non-purposeful myoclonic movements may occur. It will dilate cerebral blood vessels and should be avoided in patients with intracranial hypertension. It usually provides hemodynamic stability because both heart rate and blood pressure usually increase through sympathomimetic actions resulting from central stimulation and diminished post ganglionic catecholamine uptake. However, it does have direct myocardial depressant effects and should be used with caution in patients with limited myocardial reserve.
There are conflicting reports about the effect of ketamine on pulmonary vascular resistance.[10-14] While patients predisposed to pulmonary hypertension may demonstrate an increase in pulmonary artery pressure following ketamine administration, the response is usually minimal. On balance, therefore, ketamine can be used in patients with pulmonary hypertension, provided events such as hypoventilation and airway obstruction are avoided.
Although dose related respiratory depression may occur, patients continue to breath spontaneously after a 1-2 mg/kg bolus. Airway secretions are increased, and even though airway reflexes seem intact aspiration may occur. It is essential, therefore that patients are fasted prior to administration of ketamine and that complete airway management equipment be available. The increase in airway secretions can result in laryngospasm during airway manipulation and an agent such as atropine or glycopyrolate should be administered concurrently. The major side effect during emergence is delirium, hallucinations and nightmares. These may be ameliorated with the concurrent use of benzodiazepines.

Barbiturates

The short acting barbiturates thiopental and methohexital can be used for cardiac catheterization procedures by personnel trained in anesthesia. They can significantly depress myocardial function and venous tone. They have a rapid onset with a short duration of action, due mainly to re-distribution. The longer acting barbiturate pentobarbital can be used to sedate children for relatively short procedures, although supplemental sedation is often necessary and hypotension may occur in patients with poorly compensated cardiac failure.

Propofol

Propofol is a phenol derivative supplied in a soy emulsion and egg phospholipid to make an injectable emulsion. It is used primarily for induction or as part of a total intravenous anesthetic technique.[15,16] A major disadvantage is pain on injection, although this can be overcome by the addition of lidocaine. Because propofol has a short duration of action and rapid clearance, it has been used by infusion or repeat bolus doses with patients awakening rapidly when it is discontinued. Hypotension secondary to a decrease in systemic vascular resistance and direct myocardial depression may limit its use during cardiac catheterization.

Etomidate

Etomidate is an anesthetic induction agent with minimal cardiovascular and respiratory depression, and rapid recovery.[17] An intravenous dose of 0.3 mg/kg will induce rapid loss of consciousness with a duration of 3-to-5 minutes. It causes pain on injection and may be associated with spontaneous movements, hiccuping and myoclonus. Upper airway reflexes are increased with the potential for laryngospasm. Its use in the catheterization laboratory should be restricted to the induction of anesthesia in patients with limited cardiac reserve.

Muscle Relaxants

Muscle relaxants are either depolarizing or non-depolarizing drugs. Suxamethonium is the only available depolarizing agent available and is particularly indicated when a rapid sequence induction is necessary for airway protection during intubation. It has a rapid onset within 60 seconds but short duration of action, and is not reversible. Bradycardia is possible because of a direct effect on the SA node; this response is exaggerated in neonates and infants especially with repeat doses.

Non-depolarizing neuromuscular blocking agents vary in their onset of action, duration of action, and cardiovascular side effects. They compete with acetylcholine for binding at receptors on the motor end plate.

Pancuronium is slow in onset, but has a long duration of action and is suitable for most catheterization procedures. It causes mild tachycardia and hypertension due to delayed re-uptake of norepinephrine at receptor sites. It does not release histamine or cause ganglionic blockade and is, therefore, safe to use in patients with limited hemodynamic reserve.

Vecuronium has an intermediate duration of action of approximately 30 minutes. It is also safe in patients with limited hemodynamic reserve with minimal changes in blood pressure or heart rate. When combined with fentanyl, significant bradycardia may occur and atropine is often necessary. Newer non-depolarizing muscle relaxants that are safe during catheterization of patients with limited reserve include cisatracurium and rocuronium. Cisatracurium has an intermediate duration of action of around 30 minutes. It undergoes spontaneous pH dependent hydrolysis without requiring hepatic metabolism. Rocuronium is a fast onset non-depolarizing muscle agent with an intermediate duration of action of around 25 minutes. Neither causes histamine release.

The effect of non-depolarizing muscle relaxants can be reversed with anti-acetylcholinesterase drugs such as neostigmine and edrophonium. Their effect is not specific to the nicotinic receptors on the motor end plate, but will also act on muscarinic receptors at other sites such as the SA node, thereby causing bradycardia or even asystole. Atropine or glycopyrolate must always be administered concurrently.

Maintenance Of Anesthesia

Inhalational agents such as isoflurane, sevoflurane and halothane are commonly used to maintain anesthesia. Sevoflurane is particularly useful if an inhalational induction of anesthesia is planned as it has a rapid onset related to its solubility coefficient and a relatively safe hemodynamic profile, but can cause hypotension secondary to direct myocardial depression if an excessive concentration is used. Bradycardia and atrio-ventricular conduction blockade have been reported.

Isoflurane maintains anesthesia at an inhaled concentration of 0.5-to-1.0%. It can cause hypotension secondarily to vasodilation and at high concentrations can cause direct myocardial depression. Halothane is less commonly used because of hepatic toxicity and malignant hyperthermia. Nevertheless, it is a very useful induction agent and can be used for maintenance of anesthesia, but can cause significant hypotension secondary to direct myocardial depression. In addition, ventricular arrhythmias are more common using halothane, particularly under conditions of hypercapnea and increased endogenous catecholamine secretion.

Total intravenous anesthesia can also be used with agents such as ketamine, propofol, or the ultra short acting opioid remifentanil and all are alternatives depending on the hemodynamic reserve of the patient and the planned post procedure management.

ANESTHESIA CONSIDERATIONS FOR SPECIFIC PROCEDURE

Balloon Valvotomy

Percutaneous balloon valvotomy is palliative in mitral and aortic stenosis, and usually curative in isolated pulmonary valve stenosis.

Hemodynamic catheterization is always performed prior to valvotomy, and the majority of these procedures are done with the patient sedated, breathing spontaneously. After data have been obtained, tracheal intubation and general anesthesia may be required because of the potential hemodynamic disturbance associated with the intervention.

Pulmonary Valve Dilation

Pulmonary valve dilation is well tolerated, and is usually performed using sedation techniques.
Neonates with critical pulmonary stenosis are cyanosed at birth with a ductus dependent pulmonary circulation, and require infusion of prostaglandin E_1 and mechanical ventilation. The antegrade flow across the valve is usually low prior to dilation and therefore balloon dilation is associated with minimal hemodynamic disturbance.

Aortic Valve Dilation

Balloon valvotomy provides gradient relief but may cause a loss of cardiac output, coronary ischemia, aortic regurgitation. Nonetheless, most patients tolerate the procedure without incident and can be successfully managed using sedation techniques. The balloon remains inflated for 10-20 seconds, and although the cardiac output falls immediately, systolic blood pressure rapidly recovers provided preload is maintained.
Neonates with critical aortic stenosis may present with severe acidosis and circulatory collapse. The systemic circulation is ductus arteriosus dependent and patients require prostaglandin E_1 infusion to maintain ductal patency, along with inotrope support and mechanical ventilation. Once the patient has been resuscitated, balloon dilation is performed. Preload must be maintained, excessive tachycardia and any decrease in afterload avoided. They require close monitoring in the catheterization laboratory, often with general anesthesia and mechanical ventilation.

Mitral Valve Dilation

The hemodynamic reserve of some patients with mitral stenosis may be marginal because of pulmonary hypertension and congestive heart failure. Balloon dilation can be associated with significant hemodynamic disturbances and general endotracheal anesthesia is necessary in most cases. Balloon dilation results in an immediate fall in cardiac output and increase in pulmonary venous pressure that may precipitate pulmonary edema. In addition, dysrhythmias may compromise cardiac output. A significant complication related to dilation is mitral regurgitation resulting in pulmonary edema because of the poorly compliant left atrium and low cardiac output. Patients are best monitored in the ICU following dilation and weaned from mechanical ventilation when hemodynamically stable.

Pulmonary Artery Balloon Dilation and Stent Placement

Factors that determine whether dilation should be performed under sedation or general anesthesia include the number of required balloon dilations, anticipated complications, the duration of the procedure, and the function of the right ventricle.

During dilation, cardiac output may decrease significantly causing hypotension, bradycardia, arterial oxygen desaturation and a fall in end-tidal CO_2. When the balloon is only inflated for a few seconds, and preload is maintained, the procedure is usually well tolerated and the circulation usually recovers spontaneously. Therefore, sedation techniques are suitable for most patients requiring isolated right ventricular outflow tract or branch pulmonary artery balloon dilation, with or without stent placement.

Patients who have a hypertrophied, poorly compliant right ventricle with intra-ventricular pressures at systemic or supra-systemic levels may not tolerate the sudden increase in afterload associated with balloon dilation, even for a short period. In particular, myocardial ischemia and arrhythmias may occur causing severe acute RV failure and loss of cardiac output. General anesthesia and controlled ventilation is recommended prior to the intervention in this at risk group of patients.

Patients who have a dilated right ventricle secondary to a long standing volume load, such as chronic pulmonary regurgitation, are also at risk for arrhythmias and low output during catheter manipulations and interventions. On most occasions the changes in rhythm are short lived. Nevertheless, anesthesia and airway control are recommended if the circulation is compromised, and a defibrillator and transvenous pacing must be immediately available.

Initial hemodynamic data can be obtained under sedation, and then converted to endotracheal general anesthesia if necessary. Potential movement at the time of critical balloon dilation or stent placement must be avoided. The dilation of pulmonary arteries is painful and will often cause patients to wake from sedation and move. In addition dilation of the pulmonary arteries may induce coughing. This is usually not a problem for isolated pulmonary artery dilation; however if the patient moves during stent placement, it is possible to obstruct lobar or segmental branch pulmonary arteries inadvertently by the stent. Therefore, it is essential the patient be immobile and additional sedation may be given immediately prior to stent placement.

Dilations of multiple peripheral pulmonary artery stenoses, as in patients with Williams syndrome, are prolonged procedures and are associated with significant hemodynamic changes; endotracheal general anesthesia is usually required from the outset. Right ventricular hypertension and post-dilation pulmonary edema are additional risks. Edema usually occurs immediately following balloon dilation, but can be delayed for up to 24 hours. Endotracheal intubation and controlled ventilation are usually necessary until the edema resolves.

Additional complications from pulmonary artery dilation include pulmonary artery tears, aneurysm formation, and pulmonary artery rupture. These may manifest as immediate circulatory collapse, hemothorax, pericardial tamponade or hemoptysis, and require expert anesthetic and catheter management.

Balloon Dilation Of The Aorta

Coarctation of the aorta can be, for the most part, done using sedation techniques.

Occlusion Device Insertion

Device closure of patent ductus arteriosus (PDA), atrial septal defects (ASD) and ventricular septal defects (VSD) are commonly performed interventions in our catheterization laboratory. The placement of a PDA or ASD device is usually associated with minimal hemodynamic disturbance and can be performed in most patients using sedation techniques.[18,19] General anesthesia may be necessary for airway protection if transesophageal echocardiography is used to guide device placement.

In contrast, transcatheter VSD device closures can be prolonged procedures, often associated with profound hemodynamic instability and blood loss (Tables 12-3 and 12-4).[20]

TABLE 12-3

Complications During 70 Consecutive VSD Transcatheter Closures

	n (%)	
Blood loss requiring transfusion	38	(54)
Hypotension (20% reduction in systolic pressure)	28	(40)
Arrhythmia (with or without hypotension)	20	(26)
Pressure or nerve traction injury	4	(6)
Pleuro-pericardial effusion	3	(4)
Air embolus	1	(1)

Intensive care management is frequently required following placement. The indications for VSD device placement include closure of a residual or recurrent septal defect, preoperative closure of defects that may be difficult to reach surgically, and closure of defects following myocardial infarction. While the clinical condition of patients undergoing VSD device placement may vary considerably, in a review of 86 devices inserted in 70 patients the preoperative clinical condition or ASA status was not a predictor of hemodynamic disturbance during device placement. Rather, it is the technique necessary for deploying the occlusion device that results in significant hemodynamic compromise. All patients are therefore at risk.

Factors contributing to hemodynamic instability include blood loss, arrhythmias from catheter manipulation in the ventricles and across the septum, atrioventricular or aortic valve regurgitation from stenting open of valve leaflets by stiff walled catheters, wires or sheaths and device related factors such as malposition of the umbrella with arms impinging on valve leaflets or dislodgment from the ventricular septum.

TABLE 12-4

VSD Closure Details

	N	Mean Duration (min)	Mean Weight (kg)	Resuscitation During Procedure n(%)	
Group I	24	339 ± 112	36 ± 19.5	11	(46)
Group II	42	294 ± 98	13.3 ± 5.5	18	(43)
Group III	4	245 ± 91	70 ±	2	(50)

Group I   =   Residual or recurrent ventricular septal defect (VSD)
Group II   =   Muscular VSD: Primary defect or associated with other complex congenital cardiac defects.
Group III =   Acquired VSD after myocardial infarction or trauma.

The procedures are often prolonged (Table 12-4). In our study, the total procedure time average was 305 minutes (range 127-580 minutes). Because of the large sheath required, and the need for frequent catheter changes through the sheath, considerable blood loss may occur (often concealed by drapes) and the risk for air embolism is also increased. In our experience, transfusion was required in over 50% of patients with the amount transfused significantly greater in patients less than 10kg.

The hemodynamic instability that can occur during device placement is often unpredictable. In 40% of our patients hypotension occurred, with 12 responding to volume replacement alone whereas 16 patients required additional resuscitation with inotropes, vasopressor, transvenous pacing or cardioversion. During four procedures, external cardiac massage was required. Nonetheless, there were no deaths in this series. Arrhythmias associated with hypotension and desaturation required treatment or catheter withdrawal in 30% of procedures. The common dysrhythmias included ventricular tachycardia, junctional tachycardia and complete heart block.

Intensive Care Unit facilities must be available for this group of patients. In our series, 50% of patients were admitted directly to the CICU because of hemodynamic instability, procedure duration or concern over the position of the device.

Additional indications for general anesthesia in these patients include airway protection during transesophageal echocardiography used to guide device placement, and internal jugular venous access.

Coil Embolization of Collateral Vessels

While systemic artery to pulmonary artery collateral vessels may vary in size and result in a considerable left-to-right shunt, most patients tolerate coil embolization with sedation techniques.

Trans-catheter Radio-frequency Ablation

Pediatric patients undergoing radiofrequency ablation vary in age and diagnosis. Ablation may be necessary in the newborn with persistent re-entrant tachycardia or ectopic atrial tachycardia and cardiac failure, as well as in older children with an ectopic focus and otherwise structurally normal heart. An increasing number of patients undergo ablation following surgical repair of congenital heart defects. Patients with persistent volume or pressure load on the right atrium, and those who have required an extensive incision and suture lines within the right atrium, such as following a Mustard, Senning or Fontan procedure, may be at increased risk for tachyarrhythmias such as atrial flutter and fibrillation. Ventricular tachyarrhythmias may also develop late following repair of certain congenital heart defects, such as RV outflow tract reconstruction for tetralogy of Fallot.

Radio-frequency catheter ablations (RFCA) are often prolonged procedures. It is unreasonable to expect children to lie still for many hours, especially at the moment of ablation, and therefore endotracheal general anesthesia is preferred. For instance, if the focus is close to the AV node, inadvertent movement might displace the catheter and cause permanent AV conduction blockade. On occasions, holding the ventilation either in inspiration or expiration may be necessary to ensure adequate contact of the ablation catheter with the arrhythmic focus.

Although prolonged, these procedures are well tolerated and blood loss is minimal. During mapping, the focus is stimulated and the tachyarrhythmia induced. This may result in hypotension; however this is usually short lived and can be readily converted via intracardiac pacing. If hypotension is prolonged and intracardiac conversion unsuccessful, transthoracic cardioversion may be necessary and a defibrillator should be immediately available.
There are a few reports of the direct effects of anesthetic agents on the normal conduction pathway.[21-25] In adults, propofol has been shown to have little effect on atrio-ventricular conduction; however, isolated case reports in children have suggested that paroxysmal supraventricular tachycardia may revert to normal sinus rhythm with the use of propofol.[26] It is unclear, however, whether this is a non-

specific autonomic effect or a direct electrophysiologic affect of the drug. At Children's Hospital, Boston we recently demonstrated that neither propofol nor isoflurane anesthesia altered sino-atrial or atrio-ventricular node function.[27] A similar study, evaluating the effects of halothane and sevoflurane, demonstrated no significant effect on cardiac conduction in children with SVT undergoing RFCA (28). Because anesthetic drugs have minimal effect on intrinsic conduction, a range of techniques can be used to maintain general anesthesia during RFCA. Some tachyarrhythmias however, such as ectopic atrial tachycardia, are catecholamine sensitive, and the focus may be difficult to localize after induction of anesthesia. For this reason, it is preferable in these patients to perform the procedure under light sedation or light general anesthesia if necessary.

Additionally, long ablation procedures may cause pressure and nerve traction injuries, and urinary retention. All dependent areas and bony prominences must be well padded and protected. Intravenous fluid management should be restricted to avoid urinary retention, which may cause hypertension and considerable patient distress during emergence from anesthesia. Post procedural nausea and vomiting are common, possibly related to the duration of anesthesia and the use of isoproterenol during the ablation procedure. An anti-emetic is necessary for most patients.

CONCLUSION

Managing patients with either sedation or general anesthesia during cardiac catheterization requires a close working relationship with the cardiologist. Anesthesiologists and nurses involved with the management of these patients not only must be skilled in the conduct of pediatric sedation and anesthesia, but need to have a thorough understanding of the pathophysiology of congenital heart defects and surgical procedures previously performed. Knowledge of the planned catheterization procedure and potential complications is clearly essential and emphasizes the close liaison required between anesthesia and cardiology staff.

REFERENCES

1. Baum VC, Palmisano BW. The immature heart and anesthesia. Anesthesiology 1997;87:1529-48
2. Eichorn JH, Cooper JB, Gessner JS et al. Anesthesia standards at Harvard: A review. J Clin Anesth 1988;1:55-65.
3. American Academy of Pediatrics, Committee on Drugs. Guidelines for monitoring and management of pediatric patients during and after sedation for diagnostic and therapeutic procedures. Pediatr 1992;89:1110-1115.
4. Friesen RH, Alswand M. End-tidal CO_2 monitoring via nasal cannulae in pediatric patients: accuracy and sources of error. J Clin Monitoring 1996;12(2):155-9.

5. American Academy of Pediatrics, Committee on Drugs and Committee on Environmental Health. Use of choral hydrate for sedation in children. Pediatr 1993;92:471-473.

6. Hickey PR, Hansen DD, Wessel DL. Pulmonary and systemic hemodynamic responses to fentanyl in infants. Anesth Analg 185;64:483-486.

7. Hickey PR, Hansen DD, Wessel DL, et al. Blunting of stress responses in the pulmonary circulation of infants by fentanyl. Anesth Analg 1985;64:1137-1142.

8. Meretoja OA, Rautiainen P. Alfentanil and fentanyl sedation in infants and small children during cardiac catheterization. Can J Anesth 1990;37(6):624-8.

9. Lynn AM. Editorial. Remifentanil: The paediatric anaesthetist's opiate? Paediatric Anaesthesia 1996;6:433-35.

10. Morray JP, Lynn AM, Stamm SJ, et al. Hemodynamic effects of ketamine in children with congenital heart disease. Anesth Analg 1994;63:895-899.

11. Hickey PR, Hansen DD, Stafford MM, et al. Pulmonary and systemic hemodynamic responses to ketamine in infants with normal and elevated pulmonary vascular resistance. Anesthesiology 1985;62:287-293.

12. Berman W Jr, Fripp RR, Rubler M et al. Hemodynamic effects of ketamine in children undergoing cardiac catheterization. Pediatr Cardiol 1990;11(2):72-6.

13. Maruyama K, Maruyama J, Yokochi A et al. Vasodilatory effects of ketamine on pulmonary arteries in rats with chronic hypoxic pulmonary hypertension. Anesth Analg 1995;80:786-92.

14. Wolfe RR, Loehr JP, Scaffer MS et al. Hemodynamic effects of ketamine, hypoxia and hyperoxia in children with surgically treated congenital heart disease residing > 1200 metres above sea level. Am J Cardiol 1991;67:84-87.

15. Smith I, White PF, Nathanson M, et al. Propofol: an update on its clinical use. Anesthesiology 1994;81:1005-1043.

16. Lebovic S, Reich DL, Steinberg LG et al. Comparison of propofol versus ketamine for anesthesia in pediatric patients undergoing cardiac catheterization. Anesth Analg 1992;74:490-4.

17. Gooding JM, Wang JT, Smith RA, et al. Cardiovascular and pulmonary responses following etomidate induction of anesthesia in patients with demonstrated cardiac disease. Anesth Analg 1979;58:40-41.

18. Wessel DL, Keane JF, Parness I, et al. Outpatient closure of patent ductus arteriosus. Circ 1988;77:1068-1071.

19. Hickey PR, Wessel DL, Streitz SL, et al. Transcatheter closure of atrial septal defects: hemodynamic complications and anesthetic management. Anesth Analg 1992;74:44-50.

20. Laussen PC, Hansen DD, Perry SB, et al. Transcatheter closure of ventricular septal defect: hemodynamic instability and anesthetic management. Anesth Analg 1995;80:1076-1082.

21. Renwick J, Kerr C, Mctaggart R, et al.   Cardiac electrophysiology and conduction pathway ablation. Can J Anesth 1993;40:1053-1064.
22. Sharp MD, Dobkowski WB, Murkin JM, et al.   Alfentanyl-midazolam anesthesia has no electrophysiological effects upon the normal conduction system or accessory pathways in patients with Wolf Parkinson White syndrome. Can J Anesth 1992;39:816-821.
23. Sharp MD, Dobkowski WB, Murkin JM, et al.   The elelectrophysiological effects of volatile anesthetics and sufentanyl on the normal atrioventricular conduction system and accessory pathways in Wolf Parkinson White syndrome. Anesthesiology 1994;80:63-70.
24. Lau W, Kovoor P, Ross DL.   Cardiac electrophysiologic effects of midazolam combined with fentanyl. Am J Cardiol 1993;72(2):177-82.
25. Sharpe MD, Dobkowski WB, Murkin JM et al. Propofol has no direct effect on sino-atrial node function or on normal atrioventricular accessory pathway conduction in Wolff-Parkinson-White syndrome during alfentanil/midazolam anesthesia. Anesthesiology 1995;82:888-895.
26. Hermann T, Vettermen J. Change of ectopic supraventricular tachycardia to sinus rhythm during administration of propofol. Anesth Analg 1985;64:693-99.
27. Lavoie J, Walsh EP, Burrows FA, et al. The effects of propofol or isoflurane anesthesia on cardiac conduction in children undergoing radiofrequency catheter ablation for tachydysrhythmias. Anesthesiology 1995;82:884-887.
28. Zimmerman AA, Ibrahim AE, Epstein MR, et al. The effects of halothane and sevoflurane on cardiac electrophysiology in children undergoing radiofrequency catheter ablation. Anesthesiology 1997;87:A1066.

13. HOW TO CATHETERIZE SOME COMMON COMPLEX LESIONS

John F. Keane, M.D.

1. **SINGLE VENTRICLE (SV).**
2. **TETRALOGY OF FALLOT WITH PULMONARY ATRESIA (TOF - PA).**
3. **PULMONARY ATRESIA WITH INTACT VENTRICULAR SEPTUM (PA-IVS).**

Following the dramatic advances in surgical and interventional catheterization techniques, prolonged survival is now common in patients with complicated lesions, some heretofore considered inoperable such as hypoplastic left heart syndrome (HLHS). In the course of management of 3 such complex lesions, namely SV, TOF - PA and PA - IVS, surgery and catheterization at planned intervals are necessary. In the past 10 years at our institution, among 6,441 patients (11,593 catheterizations) were 952 patients with SV, including patients with HLHS, tricuspid atresia (TA), corrected transposition with a hypoplastic right ventricle (SLL-hypoRV), malaligned common atrioventricular canal and a straddling atrioventricular valve with hypoplasia of a ventricle. The final surgical procedure, a modified Fontan approach is preceded by staged surgeries, catheterizations and interventional procedures. These patients underwent 2,318 catheterizations and 1,198 interventional procedures. There were also 517 patients with TOF-PA in this population (1,319 catheterizations and 873 interventional procedures), the goal in these being to achieve a biventricular repair with an adequate pulmonary arterial tree [1] and 178 patients with PA-IVS (351 catheterizations and 207 interventional procedures) the desired end point in these being achievement of a biventricular repair and when not feasible a modified Fontan approach.

It is the purpose of this chapter, based on our experience to outline the catheterization methodology and interventional procedures involved in these 3 groups of patients at each of several stages. We recognize that medically indicated deviations from these schedules inevitably occur, yet the methodology, data acquisition and interventions required at these unscheduled studies are often similar to those necessary at the elective catheterizations.

1. SINGLE VENTRICLE (SV).

In this group surgery in the neonatal period is usually based on echocardiography alone; for example, a stage 1 Norwood procedure in HLHS or a pulmonary artery band placement in those with TA and unrestricted pulmonary blood flow. The subsequent surgical course in these patients usually involves a bidirectional Glenn and then a fenestrated Fontan, each preceded by a catheterization.

Cath 1: Pre Bidirectional Glenn (BDG).

This first catheterization is usually at 6 months of age just prior to a bidirectional Glenn anastomosis (BDG). In many, a single femoral venous line (5F) alone may be adequate to acquire all the necessary data - if however, aortic arch obstruction,

308

distal pulmonary artery stenosis or pulmonary artery hypertension is suspected, a small 3F pigtail [2] is placed in a femoral artery. The **Physiological Data** required include saturations and pressures in superior vena cava (SVC), right atrium(RA), left atrium (LA), ventricle (V), pulmonary vein (PV), ascending and descending aorta (AO), a PV wedge pressure and an oxygen consumption to enable precise calculation of pulmonary artery resistance. If the PV mean wedge pressure exceeds 18-20 mm with a ventricular end diastolic pressure (VEDP) less than 10, then direct pulmonary artery (PA) measurement is mandatory. This latter is acquired via the arterial route using the 3F catheter with the pigtail cut to 180^0. This catheter is first placed over a wire beyond the shunt origin in the subclavian artery, withdrawn slowly until the modified tip engages the proximal orifice. Next, an 0.018" torque wire (Mallinckrodt Medical, St. Louis, MO 63134) is advanced to a distal PA and the catheter advanced over the wire. It should be remembered that the mandril of this wire proximal to the floppy platinum coated tip is quite stiff and should thus be hand-shaped to conform to the aortic arch and shunt curves prior to insertion.

Anatomical Details necessary include visualization of the (L) innominate vein and any branches (such as an LSVC-CS/LA), RSVC, both (R) and (L) PA and their branches, (Fig. 13-1) all pulmonary veins (since occasionally one may drain anomalously or be stenotic), aortic arch, shunt origin course and insertion, ventricular size and function and atrioventricular valve competence.

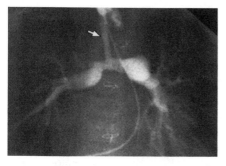

Figure 13-1: Visualization of shunt (arrow) and pulmonary arteries after stage 1 Norwood procedure for hypoplastic left heart syndrome, injecting in innominate artery proximal to distal occluding balloon: catheter course antegrade.

Interventional Possibilities: If aortic arch obstruction is identified, this should be dilated, if possible using the antegrade route (Fig. 13-2). Distal PA stenoses should also be balloon dilated (Fig. 13-3) with either a retrograde or antegrade approach using small balloons available to 8mm diameter (Boston Scientific,Watertown, MA 02172: B. Braun, Bethlehem, PA 18018), which can be advanced through a 4F sheath. Any large A-P collaterals should be coil occluded as should an LSVC-CS/LA as the latter will likely enlarge following the BDG: it is important to occlude an LSVC-CS/LA on the cardiac side of the entrance of its azygos vein (see below).

Cath 2: Post BDG Prior to Modified Fontan Procedure.

This study is usually undertaken between ages 1 and 3 years. Vascular access involves placement of two venous lines (both 5F), one in a femoral vein and the other in the (L) subclavian vein. A femoral arterial line (4F) is also required.

Physiological Data required include saturation values from SVC, (R) and (L) PA, atria, PVs, V and AO. It should be mentioned that a step up in saturation may be encountered especially in the (L) upper lobe PA due to A-P collateral flow particularly if LPA stenosis is present. Pressures are recorded in SVC, (R) and (L) PA, wedge, RA, LA, PVs, V, ascending and descending AO.

Balloon Dil. Coarct

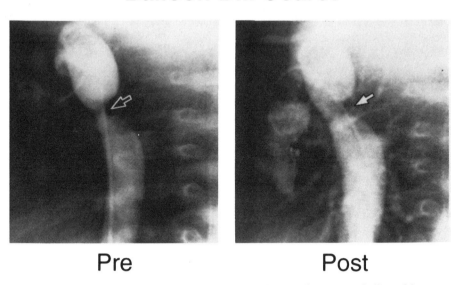

Pre   Post

Figure 13-2: Aortic coarctation pre (black arrow) and post (white arrow) balloon dilation in infant with hypoplastic left heart syndrome and stage 1 Norwood operation.

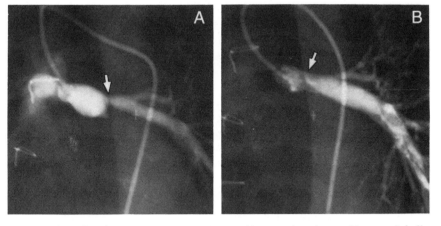

Figure 13-3: Left pulmonary artery stenosis pre (A: arrow) and post (B: arrow) balloon dilation in infant with hypoplastic left heart syndrome and stage 1 Norwood operation.

Oxygen consumption is measured for precise pulmonary blood flow and resistance calculations.

310

Anatomical Data necessary include (L) innominate vein and collateral venous channel delineation. It should be mentioned that since SVC pressure has been high following the BDG, venous collateral development to pulmonary veins of either lung or enlargement of a previously small LSVC-CS/LA vessel is quite common,[3] examples being depicted in Figs. 13-4, 5.

Details of PA, all PVs, V function and AV valve competence, and AO arch are necessary. If an interrupted IVC is present, hepatic venous drainage sites require delineation together with abdominal venous angiography to identify any other venous channels which may drain to hepatic or pulmonary veins. Pulmonary arteriovenous malformations (PAVM), confirmed by rapid transpulmonary contrast passage (< 3 beats), punctate vessel appearance and decreased pulmonary vein [4] saturation may be present especially in those with an interrupted IVC and azygos extension to an SVC.

Interventional Possibilities Any significant connections to pulmonary veins should be coil occluded as these will otherwise continue shunting right to left. An (L) SVC-CS/LA should similarly be occluded with coil placement being on the cardiac side of that vessel's azygos entry site - if the LSVC is occluded on the innominate side of this entry site, significant later (R) - (L) shunting to the LA via this azygos may increase and be unreachable by catheter (Fig. 13-4). Venous collaterals which drain to the right atrium or below the diaphragm to the IVC should also be coil occluded if the Fontan procedure is to be delayed. If a large amount of contrast is seen to pass to a PA (often LPA) on aortography, especially if associated with a significant saturation increase, then coil occlusion of the major contributing vessels (internal mammary, long thoracic artery etc.) is probably necessary. Such collateral flow should raise the suspicion of PA or PV stenosis or atresia on that side. (Fig. 13-6). Many coils (and occasionally gelfoam) may be required in these vessels since they are inter-connected, both with each other and with many of the adjoining intercostal arteries on that side. Visually significant PA stenoses, even in the absence of gradients should be balloon dilated. Aortic arch obstruction (PSEG ≥10 mg) should be similarly balloon dilated, often via an antegrade venous approach.

Cath 3: Post Modified Fontan.

Catheterization following a modified Fontan procedure is primarily used to insure an optimum hemodynamic state in this fundamentally tenuous circulation. They may be needed early or later postoperatively. **A) Early Postoperative Studies** have become very infrequent because of more accurate and precise preoperative studies with appropriate therapeutic procedures and baffle fenestration creation at the time of surgery [5]. **B) Late Postoperative Studies,** now by far the more common variety, may be associated with (a) cyanosis, including those with a known fenestration, (b) evidence of excessive right sided venous hypertension such as edema, (c) both of the above and (d) atrial dysrhythmias. Investigation and management of the latter are dealt with in Chapter 14.

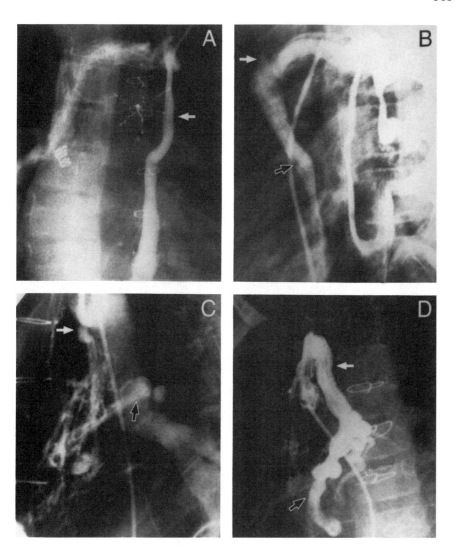

Figure 13-4:   (R)→(L) shunting venous channels seen post BDG/Fontan.
         A: A-P view: LSVC - CS (arrow) post BDG.
         B: LAT view: post Fontan, LSVC-CS ligated near innominate vein (white
            arrow): extensive R→L shunting now via (L) azygos → CS (black arrow)
            unreachable by catheter: (L)azygos subsequently closed via VATS.
         C: LAT view: vein from proximal LIV (white arrow) draining to RUPV(black
            arrow): post BDG.
         D: A-P view: patient with visceral heterotaxy, interrupted IVC post BDG, vein
            from R azygos (white arrow) draining to RLPV (black arrow).

312

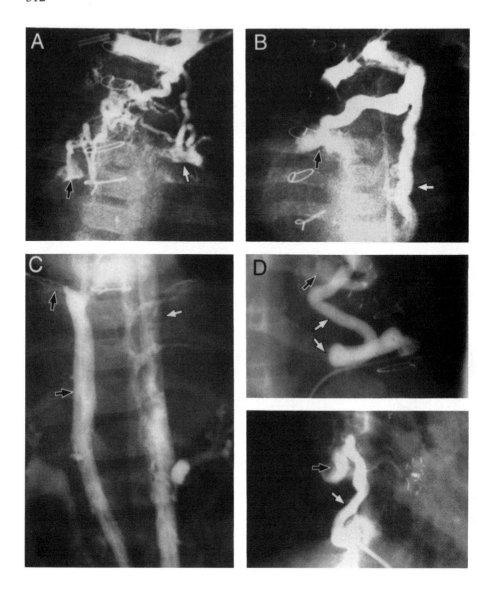

<u>*Abbreviations for Figures 13-4 & 5*</u>

*A-P = Antero Posterior: BDG = Bidirectional Glenn: IVC = Inferior Vena Cava: LAT =
Lateral: LSVC-CS = Left Superior Vena Cava to Coronary Sinus: LA = Left Atrium: LIJ Left
Internal Jugular Vein: LIV Left Innominate Vein: LUPV = Left Upper Pulmonary Vein:
RLPV = Right Lower Pulmonary Vein: VATS = Video Assisted Thoracic Surgery.*

Figure 13-5:   *(R)→(L) shunting venous channels seen post BDG/Fontan*
A: A-P view: vein from LIV divides and drains to RUPV (black arrow)
and LUPV (white arrow).
B: A-P view: vein from LIV divides and drains to RUPV (black arrow)
and via hemiazygos (white arrow) to L renal vein.
C: A-P view: patient with visceral heterotaxy, (L) azygos extension
(white arrow) draining to (L) SVC post (L) BDG: (R) IVC
(black arrows) also present draining (R) renal and hepatic
veins to RA: both systems connected inferiorly at common
iliac vein junction.
D: A-P, LAT views: vein (white arrows) from (R) hepatic vein to (R)
LPV (black arrows), post Fontan.

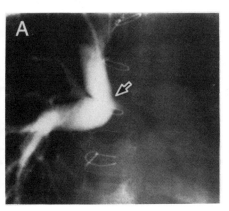
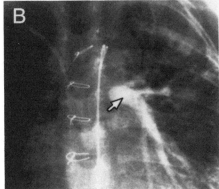

Figure 13-6:Patient, with bidirectional Glenn, with left pulmonary artery atresia (A: black arrow) with filling of left pulmonary artery by collaterals following aortography (B: white arrow).

A. Early Postoperative Catheterization

In this now unusual occurrence, a common cause has been spontaneous occlusion of the surgically created baffle fenestration, recognizable within hours of surgery by an arterial P02 > 200 mm Hg and hypotension, and confirmed by echocardiography [6]. While occasionally this may be clinically tolerated or reopen spontaneously, the more common course is one of rapid deterioration manifested by a high central venous pressure ($\geq$ 20 mm Hg), decreasing renal function and cardiac output, and increasing chest tube drainage. This condition requires urgent fenestration reopening in the catheterization laboratory.

Technique: Via a 7F femoral venous sheath following brief recordings of pressures and saturations, an angiogram in the atrial baffle is performed. Often a tiny trickle of contrast across the fenestration is seen; the latter is then crossed by an end-hole catheter through which a precurved 0.035" guidewire is passed to the LA. If there is no passage of contrast across the fenestration, probing with an angled end-hole catheter, such as a 5F multipurpose, will nearly always achieve passage across the

314

defect. In the very rare instance where this is unsuccessful, passage of a transseptal needle and sheath across the baffle may be required to reach the LA for subsequent wire placement. Sequential balloon dilations of the fenestration are then undertaken, usually to 6-8mm size,[5] monitoring arterial saturation until a value of 75-85% is achieved. These saturations usually rise in the first 6-12 hours after catheterization, often to the 85-88% range. A final baffle angiogram is recorded for fenestration patency confirmation (Fig. 13-7).

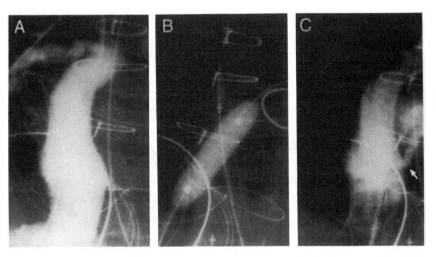

Figure 13-7: Early postoperative complete occlusion of baffle fenestration (A): balloon dilation of fenestration (B): significant post dilation right - left flow (C: arrow).

On a few occasions we have encountered extensive clot formation such that the entire baffle including the fenestration is occluded, requiring immediate reoperation (Fig. 13-8).

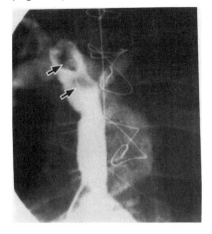

Figure 13-8: 25 yr. patient early postoperative modified fenestrated Fontan acutely ill with clots (arrows) in baffle occluding fenestration and obstructing pulmonary artery flow.

In those few post-op Fontan patients with more than 10-14 days of chest tube drainage, a complete right and left heart catheterization is required. Any pulmonary arterial stenosis distal to the recently placed suture lines should be dilated and any significant aortopulmonary collateral vessels should be coil occluded. Severe stenoses at or near suture lines are best treated with stents.

B. Late Postoperative Catheterization

Studies in this population are generally time consuming and require meticulous attention to identifying and treating with appropriate interventional procedures the legion of ever expanding causes of cyanosis and/or venous hypertension. It is important to remember that these patients with their "unnatural right heart venous pathways", in whom IVC return constitutes the major part of systemic venous return, are being catheterized while lying down. Thus obstruction anywhere in these pathways, even 1 mmHg, is of significance.

A minimum of 2 femoral lines, one venous and one arterial, are required, the former initially of 7F size. A complete right and left heart study including physiological data (pressures, saturations from all sites) together with oxygen consumption for pulmonary resistance calculation, is carried out. Angiography, in multiple locations and guided by the data acquired and by prior non invasive studies, is then undertaken. Even asymptomatic patients may have minor anatomic abnormalities which may accelerate development of atrial arrhythmias or edema. The causes of cyanosis and systemic venous hypertension are legion and some, together with appropriate catheter directed therapy, are briefly discussed.

Cyanosis

The sites of right to left shunting encountered and their management are outlined in Table 1. In general, venous collaterals from hepatic veins to pulmonary veins (Fig. 13-5D:), atrial level venous channels to LA and innominate vein connections with pulmonary veins (Figs. 13-4,5) are long and sufficiently restrictive to allow coil placement as therapy. Baffle fenestrations, large baffle suture line leaks or large septal defects encountered in the older atriopulmonary anastomoses (Fig. 13-9) require use of double umbrella devices. Any of these larger communications first require temporary balloon occlusion with baseline and occlusion recordings of atrial and systemic saturation and pressure values to identify if it is hemodynamically safe to close those permanently. For example, if temporary occlusion results in baffle pressure exceeding 20mm Hg with a significant decrease in arterial pressure and a precipitous drop in baffle saturation, closure should not be undertaken. Dehiscence of an A-V valve patch is often localized and can be closed with a CardioSEAL device (Fig. 13-10).

Pulmonary arteriovenous malformations are more common in a lung if hepatic venous return has been directed to the other lung. These are usually multiple, small and diffuse and thus not suitable for coil occlusion. Surgical redirection of hepatic flow has been curative. Rarely, one large such malformation in a small lung section may be encountered and coil occluded. The presence of these malformations is confirmed by directly sampling pulmonary veins which can be accomplished in retrograde fashion or via an atrial level defect if present.

Table 13-1   **Causes of Cyanosis**

Location Level	R - L Lesion	Interventional Therapy
Infradiaphragmatic	HV-LA: HV-PV: IVC-PV	coil, clamshell
Atrial in APA	CS-LA: ASD	coil, clamshell
Atrial Lateral Tunnel	fenestration: suture line leaks	clamshell: coil
Baffle AV valve	leak with RA-V shunt	clamshell
SVC - INNOM. V	LSVC-CS/LA: Innom. V-PV	coil
Pulmonary	PAVM: usually multiple	if single = coil

Abbreviations:
APA = Atrio Pulmonary Anastomosis: ASD = Atrial Septal Defect: AV = Atrioventricular: CS = Coronary Sinus: HV = Hepatic Vein: Innom. V = Innominate Vein: IVC = Inferior Vena Cava: LA = Left Atrium: LSVC = Left Superior Vena Cava: PAVM = Pulmonary Arteriovenous Malformation: PV = Pulmonary Vein: R-L = Right to Left: RA = Right Atrium: SVC = Superior Vena Cava: V = Ventricle

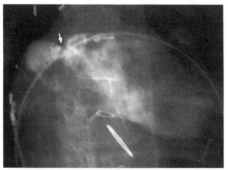

Figure 13-9: 20 yr. patient with atriopulmonary anastomosis with cyanosis due to atrial septal defect (arrow) subsequently occluded by clamshell double umbrella device.

Figure 13-10: 7 yr. patient postoperative atriopulmonary anastomosis with cyanosis; with catheter through partial dehiscence of atrioventricular valve patch (A: arrow), occluded by double umbrella device (B: arrow).

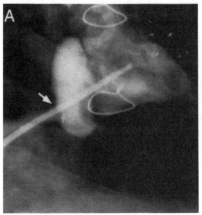
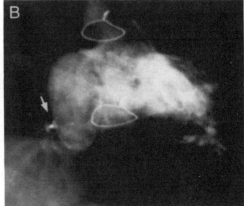

Systemic Venous Hypertension
Causes and appropriate therapies are outlined in Table 2.

Table 13-2   Causes of venous hypertension

Etiology	Therapy
Atrial baffle stenosis	BD/ Stent
Atrial - Ventricular/MPA Conduit Stenosis	BD/Stent
Giant RA compressing RPV	Surgical
Pulmonary artery stenosis	BD/Stent
Pulmonary vein stenosis	BD/Stent
Patent ventricle - MPA connection	Clamshell/coil
↑VEDP alone	Medical
AVV regurgitation	Medical/surgical
Sub-Aortic obstruction	Stent/surgical
A-P collaterals/shunt	Coil
Aortic Arch Obstruction	BD/Stent

Abbreviations
A-P = Aorto Pulmonary: AVV = Atrio Ventricular Valve: BD = Balloon Dilation: MPA = Main Pulmonary Artery: RA = Right Atrium: RPV = Right Pulmonary Vein: ↑VEDP = Elevated Ventricular End Diastolic Pressure

Angiographically significant atrial baffle stenoses, sometimes due to prosthetic material kinks should be dilated and stented even in the absence of a gradient (Fig. 13-11).

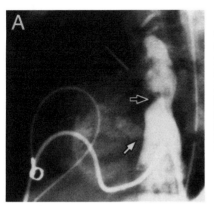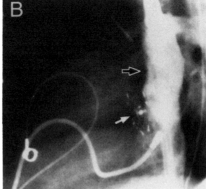

Figure 13-11: 9 yr. patient late postoperative fenestrated lateral tunnel modified Fontan procedure; lateral view (A) showing fenestration (white arrow) and stenosis of tunnel (black arrow) treated by clamshell occlusion of fenestration and stent enlargement of tunnel.

Conduit connections between the right atrium and right ventricle or main pulmonary artery are frequently obstructed often behind the sternum and are best visualized in the lateral view. These require double lumen catheters [7] to simultaneously record proximal and distal pressures to assess accurately the magnitude of the obstruction since assessing mean pressures alone will be misleading. These are managed by balloon dilation and stent placement (Fig. 13-12).

Occasionally the giant RA encountered in the older style atriopulmonary anastomoses may compress the right pulmonary veins. This is best displayed by MRI studies. In these patients, gradients between the right capillary wedge and end diastolic ventricular pressures (Rpc - VED) are often not obvious. These patients benefit from surgical conversion to a lateral atrial tunnel [8]. Angiographically significant PA or baffle stenosis, again even without any gradient should be dilated and probably stented. Pulmonary vein stenoses are sometimes encountered and similarly require dilation and stenting even though the success of this procedure is usually low.

Occasionally a patent stenotic ventricle - MPA connection has been left open at surgery and if significant requires closure with a double umbrella device in antegrade fashion (Fig. 13-13) or rarely with a coil.

Subaortic obstruction of a significant degree is occasionally encountered and may be managed by stent placement (Fig. 13-14) as an alternative to high risk surgery. Any sources of significant aorto-pulmonary flow should be coil occluded.

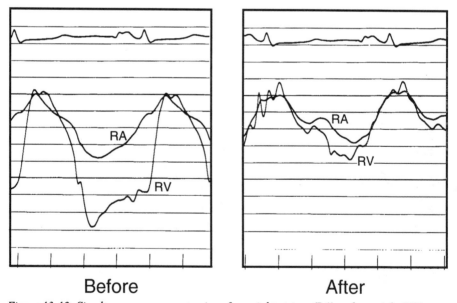

Before   **After**

Figure 13-12: Simultaneous pressure tracings from right atrium (RA) and ventricle (RV) using double lumen catheter in 26 yr. patient with tricuspid atresia with atrioventricular obstructed conduit (before) and following stent placement (after).

319

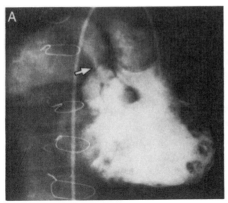
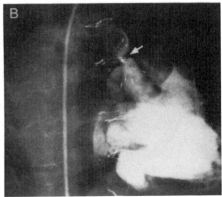

Figure 13-13: Patent stenotic ventricular - main pulmonary artery connection following modified Fontan procedure (A: arrow) with double umbrella occlusion of same (B: arrow) delivered via transvenous approach.

Again it should be noted that "significant" flow to a particular lung segment may be associated with stenosis or atresia of the pulmonary vein from that segment or to a proximal PA stenotic lesion. Any aortic arch obstruction with a gradient ≥10 mm Hg, particularly if the EDP is elevated, should be dilated or even stented.

In conclusion, the potential problems in this complex population managed as single ventricle are legion. Many catheterized patients have multiple causes for their problems, many common to both the post bidirectional Glenn and post Fontan groups. These studies require meticulous attention to detail and beneficial interventional therapeutic procedures are possible in the majority.

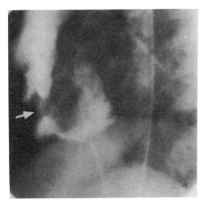
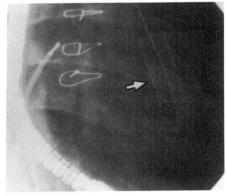

LAT   AP

Figure 13-14: Subaortic stenosis with peak systolic ejection gradient 150 mm (LAT. arrow) in 23 yr. patient following modified Fontan procedure; reduced to 5 mm by placement of 3 overlapping iliac stents (AP: arrow) dilated to 18 mm.

2. TETRALOGY OF FALLOT AND PULMONARY ATRESIA (TOF - PA).

This is a very complex lesion. Wide variations in central pulmonary artery size, intra-pulmonary connections, and collateral number and distribution are encountered. Catheterizations in this population are either preoperative or postoperative.

(1) Preoperative Most of these are undertaken in (a) neonates and young infants, with some occasionally in (b) older patients being evaluated for the first time.

(a) Neonates and Young Infants: Infants with echocardiographically displayed normal sized continuous mediastinal PAs and whose sole pulmonary blood flow (PBF) is from a patent ductus arteriosus, undergo surgical repair without catheterization. Catheterization is reserved for infants in whom there is uncertainty about central PA anatomy or VSD size and number and distribution of aortopulmonary collaterals. In these patients, a descending aortogram in a "sitting-up" view using either an occlusion technique with a 5F Berman via an antegrade venous approach or a retrograde catheter usually provides adequate anatomical central PA detail (Fig. 13-15) to allow for surgical placement of an RV-PA homograft, particularly if aortic saturation is ≤ 85%. If, however, aortic saturation is ≥ 90%, and mediastinal PAs are of adequate size, precise delineation of collateral origin and distribution is required to allow surgical repair, including ventricular defect closure with detachment and anastomoses of large collaterals to the central PA. This necessitates selective collateral angiography which may be accomplished via the umbilical artery in the newborn or via a femoral artery in those older.

(b) Older patients In this increasingly unusual group, the information required includes delineation of the central PAs and precise identification and distribution of all collateral vessels present, including pressure measurements. The most helpful initial angiogram is a rapid flow injection in the descending AO, in a "sitting up" view to separate the mediastinal "sea-gull" PAs from nearby collateral vessels.

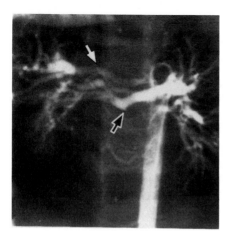

Figure 13-15: TOF-PA: descending aortogram, "sitting-up" view, showing reflux of contrast into confluent mediastinal PA (black arrow) via A-P collaterals (white arrow).

Following acquisition of these essential data, ventricular septal and coronary artery anatomy are then outlined. If surgical repair is indicated, collaterals found to be connected to the central PAs may be coil occluded to simplify the operative approach.

Collaterals with severe proximal obstructions supplying significant lung segments isolated from the central PAs should be dilated or stented to improve distal flow prior to unifocalization [9].

(2) Postoperative: This group of patients includes those (a) palliated by an RV-PA conduit or an aortopulmonary shunt and (b) following repair.

(a) Palliated: The primary purposes of an RV-PA conduit or shunt are (i) to increase systemic artery saturation, (ii) to encourage central PA growth by virtue of added flow (iii) to enable more accurate delineation of intrapulmonary connections by directly injecting into both RPA and LPA and (iv) to provide an access route to dilate any proximal or distal stenoses. The advantages of an RV-PA conduit over an aortopulmonary shunt are (a) more central pulmonary artery size increase (b) easier access to either right or left distal PA for angiographic delineation (c) more direct and technically easier route for dilation and stent placement and (d) less iatrogenic shunt induced PA distortion. Thus, in the catheterization of patients with an RV-PA conduit, 2 femoral sheaths at least 5F in size are placed, one venous and the other arterial. A standard complete right and left heart set of saturations and pressures, together with oxygen consumption, are recorded. Selective right and left PA angiograms identify the lung segments connected to each PA. In order to determine these connections more accurately, balloon occlusion of a collateral vessel to a particular lung or segment thereof while injecting into that PA or vice versa is very helpful. This allows for precise delineation of distal stenoses for balloon dilation and identification of those collaterals which because of dual segment perfusion, can be safely coil occluded. More proximal areas of stenoses in either right or left PA, particularly those considered difficult to reach surgically should be dilated and probably stented (Fig. 13-16).

At the conclusion of these often time-consuming maneuvers, repeat pressure and saturation sequences can then identify those patients in whom the VSD can be closed and a larger conduit if necessary, placed. In some where this possibility is uncertain, if significant discrete obstruction especially on the lateral view is present in the conduit or homograft, balloon dilation (not to exceed 110% of the original homograft size) and stenting should be carried out. In those palliated with an aortopulmonary shunt, modifications of the catheterization techniques described above are carried out, with an additional arterial line being required to provide simultaneous access to pulmonary arteries and collaterals.

(b) Post Repair: Patients in this group are generally being studied because of residual problems related to obstruction in the right sided circuit or residual shunts (VSD or A-P collaterals) or both. Occasionally these studies are required in the early postoperative period but are usually undertaken months or years following surgery. Vascular access requires femoral venous and arterial lines. In the early postoperative group, obstructions in the vicinity of suture lines cannot be safely dilated but any unnecessary A-P collaterals should be coil occluded. If additional apical or anterior muscular VSDs are found, consideration should be given to device closure. In those patients months or more beyond surgery, a stenotic RV-PA

322

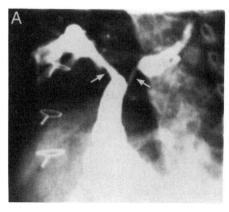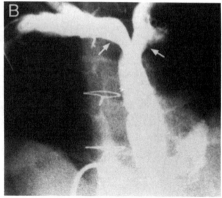

Figure 13-16: TOF-PA: stenotic right and left pulmonary arteries (A: arrows) following placement of right ventricle - pulmonary artery homograft: later after balloon dilation and stent placement (B: arrows).

homograft should be dilated with stent placement being required in many, particularly if RV pressures > 60% systemic level. Those identified with decreased lung perfusion, for example (L) lung perfusion ≤ 25% on lung scan due to (L) PA stenosis, should have the LPA dilated and then stented if dilation alone is unsatisfactory. There are occasional patients in whom the left anterior descending (LAD) arises anomalously from the right coronary artery and now passes behind the RV - PA homograft. It is important in those to first ensure the LAD is unobstructed during balloon dilation if stent placement in the homograft is being considered.

3. PULMONARY ATRESIA WITH INTACT VENTRICULAR SEPTUM (PA-IVS)

In this disease the goal is to achieve sufficient growth of the right ventricle (RV) and its structures to create a two ventricle heart. If not feasible, a modified Fontan should be attempted [10]. The usual planned approach consists of 3 catheterizations in the first two of years of life, namely (a) in the neonatal period prior to surgery, (b) at 6 months of age and (c) at 1-2 years of age.

(a) Neonatal Catheterization; At this study, usually within 24 hours of birth, two lines (umbilical venous and arterial) are required. The essential data are primarily anatomical and include the size of the RV and its outflow tract, PA anatomy and precise delineation of the coronary artery system including origins, distribution, fistulae and any stenoses or atretic sites. This crucial coronary arterial delineation can be acquired from cineangiograms in the RV and AO and, if necessary, from selective coronary artery injections using 4.5F coronary catheters. A balloon atrial septostomy should be avoided since a large defect will (a) diminish antegrade tricuspid flow and subsequent RV growth and (b) not be amenable to later device closure. The usual surgical procedure at this point includes placement of a transannular RV outflow patch and a modified right Blalock Taussig shunt in neonates who do not have an RV dependent coronary circulation.

(b) Catheterization at age 6 months; The information required at this elective study includes physiological data, anatomical details and the hemodynamic consequences of temporary balloon occlusion of the atrial defect and/or shunt. A 5F femoral venous and a 4F arterial line are required. Following acquisition of pressure (Fig. 13-17) and saturation data at all sites, angiographic details of RV size and outflow, PA, shunt and coronary arteries are obtained. If stenosis of the right PA at the shunt insertion site is identified, it should be dilated. Temporary balloon occlusion of the atrial defect is then carried out as described previously (Chapter 6). The shunt may be occluded with a 4F Berman catheter which also allows arterial pressure and saturation monitoring. It is important to avoid shunt occlusion alone as this may result in a precipitous drop in arterial saturation, as atrial pressure of a sufficient degree to open the tricuspid valve (TV) cannot then be generated. This is especially true if tricuspid stenosis is present or, as is common with pulmonary regurgitation, RV end diastolic pressure is elevated.

Interventional possibilities at this study include balloon dilation of PA or TV stenosis, or rarely stent placement for significant RV outflow obstruction.

(c) Catheterization at age 1 - 2 years
At this elective study, the aim is to close permanently the atrial defect and shunt. Femoral venous and arterial lines are placed, usually via a 7F sheath in the former and 5F sheath in the latter. Initially hemodynamic data are acquired before and during simultaneous temporary balloon occlusion of the 2 shunting sites, together with appropriate angiography.

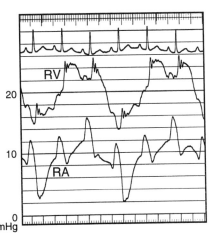

Figure 13-17: PA-IVS: Simultaneous right ventricular (RV) and right atrial (RA) pressures, age 6 months, following modified Blalock Taussig shunt and right ventricular outflow patch: RV pressure continuously higher than RA, so no antegrade flow across tricuspid valve.

Interventional Procedures:
If temporary balloon occlusion at both sites is hemodynamically well tolerated, that is cardiac output, RA and systemic pressures are satisfactory and arterial blood is fully saturated, then the atrial defect is closed with a double umbrella device. The device size, determined by balloon sizing is generally 17-23mm in diameter and is delivered via an 11F sheath. The shunt is then coil occluded via a retrograde approach with the right PA being occluded at the shunt entry site by a balloon catheter to prevent coil embolization; generally at least 2

324

coils are placed. If TV stenosis is identified this is also dilated. It is recognized that many patients with PA-IVS will not follow this ideal course. Coronary artery lesions such as those dependent on RV supply, and those with a persistently hypoplastic RV and TV, require quite different management strategies [11].

REFERENCES

1. Rome JJ, Mayer JE, Castaneda AR, Lock JE: Tetralogy of Fallot with Pulmonary Atresia:Rehabilitation of Diminutive Pulmonary Arteries. Circulation. 1993: 88:1961-8.
2. Keane JF, Fellows KE, Lang P, Fyler DC. Pediatric Arterial Catheterization using 3.2 French Catheter. Cath and Cardiovasc. Diag. 1982; 8:201-8.
3. Magee AG, McCrindle BW, Mawson J, et al: Systemic Venous Collateral Development after the Bidirectional Cavopulmonary Anastomosis Prevalence and Predictors. J Am Coll Cardiol 1998:32:502-508.
4. Srivastava D, Preminger T, Lock JE, Mandell V, Keane JF, Mayer JE, Kozakewich H, Spevak P. Hepatic Venous Blood and the Development of Pulmonary Arteriovenous Malformations in Congenital Heart Disease. Circulation 1995; 92:1217-22.
5. Gentles TL, Mayer JE, Gauvreau K, Newburger JW, Lock JE, Kupferschmid JP, Burnett J, Jonas RA, Castaneda AR, Wernovsky G. Fontan Operation in Five Hundred Consecutive Patients: Factors Influencing Early and Late Outcome. J Thorac. Cardiovasc. Surg. 1997; 114:376-91
6. Kreutzer J, Lock JE, Jonas RA, Keane JF. Transcatheter Fenestration Dilation and/or Creation in Postoperative Fontan Patients. Americ. Jour. Cardiol. 1996; 79:228-32.
7. Kreutzer J, Keane JF, Lock JE, Walsh EP, Jonas RA, Castaneda AR, Mayer JE. Conversion of Modified Fontan Procedure to Lateral Atrial Tunnel Cavopulmonary Anastomosis. J. Thorac. Cardiovasc. Surg. 1996: 111:1169-76.
8. Zeevi B, Rome JJ, Keane JF. A Newly Designed Double Pressure Balloon Catheter: Clinical use in Congenital Heart Disease. J. Inv. Card. 1989; 3:129-35.
9. Redington AN, Somerville J: Stenting of Cardiopulmonary Collaterals in Complex Pulmonary Atresia. Circulation. 1996; 94:2479-84.
10. Giglia TM, Jenkins KJ, Matitiau A, Mandell VS, Sanders SP, Mayer JE, Lock JE: Influence of Right Heart Size on Outcome in Pulmonary Atresia with Intact Ventricular Septum. Circulation 1993: 88 : 2248 - 56.
11. Gentles TL, Keane JF, Jonas RA, Marx GE, Mayer JE, Jr. Surgical Alternative to the Fontan Procedure Incorporating a Hypoplastic Right Ventricle. Circulation. 1994; 90[part 2]: II-1 - II-6.

14. INTRACARDIAC ELECTROPHYSIOLOGIC STUDIES

Edward P. Walsh, M.D.

INTRODUCTION

There have been dramatic advances in the field of cardiac electrophysiology (EP) over the past decade. Since the first edition of this text[1] was published in 1987, EP has progressed from being primarily a diagnostic and medical discipline, to become an interventional field with the potential for definitive treatment of many rhythm disorders. At many pediatric cardiology centers, transcatheter ablation of various tachyarrhythmias now accounts for the majority of EP procedures performed each year. Associated with these technological advances comes an increased responsibility for cardiologists at all levels of training to develop a solid understanding of fundamental EP principles. Even if a clinician is not directly involved with the management of complex arrhythmias, such knowledge is necessary to insure proper screening and referral of patients who could benefit from EP testing and/or ablation.

This chapter is intended as an introduction for cardiology fellows and other newcomers to the EP laboratory, and aims to provide a simple overview of equipment and basic techniques for invasive EP testing in children and young adults, along with some general discussion of the principles for radiofrequency (RF) ablation. More in-depth analysis of arrhythmia mapping and catheter ablation are beyond the scope of this text, but the interested reader is referred to several comprehensive reviews [2-4] of these topics for further information.

LABORATORY SET-UP AND PATIENT PREPARATION

The equipment used for EP testing in pediatric patients has become more sophisticated with the advent of interventional techniques. Many centers now have a dedicated laboratory suite for these studies, equipped with biplane fluoroscopy that can be delivered in a "pulsed" fashion to minimize radiation exposure for both the patient and lab personnel during potentially lengthy procedures. Standard diagnostic equipment in the EP lab includes a multichannel electrogram recorder that is capable of registering surface ECG leads along with multiple electrograms from the endocardial catheters. Commercial systems are now available for computerized digital recording of anywhere from 16 to 64 channels of electrical data. The lab must also be equipped with an electrical stimulator that is capable of cardiac pacing at finely adjustable intervals, and can be programmed to pace from one or more intracardiac sites using a constant current energy source. The stimulus amplitude and the pulse width should be carefully adjusted on the device at the beginning of each case. Generally, a pulse width of 2.0 milliseconds (msec) is used, with an amplitude (expressed in milliamperes) that is set at about twice the threshold for capture at a given pacing site.

The most important tools in the EP laboratory are the electrode catheters. As the demand for mapping accuracy has increased in the era of interventional EP procedures, some of these catheters have become quite elaborate, with higher electrode density and specialized mechanisms for deflecting and steering the tip. Complex "basket catheters" have also been developed for three-dimensional mapping[5] within cardiac chambers. For RF ablation, the distal electrode on select catheters has been further modified with a 4-8 mm tip to provide a larger surface area for RF current delivery, as opposed to the 1-2 mm tip on a standard diagnostic catheter. Examples of some commercial and investigational catheters used for pediatric EP testing are shown in Fig. 14-1.

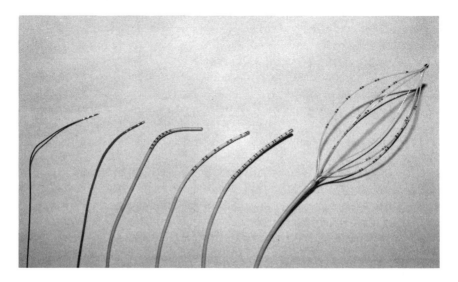

Figure 14-1. Catheters for electrophysiologic study and radiofrequency ablation.

Patient preparation for an EP study is similar to that for standard cardiac catheterization, with a few modifications. As a method of maximizing patient safety during induction of various tachycardias, it is a standard precaution to position adhesive defibrillator pads on the patient's chest at the beginning of every case. This eliminates any delay should direct current (DC) cardioversion or defibrillation become necessary during the study. Patients who are taking antiarrhythmic drugs will usually have their medications discontinued for at least 5 half-lives before an EP study. For simple diagnostic procedures, intravenous sedation with agents such as versed, morphine, or fentanyl usually provides adequate analgesia and amnesia for most young patients. For more complex procedures including ablation, many patients are given a general anesthetic using agents such as propofol or isoflurane, which have been shown to have minimal effects on EP measurements[6] and do not seem to interfere in a significant way with mapping and analysis of the common reentrant arrhythmias in young patients. However, for some "automatic" tachycardias (such as ectopic atrial tachycardia and certain forms of ventricular tachycardia), deep levels of sedation may artificially suppress the rhythm disorder to the point that it cannot be induced by any means. If such arrhythmias are suspected, it is preferable to use light levels of carefully titrated intravenous sedation[7] during the study.

Vascular access for EP testing is similar to the percutaneous technique used for routine catheterization, except that a larger number of catheters will need to be inserted. This may necessitate the use of both right and left femoral veins, and occasionally the subclavian or jugular vein. In older children, it becomes possible to position multiple vascular sheaths in a single femoral vein. After a guidewire is passed through the first femoral venous entry point, a second site is chosen about 1 centimeter below the original puncture area, and the needle can be advanced in alignment with the initial guidewire which serves as a reliable marker for the vein. As an alternative approach, several manufacturers now provide small electrode catheters[8] that are only 2 French in size. These are usually advanced to the heart through a long guiding sheath since the thin catheter shaft makes tip control in the vascular space difficult, but up to 3 of these small devices can be inserted through a single 7 French sheath as a way of minimizing venous entry requirements. In very small children, the number and size of venous catheters can be further reduced by substituting an esophageal lead as the atrial pacing and recording electrode, or by using a single endocardial catheter for combined functions such as simultaneous His bundle recording and ventricular pacing.

DIAGNOSTIC EP STUDIES

Baseline Intracardiac Recordings
All comprehensive EP studies begin with careful analysis of the baseline rhythm. Electrode catheters are positioned at standard sites within the heart that include the right atrium (RA), right ventricular (RV), His bundle electrogram area (HBE), and often the coronary sinus (CS). These 4 catheters provide a very broad view of cardiac electrical activity as it progresses from atrial depolarization, through atrioventricular (AV) conduction, and finally ends with ventricular activation. The RA catheter can be positioned either to the junction of the superior vena cava (SVC) and RA (the preferred position when evaluation of sinus node function is desired) or it can be advanced to a stable position in the right atrial appendage (the preferred position when mapping of an accessory pathway is the central concern). The HBE recording is obtained by advancing the catheter from the inferior vena cava (IVC) across the superior and medial aspect of the tricuspid valve. It is important that a catheter be chosen which has a gentle curve (about 90 degree) at its distal end to promote stability at this position. This places the tip in the commissure between the anterior and septal leaflet of tricuspid valve, adjacent to the membranous septum at the crux of the heart. The recording electrodes will straddle the AV groove, and should thus register a signal which contains an atrial

component, a small discrete His bundle deflection, and a large ventricular component. The RV catheter is usually positioned from the IVC to the ventricular apex, where it will usually remain stable with low pacing thresholds throughout long studies. It is again important that the catheter be chosen with a gently curved distal end (about 120 degrees) to facilitate apical positioning. The CS catheter can be inserted by several techniques. In more than 70% of cases, it is possible to cannulate the coronary sinus from an IVC approach using a deflectable tip catheter, which is curved down to enter the proximal portion of the CS, and is then subsequently straightened to permit advancement far out along the left AV groove. Alternatively, the CS can usually be entered easily from an SVC approach, even with a non-deflectable catheter, using an entry site in the jugular, subclavian, or antecubital vein (Fig. 14-2).

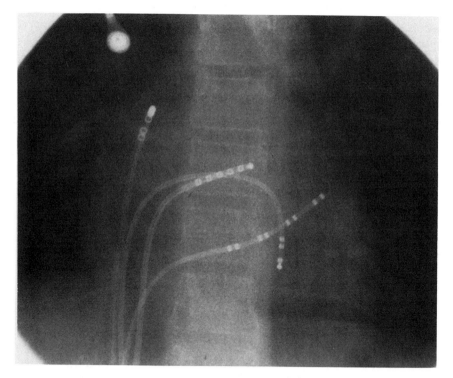

Figure 14-2. Catheters in the 4 standard positions for EP testing.

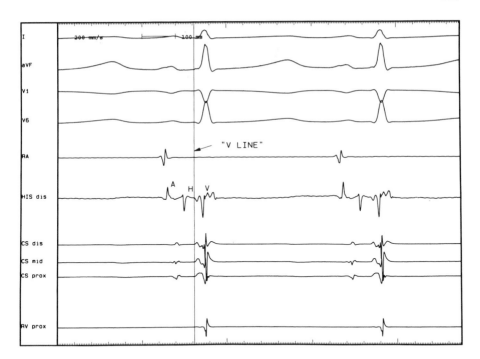

Figure 14-3. Baseline recordings during sinus rhythm.

Intracardiac electrograms are recorded from these 4 standard sites during baseline rhythm, along with several standard ECG leads, as shown in an example of sinus rhythm in Fig. 14-3. The atrial signals from the RA, HBE, and CS catheters are used to examine the sequence of atrial activation, which for sinus rhythm should proceed from high to low within the right atrium, and should then be followed by the left atrium, proceeding from the proximal electrode pair toward the distal electrode pair on the CS catheter. Subsequent to these atrial events, AV nodal and His-Purkinje conduction occurs, which is best examined on the HBE catheter. Atrioventricular conduction time can be quantified on the HBE signal as 2 phases, referred to as the AH and HV interval. The AH interval is measured as the time from the onset of local atrial activation on the HBE catheter to the onset of the rapid His deflection, and represents primarily the conduction time within the AV node. The HV interval evaluates conduction time through the His-Purkinje system and is measured from the onset of the rapid His deflection, to the so-called "V line" which is marked as the earliest evidence of ventricular activity in any lead (including all surface ECG and intracardiac leads). Prolonged HV intervals suggest impaired His bundle conduction, while short HV intervals usually suggest the presence of preexcitation from an accessory pathway (AP). Ventricular depolarization finally occurs, beginning with the RV apex, followed by the upper ventricular septum (best seen on the HBE catheter) and finally the left ventricular base (best seen on the CS catheter).

The gross atrial and ventricular activation patterns recorded at baseline provide important clues to the site of origin for abnormal arrhythmia foci and APs. For example, if a patient has active tachycardia from an ectopic atrial focus or another form of SVT, the normal atrial sequence will be disturbed since the rhythm is not generated by the sinus node, and earliest atrial activity is shifted instead toward the site of the arrhythmia focus or pathway. Similarly, if the pattern of ventricular activation is distorted by preexcitation from an AP, or a primary ventricular arrhythmia, the normal sequence of apex -> septum -> base is usually lost, and the pattern will shift to earliest ventricular activity near the region of the electrical pathology.

Evaluation of Sinus Node Function
It must be admitted that formal electrophysiology testing is a suboptimal way to evaluate sinus node function. Routine ECG, Holter monitoring, and exercise testing probably provide much better measures of sinus node performance than any diagnostic maneuvers available in the EP lab. However, it is still useful to discuss the basic EP techniques for sinus node evaluation as an introduction to the concept of pacing/stimulation of the heart.

Apart from measuring the baseline sinus rate, sinus node function can be assessed with two types of pacing maneuvers, one being a fairly straightforward technique[9] known as sinus node recovery time (SNRT), and the second a more involved technique[10] known as sinoatrial conduction time (SACT). Neither of these are perfect tests, but occasionally they can produce some dramatic and useful data. We will comment only on SNRT for this chapter, which is measured by pacing the right atrium at a rate slightly faster than the baseline sinus rate for 30 to 60 seconds, and then abruptly terminating the pacing. The time from the last paced atrial beat until reappearance of the first sinus beat is measured in msec as the SNRT. This value is then adjusted for the underlying heart rate by subtracting the cycle length of sinus rhythm from the SNRT value to yield a "corrected" sinus node recovery time (CSNRT), or alternatively, it may be standardized as a percentage of the resting sinus cycle length (%SNRT):
CSNRT = recovery time – sinus cycle length
or

%SNRT = recovery time / sinus cycle length
In the normal heart, there is always a slight pause following prolonged pacing before sinus node activity resumes, but the normal recovery time in the pediatric population is usually less than a CSNRT value of 275 msec, or less than a %SNRT of 166%. Unfortunately, using these techniques there are still many false negative studies in patients with known sinus node dysfunction, as well as some borderline or false positive studies in patients with normal sinus node function. The test is really most useful only when the recovery time is prolonged to a dramatic degree.

Evaluation of AV Nodal conduction

Atrioventricular conduction is examined using a combination of baseline measurements (PR, AH, and HV intervals), along with pacing maneuvers which measure the refractory period of the tissues involved in the AV conduction process. Refractory periods are determined by placing a carefully timed premature beat into either sinus rhythm, or at the end of an 8 beat "drive train". The use of drive trains before extrastimuli is generally preferred for clinical EP measurements, since it eliminates any variation caused by sinus arrhythmia, and allows refractory measurements to be standardized for a fixed heart rate (e.g. 120 beats/min or 500msec) that can be compared from patient to patient. The initial extrastimulus is initially placed at about 400 msec after the drive train, but is then made progressively early by 10 msec increments on each subsequent stimulation sequence. In this fashion the premature beat is scanned until it fails to conduct or excite cardiac tissue, which indicates refractoriness at the site of the block.

The typical response to initial extrastimuli in the range of 400 msec is normal capture of atrial muscle, normal conduction through the AV node and His-Purkinje system, and then normal ventricular activation. As the degree of prematurity is increased on subsequent sequences, delay within the AV node is encountered so that the AH interval begins to lengthen (Fig. 14-4).

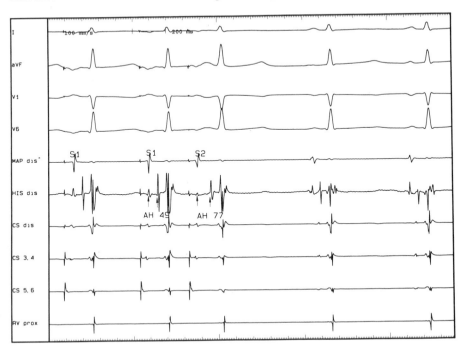

Figure 14-4. Placement of a single extrastimulus (S2) at the end of an 8 beat drive train (S1's), causing mild delay in the AV node (prolongation of AH interval).

The degree of AH increase is usually gradual and progressive as the stimulus is made more premature, but there can occasionally be "jumps" in the AH interval which suggest a phenomenon in the AV node known as "dual AV node pathway" physiology[11].

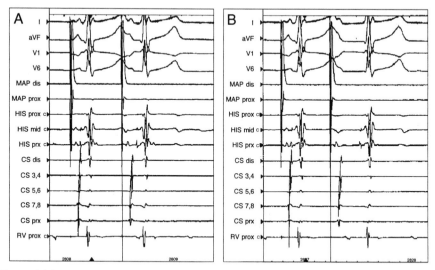

Figure 14-5. Dual AV node pathway physiology demonstrated during extrastimulus testing: there is an abrupt jump of the AH interval with only a 10 msec decrease in the premature beat between A and B.

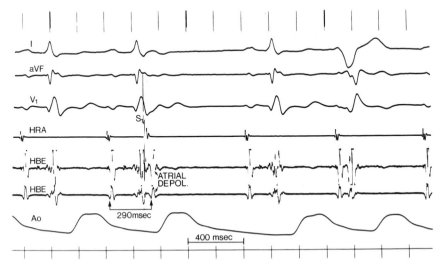

Figure 14-6. Effective refractory period (ERP) of the AV node.

This can frequently be seen as a normal variant, but may also be a clue to the origin of tachycardia in some patients who have SVT due to reentry within the AV node. Eventually, the premature beat is delivered early enough that block occurs within the AV node. This is registered on the surface ECG as a paced P wave with no subsequent QRS, and more specifically on the HBE as a paced atrial electrogram with no subsequent His or ventricular deflection (Fig. 14-6). On rare occasions, the block may occur below the AV node at the His bundle itself, in which case the HBE will still show a paced atrial electrogram, now followed by a His signal, but no ventricular deflection (Fig. 14-7).

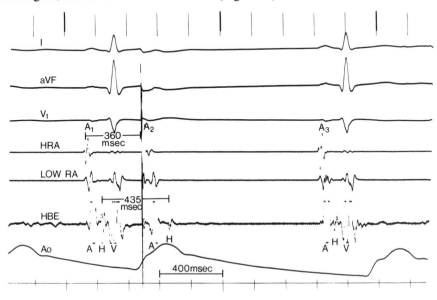

Figure 14-7. Effective refractory period (ERP) of the His bundle.

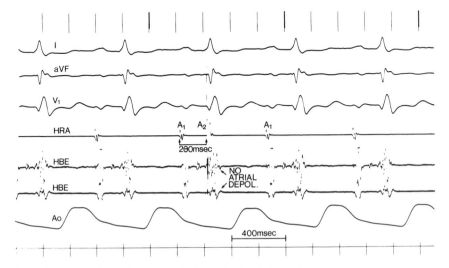

Figure 14-8. Effective refractory period (ERP) of atrial muscle.

As the premature atrial stimulus is made even more early, it will finally reach a point where it is too premature to capture atrial muscle, and this will register as a pacing artifact without atrial excitation (Fig. 14-8).

The point at which the AV node blocks, or the His bundle blocks, or the atrial muscle fails to capture, is known as the effective refractory period (ERP) for that tissue. The ERP's measured during a study can be compared to established normal values for the patient's age (Table 1).

TABLE 1. NORMAL VALUES FOR SELECT EP MEASUREMENTS IN PEDIATRIC PATIENTS

AH interval	40 – 120 msec
HV interval	30 – 55 msec
RV apex activation	10 – 35 msec
CSNRT	< 275 msec
%SNRT	< 166 %
Onset Wenckebach	< 380 msec
Atrial ERP	170 – 250 msec
AV Node ERP	200 – 300 msec
Ventricular ERP	200 – 260 msec

Another technique to evaluate AV conduction is to pace the atrium for short sequences of 8 beats at progressively faster rates, and monitor the pacing rate at which AV block occurs. The typical pattern to see during this exercise is gradual prolongation of the PR and AH intervals as the atrial pacing rate is increased, until finally 2nd degree AV block (usually Mobitz I type) develops. The rate at which Wenckebach occurs can be compared to normal values for age as a quick but fairly reliable method of evaluating AV conduction.

Basic Measurements of His-Purkinje and Ventricular Conduction

The baseline pattern of ventricular activation during sinus rhythm provides data regarding the status of His-Purkinje conduction, as well as clues for the detection of anterograde preexcitation pathways such as WPW syndrome. With catheters in the 4 standard positions, the pattern for normal ventricular conduction should involve earliest activation at the right ventricular apex (Fig. 14-9) which usually occurs within 35 msec of the "V line".

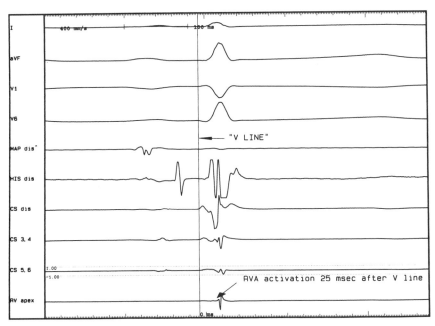

Figure 14-9. Normal activation of the right ventricular apex.

In patients who have damage to the right bundle branch, the activation time at the apex is typically prolonged to the range of 50 milliseconds or more, a situation referred to as "central" right bundle branch block. In some patients following congenital heart surgery, the integrity of the right bundle branch is preserved, but the surface electrocardiogram still shows delayed ventricular activation due to scars or patches along the anterior surface of the right ventricle and infundibulum. The surface ECG pattern is indistinguishable from that seen with central right bundle branch block, but the intracardiac recordings show that activation at the apex is still within the normal range of less than 35 milliseconds. This pattern is often referred to as "peripheral" right bundle branch block.

Close examination of the HV interval reveals additional information regarding His-Purkinje and ventricular conduction. Although there is wide variation in the range of the normal AH intervals in children, the range for a normal HV interval is narrowly defined at 30-55 msec. Prolonged HV intervals beyond 55 msec

336

usually indicate damage or disease in the His-Purkinje system. It is more common
to see long HV intervals in patients who have left bundle branch block as opposed
to patients with right bundle branch block. In the latter case, the HV interval is
typically normal, and it is only RV apex activation that is delayed. At the other
end of the spectrum is the phenomenon of a short HV interval which is
encountered in patients with preexcitation, such as WPW syndrome. Because
part of the ventricle is activated ahead of conduction through the normal AV node,
the HV interval is short, and the approximate location of the AP can usually be
inferred by examining which of the ventricular electrograms has earliest activity
relative to the "V line". For example, an accessory pathway along the left lateral
AV groove would result in an early ventricular electrogram on the CS catheter,
that clearly precedes the right ventricular apex and the ventricular septum near the
His bundle (Fig. 14-10).

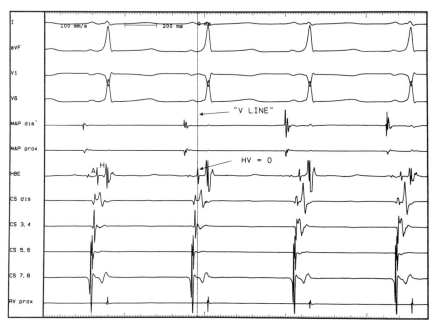

*Figure 14-10. Preexcitation with early left ventricular activation (seen on the CS catheter)
and a short HV interval in a patient with WPW syndrome.*

Evaluation of Supraventricular Tachycardia (SVT)
The primary goal of an SVT study is to record multiple intracardiac signals during
the baseline state, and also during a tachycardia episode, which allows the SVT
mechanism to be deduced. In addition, if an AP or an automatic focus are
discovered, their location can be mapped precisely to allow for the possibility of
an ablation procedure. The tachycardia of interest can occur either spontaneously,
during catheter manipulation, during baseline stimulation such as measurements of
refractory periods, or may sometimes require aggressive stimulation with rapid

pacing during infusion of isoproterenol. An optimal SVT study requires 4 catheters located at the RA, HBE, CS, and RV.

Testing begins with a thorough evaluation of all components of the conducting system, starting with baseline intervals. The atrial activation pattern in resting rhythm is first examined to be sure that the focus of atrial depolarization is originating in the vicinity of the sinus node. The resting HV interval is also carefully scrutinized looking for any evidence of a shortened interval suggestive of a preexcitation syndrome. The ventricular activation pattern is likewise examined to be sure there are no eccentric or early areas of depolarization, which would further support preexcitation.

If tachycardia is not present spontaneously during baseline measurements, it is necessary to induce the tachycardia with pacing maneuvers or pharmacologic intervention. Pacing maneuvers are nearly always successful in inducing the common forms of SVT due to reentry circuits. However, some rare forms of SVT are caused by focal automaticity rather than reentry, and the effect of pacing maneuvers for these unusual arrhythmias is unpredictable. Often, catecholamine stimulation with an infusion of isoproterenol is the only way to initiate an automatic tachycardia. The stimulation protocol for SVT studies usually begins with pacing from the right atrium, starting with a single premature beat delivered at the end of an 8 beat drive train, that is scanned until atrial refractoriness as previously described. This allows one to examine ERPs and other conduction phenomena which will help pinpoint the mechanism for the arrhythmia. If reentry SVT is not easily induced, double or triple extrastimuli can then be delivered at the end of the 8 beat drive train, or the cycle length for the drive train can be changed. Finally, burst rapid atrial pacing can be performed. If reentry tachycardia is not induced with these maneuvers, the sequence can be repeated during graded doses of isoproterenol, and after atropine administration.

It is also important to perform some simple ventricular pacing maneuvers during SVT studies, since it allows one to examine the pattern of retrograde VA conduction, and will sometimes be successful in starting the tachycardia even when atrial pacing fails. A fairly simple protocol is used involving single extra stimuli after an 8 beat drive train, looking to see if retrograde VA conduction is present, and if so, examining the site of earliest retrograde atrial activation (Fig. 14-11 AandB) to determine whether such conduction occurs via the AV node (in which case earliest atrial activity is seen on the HBE) or over an AP (in which case earliest atrial activation can be observed at an eccentric location such as the CS catheter). Aggressive ventricular stimulation protocols of the type used during formal ventricular tachycardia studies are usually not necessary during the study of SVT.

338

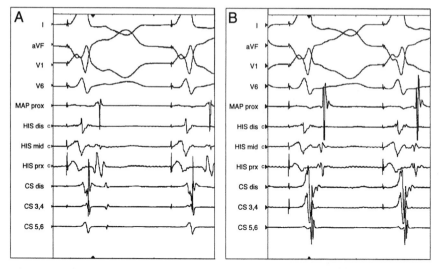

Figure 14-11. Comparison of retrograde VA conduction during ventricular pacing, showing the usual pattern for atrial activation over the AV node (A) characterized by earliest activity on the HBE catheter, versus a left sided accessory pathway (B) with earliest activity on the CS catheter.

Once tachycardia is induced, careful attention is paid to the following features:

1) <u>Mode of induction:</u> As mentioned, tachycardias induced by pacing maneuvers usually involve a reentrant mechanism. There are several varieties of reentry SVT, including atrial muscle reentry ("atrial flutter"), AV nodal reentry, and reentry via an accessory pathway. Induction of atrial flutter usually requires fairly aggressive atrial stimulation, and is not critically related in any way to the timing of the His bundle or ventricle. Often, one can observe clear instances of AV block without interruption of the atrial rhythm (Fig. 14-12), and this is usually a clear indication that the reentry circuit is isolated to atrial muscle. The more difficult differential diagnosis involves the distinction between AV nodal reentry and AP-mediated SVT. In WPW syndrome, where anterograde preexcitation in evident during sinus rhythm, the prior probability that SVT is due to the pathway is quite high, and the diagnosis is generally not very difficult. However, there are many accessory pathways which conduct in the retrograde direction only without producing a delta wave on ECG (so-called "concealed" AP's). Reentry tachycardia due to a concealed AP can be more difficult to distinguish from AV nodal reentry. Close examination of the mode of induction becomes quite important in such cases. For AV nodal reentry, one usually sees evidence of dual AV nodal pathway physiology during extrastimulus testing, involving a sudden jump of 40 msec or more in the PR and AH interval when conduction switches to the "slow pathway".

At the moment of switch to the slow pathway, there is often retrograde return over the fast pathway, at which point tachycardia is induced[11]. For most patients with a concealed accessory pathway, induction of tachycardia is not critically dependant upon this abrupt jump in AH interval.

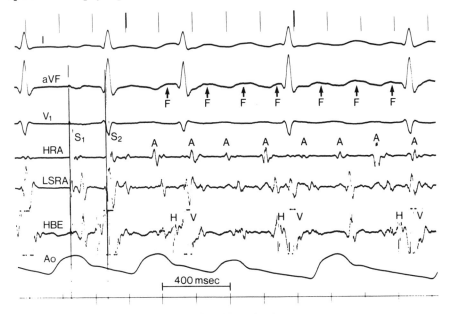

Figure 14-12. Atrial "flutter" with variable AV conduction.

2) <u>AV relationship during SVT</u>: The observation of AV block or AV dissociation without interruption of SVT is fairly good evidence that the arrhythmia circuit is not dependent on the AV node, ventricle, or an accessory pathway. This usually indicates a primary atrial tachycardia such as atrial flutter or an automatic atrial mechanism. When there is a fixed 1:1 AV ratio during tachycardia, and tachycardia terminates abruptly whenever this ratio is disturbed, it usually indicates a mechanism of reciprocating reentry between the atrium and ventricle, such as AV nodal reentry, or AP-mediated reentry. The timing of the atrial signal relative to the ventricular signal (so-called "VA interval") is another helpful differential clue in these cases[12]. During classic AV node reentry, the atrium and ventricle activate nearly simultaneously, so that the VA interval is short (0-70 msec). On the other hand, when SVT involves an AP there is built-in delay between atrial and ventricular activity as the circuit travels through the ventricle and retrograde back up the AP, resulting in a longer VA interval that typically exceeds 70 msec (Fig. 14-13 AandB). There are in addition some advanced stimulation techniques (including premature ventricular and atrial beats during SVT) that are employed routinely to confirm the SVT mechanism, but a good working diagnosis can usually be made using just the basic features described here.

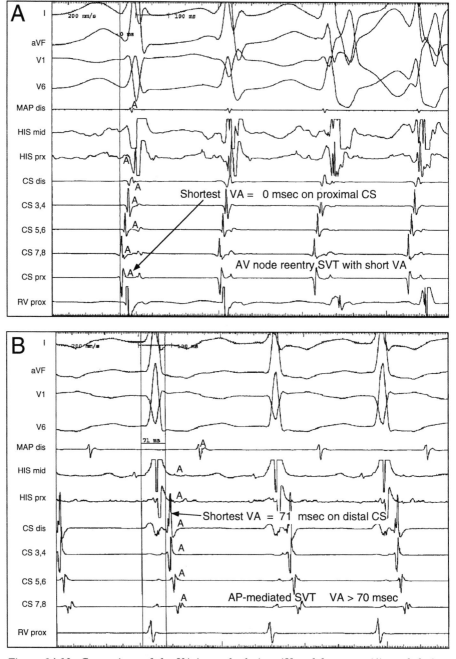

Figure 14-13. Comparison of the VA intervals during AV nodal reentry (A), and during accessory pathway-mediated tachycardia (B).

3) <u>Atrial Activation Sequence During SVT:</u> Careful attention to the atrial activation sequence during SVT will usually help localize the site of tachycardia origin. In AV nodal reentry, for example, the earliest retrograde atrial activation time is predictably found near the His bundle region. For APs, the earliest atrial activation is dependant upon the atrial insertion point of the pathway and can be found anywhere along the left or right AV valve rings. Careful mapping along both the tricuspid and mitral valve should allow one to pinpoint the AP insertion point.

In atrial flutter, the reentry circuit is usually restricted to right atrial tissue. The activation sequence for this arrhythmia is complex, since these large macroreentry circuits travel around the entire RA. During this circular motion, there is usually no clear beginning or ending electrogram, but one can often identify a critical region[13] within the RA where conduction is delayed with very fractionated signals (Fig. 14-14) referred to as the "zone of slow conduction".

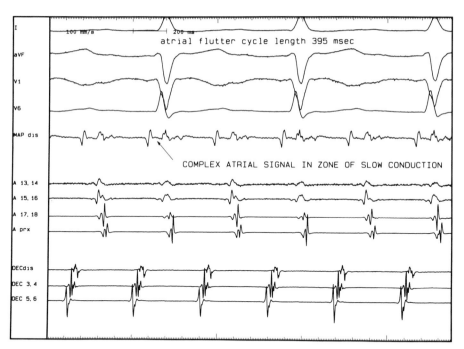

Figure 14-14. Atrial electrogram recorded on the MAP catheter at the zone of slow conduction in a patient with atrial flutter.

For a discrete ectopic focus of automatic atrial tachycardia, one is usually able to index atrial activation times against the onset of the surface P wave to identify the site of origin (Fig. 14-15).

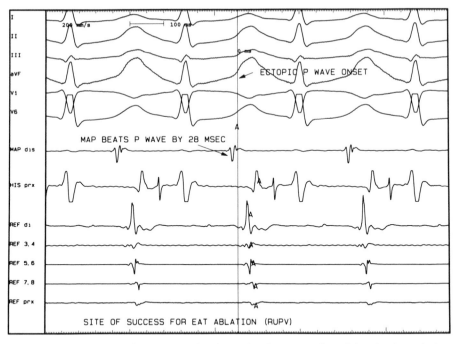

Figure 14-15. Mapping of ectopic atrial tachycardia showing early atrial activation relative to the P wave onset at the site of successful ablation.

Atrial sites which activate far in advance of the surface P wave will represent the epicenter of the automatic focus[14]. Typically, electrograms recorded from these sites will precede the P wave by 20-60 milliseconds.

Evaluation of Ventricular Tachycardia (VT)

The goals of EP testing for a suspected ventricular arrhythmia include ruling out a wide-QRS variety of SVT as the mechanism for the clinical arrhythmia, and determining if a sustained ventricular arrhythmia can be induced with a standard stimulation protocol. Sometimes patients will be retested with repeat ventricular stimulation after intravenous antiarrhythmic drug loading to evaluate efficacy, or if the tachycardia is sustained and supports stable hemodynamics, the site of VT origin can be mapped for potential surgical or transcatheter ablation.

It must be remembered that even a normal ventricle can be put into fibrillation if the stimulation is sufficiently aggressive. Thus, very strict protocols for ventricular pacing must be adhered to, and sound clinical judgement must be exercised when interpreting the results of all such studies. The indications for EP studies in patients with ventricular arrhythmias vary between institutions, and it is not firmly established that testing in the EP lab is superior to noninvasive monitoring in all forms of VT. Nonetheless, for patients who have had serious symptoms from sustained VT, or those who have a wide-QRS tachycardia where the mechanism is uncertain, EP testing has proved useful in elucidating the mechanism, and may offer therapeutic options in the form of ablation.

A complete ventricular study involves a minimum of 3 catheters, located at the RA, HBE, and RV sites. Baseline intervals are first measured, and a limited atrial stimulation protocol is then performed to rule out an unusual SVT as the mechanism for the patient's arrhythmia. Aggressive ventricular stimulation is next carried out according to the institution's established protocol. At most centers, stimulation begins at the RV apex, and premature beats are delivered at intervals which are sequentially decreased by 10 msec increments until the local ventricular muscle is refractory. The protocol starts with single premature beats at several different paced cycle lengths (usually 600, 500, and 400 msec). Next, double extrastimuli are delivered at 3 paced cycle lengths, and finally triple extra stimuli at 3 paced cycle lengths. If no tachycardia is induced, the RV catheter is moved to the outflow tract where an identical sequence is repeated. If there is still no response, the patient is begun on isoproterenol, and stimulation is repeated at both the outflow tract and apex. been adopted to describe the final result. The production of 0-4 ventricular response beats (which are referred to as "repetitive ventricular responses" or RVRs) is generally benign.

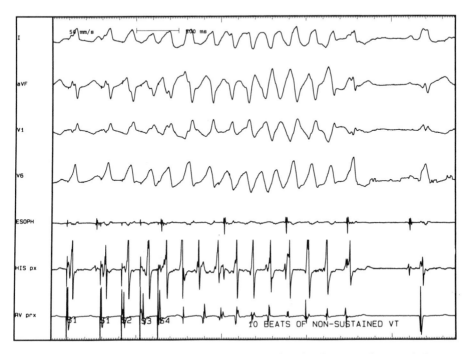

Figure. 14-16. Nonsustained ventricular tachycardia induced with ventricular stimulation.

344

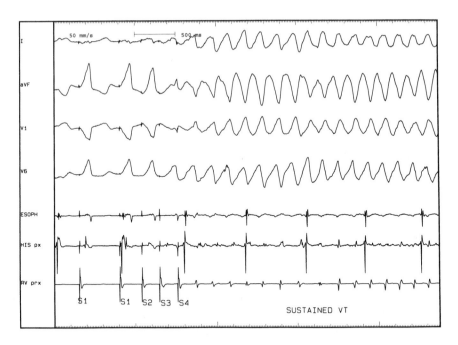

Figure 14-17. Sustained monomorphic ventricular tachycardia induced with ventricular stimulation.

The response to ventricular stimulation can be varied, and rigid definitions have If a ventricular arrhythmia is induced which lasts more than 4 beats but less than 30 seconds and does not require intervention (Fig. 14-16) it is defined as "nonsustained VT". If the induced VT lasts more than 30 seconds, or requires prompt intervention with pacing or cardioversion because of hemodynamic instability (Fig. 14-17) it is defined as "sustained VT". Any induced VT is further characterized as polymorphic or monomorphic depending upon QRS morphology. Finally, ventricular fibrillation (VF) might be induced.

Whenever VT or VF is induced in the EP lab, the team must be prepared to intervene with either bursts of rapid ventricular pacing or an external DC shock to correct the rhythm. This must be done immediately for any patient with hemodynamic instability. Some patients with slow monomorphic VT can be observed carefully in the EP lab for a period of time without intervention, and this allows the opportunity for mapping of the circuit or focus for purposes of ablation. However, any patient who is left in sustained VT for mapping must have continuous monitoring of arterial blood pressure and other hemodynamic parameters, and the arrhythmia should be terminated promptly at the first sign of deterioration.

THERAPEUTIC TECHNIQUES IN THE EP LABORATORY

Placement of an Emergency Pacing Wire for Bradycardia

The capacity for emergency transvenous pacing is a standard safety precaution in every catheterization lab, and the procedure should be well rehearsed by all members of the lab team. During any catheterization study, particularly in patients with complex congenital heart disease and preexistent conduction problems (e.g. corrected transposition or AV canal defects), one must be prepared for the possibility of catheter induced AV block, or even drug-resistant sinus bradycardia, which might require emergency pacing support. Various sized electrode catheters, sterile connecting cables, as well as a temporary pacemaker device, should be readily available in all cardiac catheterization suites.

The technique for placement of a temporary pacing catheter is relatively simple. Vascular entry is achieved at any convenient venous site, and a standard introduction sheath is placed. A bipolar or quadrapolar electrode catheter is then introduced, and is positioned in either the atrium (for sinus bradycardia) or the ventricle (for AV block). The distal electrodes on the pacing wire must be in good contact with myocardium, and should be in a stable anatomic position where abrupt dislodgment is unlikely to occur. The RA appendage is usually the most suitable site for an atrial pacing catheter, while the RV apex is the preferred site for ventricular leads. The two distal electrodes from the catheter are then attached to a temporary pacing device. The more distal tip electrode should be used as the cathode (or negative pole) for pacing, and the more proximal electrode as the anode (positive pole). Pacing is begun at the desired rate, and the "threshold" is checked by gradually decreasing the current to determine the lowest energy that provides reliable capture. The threshold value for a well positioned wire should be less than 2 milliAmperes. The pacemaker is then set for a wide margin of safety which is 3-5 times this threshold value. If the wire is to be left in place for a long period of time, the threshold should be rechecked any time the patient is moved from the cath table to a bed or stretcher, and on a twice daily basis thereafter to make sure the tip does not become dislodged from the original location.

Overdrive Pacing for Termination of Reentry Tachycardia

It is often desirable to convert patients from SVT, or some types of VT, without resorting to external cardioversion or intravenous medications. A good example would be a patient undergoing routine cardiac catheterization where manipulation in the heart causes repeated bouts of reentrant SVT. In order to complete the intended procedure, there should be a reliable technique that can be used on a repeated basis to terminate the arrhythmia. Overdrive pacing through a transvenous catheter is a useful tool in such situations.

The principle of overdrive pacing is to stimulate cardiac tissue involved in reentry at a rate that is faster than the conduction velocity or refractoriness of the circuit, and thereby force collision of electrical wavefronts which will promptly terminate reentry. However, if one stimulates the heart too rapidly or for prolonged periods of time, fibrillation can be induced. There is often a narrow range of pacing rates that can interrupt reentry without causing fibrillation, and thus, overdrive pacing should begin with relatively non-aggressive sequences that are escalated very gradually. Before attempting overdrive pacing, equipment must be on hand for a standard external DC conversion in the event that the technique proves unsuccessful, or should fibrillation develop.

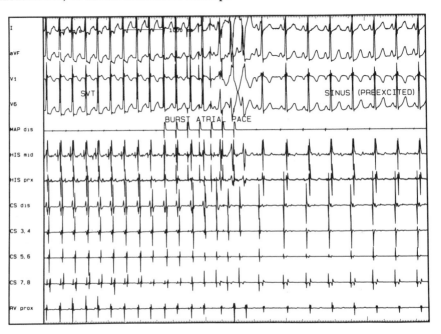

Figure 14-18. Prompt termination of reentry SVT with overdrive atrial pacing.

Initially, a pacing rate is chosen that is just slightly faster than the tachycardia, and is delivered for 3-5 beats or so (Fig. 14-18). If unsuccessful, the pacing rate is made slightly faster on subsequent attempts, and if still unsuccessful, longer pacing trains of 10-20 beats can be delivered. This scheme works well to terminate most of the common forms of SVT, including[15] atrial flutter, AV node reentry, and reentry due to an AP. It is not useful for SVT involving an automatic focus, nor will it have any effect on a patient who is already in atrial fibrillation. When overdrive pacing is attempted in the ventricle, it should only be performed by an experienced individual who is well trained in EP techniques. The major concern is that ventricular tachycardia can be accelerated with pacing maneuvers, or may degenerate into ventricular fibrillation, requiring prompt external DC conversion.

Basic Principles of Transcatheter RF Ablation

The most significant advance in clinical EP over the last decade has been the introduction of reliable methods for transcatheter ablation of arrhythmia foci and pathways. These procedures are accomplished by carefully mapping the target site, followed by delivery of some energy form through the catheter tip which causes destruction of the small area of cardiac tissue responsible for the arrhythmia, while trying to minimize collateral damage to uninvolved cardiac structures. Several energy forms have been used for catheter ablation (including DC electrical current, microwave energy, chemical infusion, and freezing with a cryocatheter) but by far the most popular energy form in recent years has been radiofrequency (RF) electrical current. The RF current used in the EP lab is similar in many ways to the familiar electrical energy used for electrocautery during surgical procedures, although the applied power used in the heart is considerably less. When RF energy is passed through a catheter tip, it causes local heating of tissue under the electrode, resulting in a small area of coagulation necrosis.

Radiofrequency ablation has now been performed in thousands of children and adults, with success rates exceeding 90-95%, and a low complication rate. For the pediatric population, the technique has been highly successful[16] for all varieties of accessory pathways, as well as AV nodal reentry and ectopic foci in the atrium or ventricle. Furthermore, there is growing experience with the use of RF ablation for treatment of both reentrant atrial tachycardias[13] (atrial flutter) and reentrant VT[17] in patients following congenital heart surgery.

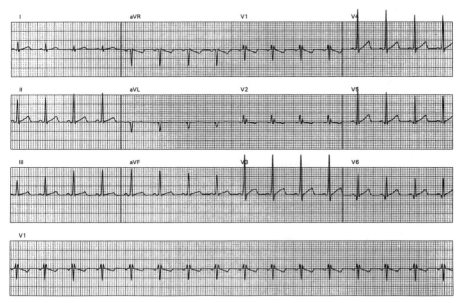

Figure 14-19. Pre-ablation ECG showing a delta wave pattern most consistent with a left sided accessory pathway.

The experience with these latter arrhythmias is still limited, but the early and midterm results have been encouraging.

Discussion of precision mapping and RF ablation has occupied entire textbooks[3], but as a basic introduction to the technique, this section will present an illustrative case example involving a patient with WPW syndrome. Prior to EP study, the patient's records are carefully reviewed for all ECG's that show examples of the clinical arrhythmia, as well as sinus rhythm recordings of the delta wave pattern. The polarity of the delta wave on a surface ECG will often provide some useful clues to the possible position of the AP along the mitral or tricuspid valves[18]. In our case example, the ECG suggests a location near the lateral mitral ring (Fig. 14-19). The clinical tachycardia in this patient had a narrow QRS, indicating "orthodromic" reentry with anterograde conduction over the AV node, and retrograde return to the atrium over the AP (Fig. 14-20).

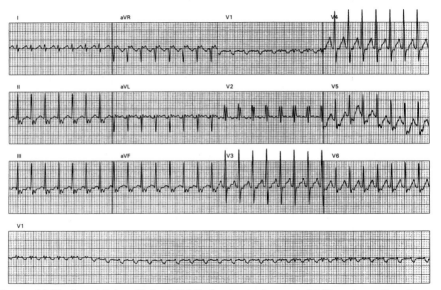

Figure 14-20. Pre-ablation 12-lead ECG showing a "normal QRS" tachycardia, due to orthodromic reentry.

In the EP lab, catheters are induced to the 4 standard sites of RA, HBE, RV, and CS. In this case with anterograde preexcitation, the baseline measurements in sinus rhythm are particularly revealing, since the site of earliest ventricular activation provides a good indication of the ventricular insertion for the AP. Note that earliest ventricular activity is seen in the distal CS catheter located along the lateral mitral ring (Fig. 14-21). Orthodromic tachycardia is then induced with atrial stimulation (Fig. 14-22), during which the circuit travels over the AP in the retrograde direction. The earliest atrial activation during SVT will also be seen in the distal CS catheter, confirming an atrial insertion of the AP along the lateral mitral ring.

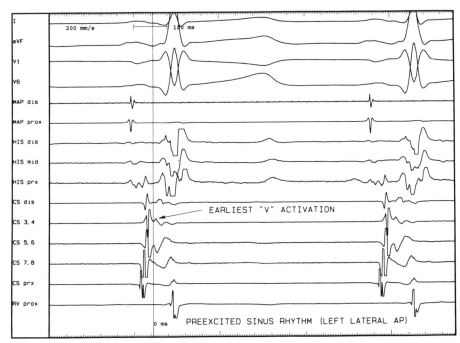

Figure 14-21. Baseline EP recordings showing earliest ventricular activation on CS catheter consistent with a left lateral accessory pathway.

Once the pathway is localized in this fashion, one must then decide on a catheter approach to position the ablation tip electrode at the region of interest. There are two conventional approaches[19] to a left lateral AP. One involves a transseptal technique where the catheter is advanced through either a PFO, or through a long vascular sheath following Brockenbrough transseptal puncture (Fig. 14-23).

The second method is to advance the catheter retrograde from the femoral artery back through the aortic valve, and tuck the tip of the catheter under the mitral leaflet in the region of interest along the AV groove. Both techniques have proved highly successful. After reaching the general target area, more precise mapping is done with the tip of the ablation catheter. In addition to reconfirming the atrial and ventricular insertion points, it is often possible to observe a sharp discrete electrical potential that may be generated by the AP itself (Fig. 14-24).

350

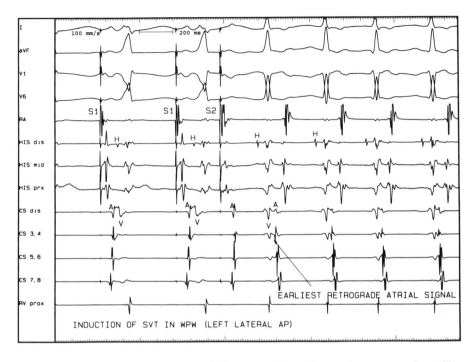

Figure 14-22. Induction of orthodromic SVT with atrial stimulation: the premature beat (S2) blocks in the accessory pathway, and conducts anterograde exclusively over the AV node with a normal QRS. The circuit then reenters back to the atrium over the accessory pathway. Earliest atrial activity is observed on the CS recording, consistent with a left lateral accessory pathway.

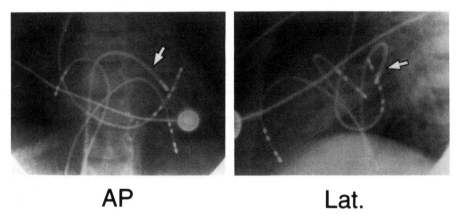

AP   Lat.

Figure 14-23. Catheter advanced across the atrial septum for ablation of a left lateral accessory pathway (arrow, AP, LAT).

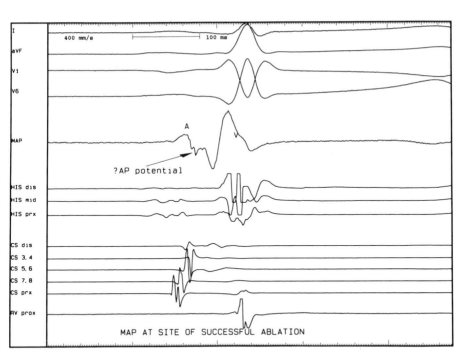

Figure 14-24. Recording from a well positioned ablation catheter (MAP) showing preexcited sinus rhythm, with a sharp signal between the atrial and ventricular components which may be a potential from the accessory pathway itself.

Once ideal electrograms are found, RF energy is delivered from the generator through the distal tip electrode. If the catheter is in good position, there should be clear evidence for block of AP conduction within 1-5 seconds[20] of starting the application (Fig. 14-25), in which case the lesion is continued for 30-60 seconds which will usually cause permanent interruption of AP conduction. If the pathway does not appear to be interrupted within the first 5-10 seconds, the RF application is usually terminated and the tip of the catheter must be repositioned slightly to a better location. Following a successful RF application, the patient is observed carefully in the EP lab for at least 30 minutes with repeat atrial and ventricular stimulation to be sure there is no recovery of AP conduction. If all testing looks optimistic after this waiting period, the procedure is terminated.

The success rates for radiofrequency ablation in the pediatric and adult populations have been quite impressive, but like any type of catheterization procedure, there are measurable risks involved[21]. This is particularly true when ablation is performed in very small children, or when the RF applications need to be made in close proximity to the AV node. In the later scenario, there is a small chance of damaging normal conduction, necessitating implantation of a permanent pacemaker.

352

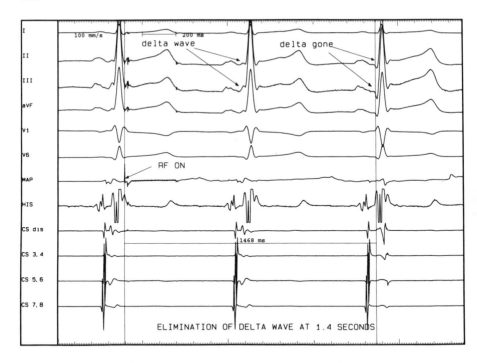

Figure 14-25. Successful interruption of accessory pathway conduction early into an RF application.

However, as more experience has been gained with the technique, it is now possible to perform successful ablation within a few millimeters of the normal conducting system without jeopardizing the AV node or bundle of His. For patients with recurrent tachycardia in the current era, RF ablation has become an early management option, and for those with serious symptoms, is now considered the treatment of choice.

REFERENCES

1. Walsh EP, Keane JF. Electrophysiologic studies and related procedures in congenital heart disease. In: Diagnostic and Interventional Catheterization in Congenital Heart Disease, Eds: Lock JE, Keane JF, Fellows KE. Boston, Martinus Nijhoff Co, 1987, pp 161-181.
2. Josephson ME. Clinical Cardiac Electrophysiology. Philadelphia: Lea and Febiger, 1993.
3. Huang SKS. Radiofrequency Catheter Ablation of Cardiac Arrhythmias. Armonk NY: Futura, 1995.
4. Walsh EP. Ablation therapy. In: Current Concepts in Diagnosis and Management of Arrhythmias in Infants and Children, Deal B, Wolff G Gelband H, (eds.) Armonk NY, Futura, 1998, pp 329-367.

5. Triedman JK, Jenkins KJ, Colan SD, et al. Intra-atrial reentrant tachycardia after palliation of congenital heart disease: Characterization of multiple macroreentrant circuits using fluoroscopically based three-dimensional endocardial mapping. J Cardiovasc Electrophysiol 1997, 8:259-270.
6. Lavoie J, Walsh EP, Burrows FA, et al. Effects of propofol or isoflurane anesthesia on cardiac conduction in a pediatric population. Anesth 1995, 82:884-887.
7. Walsh EP. Transcatheter ablation of ectopic atrial tachycardia using radiofrequency current, in Huang SK (ed): Catheter Ablation for Cardiac Arrhythmias. Mt. Kisco, Futura, 1994, pp. 421-443.
8. Stabile G, DeSimone A, Turco P, et al. Feasibility and safety of 2 French electrode catheters in the performance of electrophysiological studies. PACE 1998, 21:2506-2509.
9. Narula OS, Samet P, Javier RP. Significance of the sinus node recovery time. Circulation 1972, 45:140-158.
10. Kugler JD, Gillette PC, Mullins CE, et al. Sinoatrial conduction time in children: an index of sinus node function. Circulation 1979, 59:1266-1276.
11. Kadish A, Goldberger J. Ablative therapy for atrioventricular nodal reentry arrhythmias. Prog Cardiovasc Dis 1995, 37:273-294.
12. Walsh EP, Saul JP. Cardiac arrhythmias. In Fyler DC (ed), Nadas' Pediatric Cardiology. Philadelphia: Hanley and Belfus, 1992, pp 377-433.
13. Triedman JK, Saul JP, Weindling SN, et al. Radiofrequency ablation of intraatrial reentrant tachycardia following surgical palliation of congenital heart disease. Circulation 1995, 91:707-714.
14. Walsh EP, Saul JP, Hulse JE, et al. Transcatheter ablation of ectopic atrial tachycardia in young patients using radiofrequency current. Circulation 1992, 86:1138-1146.
15. Rhodes LA, Walsh EP, Saul JP. Conversion of atrial flutter in pediatric patients using transesophageal atrial pacing: A safe, effective, and minimally invasive technique. Am Heart J 1995, 130:323-327.
16. Tanel RE, Walsh EP, Triedman JK, et al. A five year experience with radiofrequency catheter ablation: Implications for arrhythmia management in the pediatric and young adult patient. J Peds 1997, 131:878-887.
17. Gonska BD, Cao K, Raab J, et al. Radiofrequency catheter ablation of right ventricular tachycardia late after repair of congenital heart defects. Circulation 1996, 94:1902-1908.
18. Chiang CE, Chen SA, Teo WS, et al. An accurate stepwise electrocardiographic algorithm for localization of accessory pathways in patients with Wolff-Parkinson-White syndrome from a comprehensive analysis of delta waves and R/S ratio during sinus rhythm. Am J Cardiol 1995, 76:40-46.
19. Saul JP, Hulse JE, De W, et al. Catheter ablation of accessory atrioventricular pathways in young patients: Use of long vascular sheaths, the transseptal approach, and a retrograde left posterior parallel approach. J Am Coll Cardiol 1993, 21:571-583.

20. Laohaprasitiporn D, Walsh EP, Saul JP, et al. Predictors of permanence of successful radiofrequency lesions created with controlled catheter tip temperature. PACE 1997, 20:1283-1291.
21. Kugler JD, Danford DA, Deal B, et al. Radiofrequency catheter ablation in children and adolescents: Early results in patients from 24 centers. New Engl J Med 1994, 330:1481-1487.

15. ECHOCARDIOGRAPHY IN THE CATHETERIZATION LABORATORY.

Mary E. van der Velde, M.D.

INTRODUCTION

Advances in echocardiographic technique have reduced the importance of angiography for diagnosis and delineation of the anatomic details of congenital heart lesions, and have eliminated the need for hemodynamic catheterization in many cases. Simultaneously, however, the expanded role of interventional catheterization in the care of patients with congenital heart disease has more than filled the gap left by the dwindling need for diagnostic catheterization. Echocardiography has become invaluable in determining the morphology of a lesion and in assessing candidacy and likelihood of success of many interventional procedures. In addition, interventional procedures can be complicated by cardiac perforation, vessel and valve injury, and migration of catheter-delivered devices. Echocardiographic monitoring during interventional procedures helps guide balloon and device positioning, while providing immediate assessment of results and identification of complications. Potential for reduced radiation exposure and contrast load is an added benefit of echocardiographic monitoring during interventions. For these reasons, echocardiography has become an integral part of cardiac catheterization in many children and adults with congenital heart disease.

TECHNIQUE

Echocardiography in the catheterization laboratory can be transthoracic (TTE), transesophageal (TEE), or intravascular. Transthoracic imaging can be difficult due to transducer and patient positioning constraints, and may interfere with the sterile field and image intensifiers. Transthoracic imaging also obscures to varying degrees the fluoroscopic image while subjecting the operator to direct irradiation. For these reasons, transthoracic imaging is of limited value. In contrast, transesophageal imaging rarely interferes with fluoroscopic imaging, does not risk contaminating the sterile field, and exposes the operator to little if any direct irradiation, while providing superior images of most cardiac structures without the need to reposition the patient (1-3).

Intravascular ultrasound proved to be useful in defining the mechanisms of balloon angioplasty, although its routine value appears to be less than initially predicted. Three-dimensional echocardiography, although initially of limited value because of low resolution and unacceptably long image reconstruction times, is fast becoming more practical and accurate, and is likely to prove valuable during interventional procedures such as device closure of intracardiac defects.

Optimally, the echo machine is positioned so that both echocardiographer and catheterizer can view the image. Projection of the image on an additional monitor is often necessary. Because the echocardiographer must provide highly accurate information within a short period of time, often under stressful and rapidly changing conditions, the role of cath lab echocardiographer should be reserved for more experienced personnel.

Additional patient sedation and/or intubation may be necessary when transesophageal echocardiography is employed, in order to prevent patient movement during the interventional procedure.

BALLOON DILATION
Valvuloplasty

Balloon valvuloplasty often involves repeated dilations with successively larger balloons to achieve optimal results. An assessment of transvalvar gradient and regurgitation is necessary between dilations, but repeated direct pressure measurements and angiography can be impractical (especially if the catheter must remain in position across the valve) and increases the duration of a procedure, contrast load, and radiation exposure. Echocardiographic evaluation of valve status can be achieved relatively rapidly, with catheters in place and without added risk to the patient. TEE allows imaging during the dilation, and can assist with balloon positioning as well as providing nearly instantaneous assessment of regurgitation and gradient. Echocardiography has proved to be most useful during valvuloplasty of the mitral valve, when repeated assessments of the degree of mitral regurgitation and precise balloon sizing appear integral to achieving optimum results (4-7).

Angioplasty

The value of transthoracic or transesophageal echocardiography during balloon dilation of vascular stenoses is comparatively low given the simple anatomy of these lesions. TEE may occasionally be helpful in assessing lumen diameter and evaluating aneurysm or dissection after coarctation dilation (3).

Other Obstructions

TEE has proven useful during dilation of venous pathways after atrial baffling procedures for transposition of the great arteries (TGA). It is very helpful in guiding stent placement in obstructed subaortic outflow tracts, particularly after Rastelli repair of TGA with ventricular septal defect (VSD), and in tricuspid atresia with TGA and a restrictive bulboventricular foramen. During positioning and dilation of stents in these subaortic outflow tracts, TEE guidance has been very useful in assessing the anatomic effects of test balloon dilation, to prevent subsequent impingement of the stent on aortic or mitral valve structures. Similarly, during balloon dilation and stenting of obstructed pulmonary veins, stents can block the orifices of adjacent veins (8,9); TEE during test dilation can identify adjacent veins at risk and prompt modification of the stent implanting procedure.

DEVICE CLOSURE
Atrial Septal Defects

Device closure of uncomplicated atrial septal defect (ASD), patent foramen ovale (PFO), and of other interatrial communications is an attractive alternative to surgery, particularly for small to moderate defects and for patients considered high risk surgical candidates. Several devices developed for these indications are undergoing evaluation of their respective efficacy and potential complications (Chapter 8).

TEE is not only useful, but in many cases is mandatory, during several stages of device closure. Assessment of candidacy for device closure, and selection of the appropriate device size, require measurement of the defect in several planes, and assessment of rim width, distance to valves and pulmonary veins, and atrial dimensions. Adequate images for making these measurements are often difficult to obtain transthoracically, particularly in larger patients, making TEE necessary (10). The presence, size, and location of additional defects must also be documented, to determine if a single device, properly positioned, can cover all defects. The stretched diameter of the defect can be measured echocardiographically as the sizing balloon is withdrawn across it during subsequent catheterization.

The technique of device closure is described in Chapter 8. Since angiography cannot be easily performed during positioning of the delivery system and device, the interventionalist relies on earlier angiograms in combination with TEE and fluoroscopic landmarks such as bony structures, the cardiac silhouette, and sternal wires, to determine the approximate location of the defect and other intracardiac structures. Transesophageal echocardiography can be performed continuously during device placement, to assess positioning of the delivery system and the device itself prior to release (1,2,11).

For most closure devices currently in use, the distal portion or arms are deployed in the left atrium, after which the device is pulled back towards the septum. It is at this point that assessment of position is most crucial. Because of the angle of the delivery system with respect to the septum, the superior left atrial arms or ridge of most devices come in contact with the septum first, and are prone to being pulled across to the right atrial side in an attempt to bring the inferior left atrial components closer to the septum and insure that the right atrial components of the device are deployed on the correct side of the septum. Without TEE guidance, the interventionalist must rely on the fluoroscopic appearance of the arms or other device components, which move in predictable ways as they are pulled back against and put tension on the septum. The disadvantage of this method is that arms caught on other cardiac structures may mimic properly positioned arms, and properly positioned arms may be dislodged in an attempt to confirm their position through device manipulation.

Device arms are easily imaged by TEE, providing continuous assessment of arm position during deployment of the device. In addition, device interference with AV valves or venous orifices can be detected prior to device release. Evaluation of device position is best achieved by imaging in multiple planes, preferably using a biplane or multiplane transducer. By advancing and withdrawing the probe the device can be imaged along its entire length in the horizontal, or transverse view, but additional imaging sweeps in the vertical or longitudinal plane improve the ability to detect arm malposition. In order to

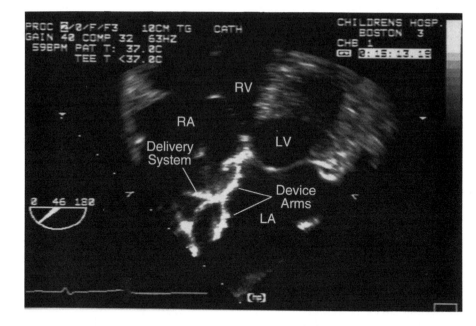

Figure 15-1: Transesophageal echocardiographic (TEE) image after deployment of the left atrial arms of a CardioSeal device during ASD closure. An anterior arm is in contact with the left atrial surface of the septum; a posterior arm is further from the septum, as is typical because of the angle of delivery with respect to the septum. LA=left atrium; LV=left ventricle; RA=right atrium; RV=right ventricle.

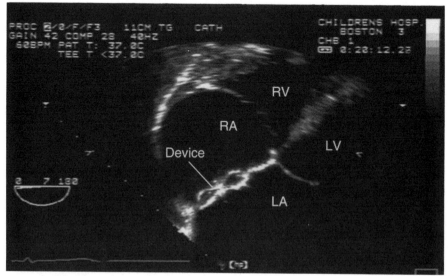

Figure 15-2: TEE image after release of a properly-positioned ASD CardioSeal device. Abbreviations as in Figure 15-1.

provide as accurate an assessment of device position as possible, the echocardiographer should preferably have had an opportunity to image the defect prior to device insertion, be very familiar with the normal appearance of the particular device being used, and should perform methodical, complete sweeps of the device in at least two planes. In the case of an umbrella or CardioSEAL device, each individual arm should be imaged from the center of the device out to the tip, and its relationship to the septum determined. Assessment of arm position is most easily achieved if the interpreting physician is actually manipulating the TEE probe, so that changes in the image resulting from small movements of the probe can be integrated immediately to allow mental reconstruction of three-dimensional relationships. Because of the potential ramifications of malposition of even the tip of one arm, the importance of this echocardiographic evaluation cannot be overemphasized (Figs. 15-1, 15-2)

When using a CardioSEAL device, if arm malposition is suspected prior to deployment of the right atrial arms, and malposition is confirmed by TEE, the device can be withdrawn into the delivery sheath and immediately reexpanded in the left atrium. This specific step has proven to be the most valuable contribution of TEE during device placement.

Once the right atrial arms are deployed, however, the device has to be removed from the body via the sheath and the procedure begun again using a new device. This may result in damage to vascular and valvar structures in addition to the device itself. When using the Amplatzer device, the device can be retracted and redeployed up until the moment of final release. After final release, if either device is found to impinge on valvar structures, the CardioSEAL can be retrieved relatively easily, and the Amplatzer with more difficulty. Finally, the efficacy of closure can be assessed both echocardiographically and angiographically.

Ventricular Septal Defects
The principles of echocardiographic guidance of device closure of VSDs are similar to those for ASDs, but several factors make this procedure more complicated. VSDs often have irregular shapes, and may divide into several channels within the septum; right ventricular openings are obscured by muscle trabeculations in many instances. Multiple VSDs present a particular challenge to the interventionalist and echocardiographer. Identification, sizing, and localization of multiple defects are currently best achieved using a combination of transthoracic and transesophageal two-dimensional echocardiography and angiography using multiple camera angles. Once again, for both TTE and TEE, the importance of slow, methodical imaging sweeps of the ventricular septum in the evaluation of multiple VSDs is paramount. Careful mapping with color Doppler, decreasing the color velocity scale if necessary to improve detection of low-velocity flow (in the case of equal ventricular pressures) improves detection of smaller or tortuous defects. Because of the availability of more imaging windows,

if the patient's windows are good transthoracic imaging is often better than TEE for the pre-catheterization evaluation, particularly for evaluation of the anterior and apical portions of the muscular septum. The advantage of direct hands-on imaging by the echocardiographer who will interpret the study must be emphasized. Three-dimensional echocardiography is particularly attractive as a potential means of improving the assessment of multiple ventricular septal defects.

Muscular VSDs may be close to atrioventricular (AV) or semilunar valve leaflets and attachments, which complicates device positioning. Ventricular septal defect anatomy may also be complex, as with malalignment of the apical muscular septum (12), left ventricle to right atrium shunt, post-infarction VSD, and postoperative "intramural" defects through right ventricular free wall trabeculations (13).

After determination of number, size and position of VSDs, TEE can be useful to guide a catheter through the defect designated for device closure. In the case of multiple muscular VSDs, proper positioning of a device in a centrally-located defect may allow the device to occlude several VSDs at once if the CardioSEAL device is being used. Depending on the position of the VSD and catheter course, the initial set of arms may be deployed on either side of the septum. As during ASD device closure, the distal arms or occluder are deployed, the device is pulled back until it is flush with the septum, and the proximal side of the device is then deployed.

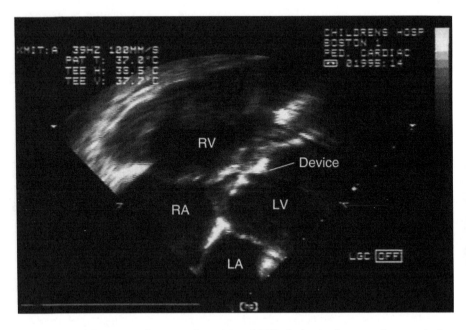

Figure 15-3: TEE image of a properly-positioned VSD device in the muscular ventricular septum. Two other devices in the muscular septum are not imaged in this particular plane. Abbreviations as in Figure 15-1.

TEE imaging provides valuable information regarding the position of the device at each stage of deployment, detecting whether the device interferes or comes in contact with valve structures (14). During closure of apical and anterior muscular VSDs, distal device arms may "hang up" on muscle trabeculations, giving the impression fluoroscopically that they are being pulled against the septum when in fact they are not.

After both sides of the device are deployed, position and residual flow can be assessed prior to and after release from the delivery system (Fig. 15-3).

In the case of multiple VSDs, the site(s) of most significant residual flow can be assessed after placement of one or more devices, to determine which if any residual defects should be addressed with additional devices. Since many such patients have outflow tract obstruction or have undergone previous pulmonary artery banding, and in some cases have no shunt or a net right-to-left shunt, hemodynamic assessment of Qp:Qs may not be helpful in assessing the size of residual defects. Additionally, in situations where multiple muscular VSDs coexist with a large membranous or malalignment VSD, angiographic evaluation of the muscular septum may be difficult because of the large quantity of contrast opacifying the conoventricular defect. In both of these circumstances, TEE can be invaluable. Finally, we have found TEE to be mandatory during closure of fenestrated VSD patches. These defects are always close to the aortic valve, and documentation of aortic valve competence prior to device release has become an essential part of these procedures.

Other Device Closures

Other defects that have been closed with umbrella or CardioSEAL-type occluder devices include perivalvar leak, Potts shunt, leaks at the margin of a patch closing an AV valve as part of a modified Fontan procedure, left superior vena cava to the left atrium, dilated azygous vein after classic and bidirectional Glenn shunt, hepatic vein purposefully left on the pulmonary venous side after a Fontan procedure. Yet other defects as managed include right ventricular outflow tract or apical aneurysm with a "neck", residual right ventricle to pulmonary artery communication after a Fontan or Glenn operation, left ventricular apex to descending aorta conduit, large pulmonary arteriovenous fistula, and aorto-pulmonary fistula. TEE imaging can help direct the catheter to the defect, assist with device positioning, and assess residual patency.

Closure of defects such as Fontan baffle fenestration, patent ductus arteriosus (PDA), coronary fistula, and arterial or venous collaterals with coils, umbrellas, or other closure devices does not routinely require echocardiographic guidance, although in the case of PDA and fistulae, efficacy of closure is easily assessed echocardiographically prior to discharge.

BALLOON AND BLADE SEPTOSTOMY

Successful balloon septostomy in neonates with TGA using echocardiographic guidance, with or without fluoroscopy, has been extensively reported (15,16). Transthoracic echo is usually adequate for this purpose, although TEE guidance has been reported (17), and might be preferable if simultaneous fluoroscopic and echocardiographic imaging are used. However, given the size and clinical status of infants with TGA, TEE is rarely indicated for a balloon septostomy.

TEE has been invaluable in guiding Brockenbrough transseptal puncture and dilation septostomy in patients with a small left atrium, thickened septum, or unusual septal anatomy or orientation. Immediate echocardiographic assessment of defect size and gradient can be obtained, allowing the catheter or wire to remain in position through the defect in case further enlargement of the ASD is indicated.

BIOPSIES

Echocardiographic guidance of endomyocardial biopsy has been reported often and well. By both TTE and TEE (18), the open bioptome can be imaged and its position (septal surface or free wall) can be determined prior to sampling. Echocardiographic guidance probably reduces the risk of myocardial perforation and damage to valve structures during biopsy, and in our laboratory has been especially useful in infants or when cardiac anatomy or position is distorted. Echocardiographic guidance is particularly helpful if biopsies of a particular structure, such as a cardiac tumor, are desired. It is not unreasonable to expect that echo will supplant fluoroscopy as the imaging modality of choice during many cardiac biopsies in the future.

RADIOFREQUENCY ABLATION

Several investigators have reported the utility of echocardiographic imaging (intracardiac or transesophageal) during ablation procedures, primarily to assist with catheter localization, assessment of lesion size, early identification of complications such as perforation, and reduction of fluoroscopy time (19,20).

EFFUSION

Echocardiography is often invaluable as an adjunct to fluoroscopy during elective evacuation of pericardial or pleural effusions, particularly when the fluid collection is "loculated" (as opposed to free flowing), or non-circumferential. Surface imaging demonstrates the location of the fluid pocket and its distance from the anticipated needle puncture site below the xiphoid process or on the chest wall, and should be used, with few exceptions, during access to loculated pericardial collections.

VASCULAR ACCESS

Etheridge (21) found that ultrasound guidance increased the success rate of percutaneous cannulation of the internal jugular vein (IJ) for endomyocardial biopsy or cardiac catheterization in pediatric patients. The technique reduced complications and vessel injury, and was felt to be most useful in transplant patients needing repeated cannulation of the IJ for biopsies.

SUMMARY

Echocardiography is useful during many interventional procedures, for delineation of anatomic details, assistance with device or balloon positioning, assessment of results, and early detection of complications. Transesophageal echocardiography is preferable because it allows continuous imaging during intervention without interfering with the procedure. The use of echocardiography reduces radiation exposure and contrast load, which in turn increases the amount of information that can be obtained, and the number of interventions that can be performed, if necessary, during a single catheterization.

REFERENCES

1. van der Velde ME, Perry SB. Transesophageal echocardiography during interventional catheterization in congenital heart disease. Echocardiography 1997;14:513-8.
2. van der Velde ME, Perry SB, Sanders SP. Transesophageal echocardiography with color Doppler during interventional catheterization. Echocardiography 1991;8:721-30.
3. Stumper O, Witsenburg M, Sutherland G, Cromme-Dijkhuis A, Godman MJ, Hess J. Transesophageal echocardiographic monitoring of interventional cardiac catheterization in children. JACC 1991;18:1506-14.
4. Kronzon I, Tunick PA, Schwinger ME, Slater J, Glassman E. Transesophageal echocardiography during percutaneous mitral valvuloplasty. J Am Soc Echo 1989;2:380-5.
5. Ramondo A, Chirillo F, Dan M, Isabella G, Bonato R, Rampazzo C, Razzolini R, Andriolo L, Mazzucco A, Chioin R. Value and limitations of transesophageal echocardiographic monitoring during percutaneous balloon mitral valvotomy. Int J Cardiol 1991;31:223-34.
6. Vilacosta I, Iturralde E, San Roman JA, Gomez-Recio M, Romero C, Jimenez J, Martinez-Elbal L. Transesophageal echocardiographic monitoring of percutaneous mitral balloon valvulotomy. Am J Cardiol 1992;70:1040-4.
7. Goldstein SA, Campbell A, Mintz GS, Pichard A, Leon M, Lindsay J. Feasibility of on-line transesophageal echocardiography during balloon mitral valvulotomy: Experience with 93 patients. J Heart Valve Dis 1994;3:136-148.

8. Driscoll DJ, Hesslein PS, Mullins CE. Congenital stenosis of individual pulmonary veins: Clinical spectrum and unsuccessful treatment by transvenous balloon dilation. Am J Cardiol 1982;49:1767-72.

9. Mendelsohn AM, Bove EL, Lupinetti FM, Crowley DC, Lloyd TR, Fedderly RT, Beekman RH. Intraoperative and percutaneous stenting of congenital pulmonary artery and vein stenosis. Circulation 1993;88(pt 2):210-7.

10. Rosenfeld HM, van der Velde ME, Sanders SP, Colan SD, Parness IA, Lock JE, Spevak PJ. Echocardiographic predictors of candidacy for successful transcatheter atrial septal defect closure. Cathet Cardiovasc Diag 1995;34:29-34.

11. Hellenbrand WE, Fahey JT, McGowan FX, Weltin GG, Kleinman CS. Transesophageal echocardiographic guidance of transcatheter closure of atrial septal defect. Am J Cardiol 1990;66:207-13.

12. Kumar K, Lock JE, Geva T. Apical muscular ventricular septal defects between the left ventricle and the right ventricular infundibulum: Diagnostic and interventional considerations. Circulation 1997;1207-13.

13. Preminger TJ, Sanders SP, van der Velde ME, Castaneda AR, Lock JE. "Intramural" residual interventricular defects after repair of conotruncal malformations. Circulation 1994;89:236-42.

14. van der Velde ME, Sanders SP, Keane JF, Perry SB, Lock JE. Transesophageal echocardiographic guidance of transcatheter ventricular septal defect closure. J Am Coll Cardiol 1994;23:1660-5.

15. Perry LW, Ruckman RN, Galioto FM, Shapiro SR, Potter BM, Scott LP. Echocardiographically assisted balloon atrial septostomy. Pediatrics 1982;70:403-8.

16. Lin AE, DiSessa TG, Williams RG. Balloon and blade atrial septostomy facilitated by two-dimensional echocardiography. Am J Cardiol 1986;57:273-7.

17. Boutin C, Dyck J, Benson L, Houde C, Freedom RM. Balloon atrial septostomy under transesophageal echocardiographic guidance. Pediatr Cardiol 1992;13:176-7.

18. Kawauchi M, Gundry SR, Boucek MM, de Begona JA, Vigesaa R, Bailey LL. Real-time monitoring of the endomyocardial biopsy site with pediatric transesophageal echocardiography. J Heart Lung Transplant 1992;11:306-10.

19. Kalman JM, Olgin JE, Karch MR, Lesh MD. Use of intracardiac echocardiography in interventional electrophysiology. PACE 1997;20(Pt. I):2248-62.

20. Goldman AP, Irwin JM, Glover MU, Mick W. Transesophageal echocardiography to improve positioning of radiofrequency ablation catheters in left-sided Wolff-Parkinson-White Syndrome. PACE 1991;14:1245-50.

21. Etheridge SP, Berry JM, Krabill KA, Braunlin EA. Echocardiographic-guided internal jugular venous cannulation in children with heart disease. Arch Pediatr Adolesc Med 1995;149:77-80.

INDEX